Props for Yoga

A Guide to Iyengar Yoga Practice with Props
Volume I: Standing Asanas

Eyal Shifroni, Ph.D.

Co-Author: *Michael Sela*

Based on the teachings of
Yogacharya B.K.S.. Iyengar, Geeta S. Iyengar and Prashant S. Iyengar
at the Ramamani Iyengar Memorial Yoga Institute (RIMYI), Pune, India.

Photography Aviv Naveh
Text Editing Nancy Gardosh
Models Ravit Moar, Eleanor Jacobovitz, Michael Sela & Eyal Shifroni
Graphic Design Aviv Gros-Allon, ViV design
Props Illustrations Kym Ben-Yaakov

No part of this publication may be reproduced, stored in a retrieval system, or transmitted in any form or by any means, electronic, mechanical, photocopying, recording, scanning, or otherwise, without the prior written permission of the author.
Copyright © 2015 (2nd Printing) by Eyal Shifroni

The author of this book is not a physician and the instructions, procedures, and suggestion in this guide are not intended as a substitute for the medical advice of a trained health professional. All matters regarding your health require medical supervision. Consult your physician before adopting the procedures suggested in this guide, as well as about any condition that may require diagnosis or medical attention. The author and the publisher disclaim any liability arising directly or indirectly from the use of this guide.
All rights reserved © 2015 (2nd Printing)

Acknowledgments and Gratitude

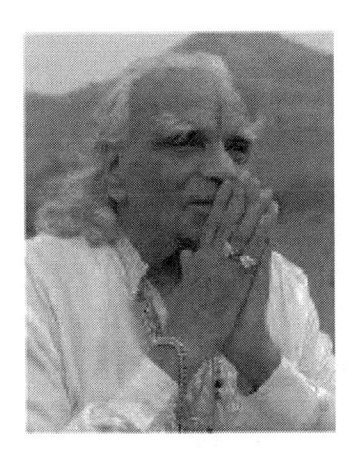

1918 - 2014

The source of all the knowledge presented in this guide is my Guru, the late Yogacharya B.K.S. Iyengar, Guruji as we had fondly used to call him, the founder of the Iyengar Yoga method. The use of props in yoga practice was introduced by Mr. Iyengar. The various apparatus which he invented and adapted over the years were created to enrich practice and to enable every person to benefit from the gift of Yoga. I wish to express my deepest admiration and gratitude to my beloved Guruji, not only for being my personal teacher, but also for making yoga accessible to millions worldwide.

Guruji was so kind to go over the manuscript of my previous book, *A Chair for Yoga*, and to give insightful comments and suggestions. When I visited RIMYI[1] in August 2014, I had planned to show him the manuscript of this volume. Unfortunately this was deemed impossible because of his failing health. I was, however, privileged to be present in Pune on the 20th of August, the day B.K.S. Iyengar left his body and to have the chance to say a last good-bye to my Guru before he travels onward, and to participate in his funeral. I will always be grateful to this man for touching my life so deeply and for offering the gift of yoga to the world through the ingenious method he developed. I wish to humbly dedicate this book to his memory!

I have been very fortunate to have come across many inspiring teachers who have shared their deep knowledge with me and who have shed light on Yoga in general and on the use of props in particular. First and foremost are Prashant and Geeta Iyengar, I wish to thank them for their ongoing guidance and inspiration in their teaching in RIMYI. Second, I wish to thank my teacher and friend Jawahar Bangera from Mumbai, who was so kind to go over the draft of this guide and contribute many helpful comments and suggestions.

I learned a lot from many other teachers - too many to list their names here. However, I am indebted to each and every one of them and wish to express my deep gratitude to them all.

A Chair for Yoga has received enthusiastic responses from many people in all parts of the world, students and teachers alike. It was indeed heartwarming to experience firsthand how yoga is relevant for all human beings, regardless of national, cultural, religious and age differences. This network of comments and responses demonstrated in simple and real terms the truth held by yoga that all

[1] Ramamani Iyengar Memorial Yoga Institute – the home and teaching site of the Iyengars in Pune, India.

of us share a Universal Consciousness (or *Mahat*). The feedback and requests I received from you was a strong motivator for writing this present book!

This second printing of Props for Yoga contains minor improvements relative to the first printing (November 2014); the most significant change is in the titles of the variations, which are now more informative.

This Guide owes its conception and delivery to my friend and colleague, Michael Sela, who helped conceive it and formulate its structure. Michael went through the text over and over again and contributed substantially to its clarity and flow. I wish to express deep appreciation for his collaboration on this project.

Thanks to Ravit Moar and Eleanor Jacobovitz, who teach with me at the Zichron-Ya'akov Center, for spending so many hours modeling for the photos in this guide.

All the teachers at our center have also contributed many beneficial ideas and feedbacks – I wish to thank all of them. Thanks also to my colleagues, Ephrat Michelson, Sara Tal, Nancy Gardosh and Noa Zweig for reading the manuscript of this guide and for providing many useful comments and suggestions. Nancy also went through the text carefully to correct my English and provided encouraging feedback.

I extend many thanks to my students who helped test and develop new ideas of using props during classes and workshops. Their willingness to try out these ideas and their enthusiastic feedback encouraged me to write this guide.

And, last but not least, thanks to my wife, Hagit, for her continuous love and support which made this guide (and many other things) possible.

Table of Contents

Acknowledgments and Gratitude / III
Introduction / IX
About the Use of Props / X
About this Guide / XII
The Structure of the Guide / XIII
How to Use this Guide / XIV

Chapter 1: Understanding the Standing Asanas / 1

Appendix 1: A Practice Sequence / 143
Index / 157

Detailed Contents of Chapter 1: Understanding the Standing Asanas (Utthistha Sthiti)

About Standing asanas	3
Tadasana	4
About Tadasana	4
Feet and Legs	4
1. Activating the feet: Block between feet	5
2. Activating the knees: Block between knees	6
3. Activating the thighs: Block between thighs	7
4. Turning the upper thighs in: Belt on each groin	8
5. Stabilizing the pelvis: Belt around pelvis	9
6. Moving the sacrum in: Block between sacrum and wall	10
7. Thighs back, buttocks in: Two opposite pulls	11
8. Sensing the bones of the legs: Standing on two blocks	12
9. Extending the calves: Standing on a slant	13

Arms and Chest	14
10. Activating the arms: Belt around forearms	14
11. Moving the trapezius down: Shoulder traction	15
12. Sensitizing the top chest: Belt around chest	17
13. Aligning the spine: Spine on a wall edge	18
Urdhva Hastasana	19
1. Stretching the sides: One arm stretches the other	20
2. Activating the arms: Belt around forearms, block between palms	21
3. Extending the armpits: Facing the wall, palms on blocks	22
4. Extending the entire body upward: Holding a ceiling rope	23
Vrksasana	24
Opening the Pelvis	24
1. Moving the femur head in: Bent leg against the wall	25
2. Increasing the movement of the hip joint: Back against the wall	26
3. Widening the pelvis: Facing the wall	27
Stretching Up	28
4. Extending the body upward: Holding a ceiling rope	28
Adho Mukha Svanasana	29
About Adho Mukha Svanasana	29
General Structure of the Pose	29
1. Finding the distance between feet and palms	30
2. Ensuring symmetry: Using a middle line	31
Raising the Palms	32
3. Shifting weight to the legs: Supporting the palms	32
Working with a Partner	34
4. Stretching back and up: Partner pulls backward with belt	34
5. Rooting the heels: Sitting on the "dog"	36
6. Moving in the sacrum: "Two dogs"	37
7. Action and counter-action: Partner pushes against back groins	38

Lifting the Feet — 39
  8. Sensitizing the buttocks: Elevating the feet — 39
  9. Lifting the entire pose: Feet and palms on blocks — 40
  10. Activating the front thighs: Heels on blocks' edges — 41

Activating the Arms and Shoulders — 42
  11. Widening the shoulder girdle: Partner helps to turn the arms — 42
  12. Releasing the neck: Partner pulls the trapezius muscles — 43
  13. Spreading the fingers: Using wall and blocks — 44
  14. Relieving wrist pain: Palms on a slant — 45
  15. Flexing the wrists: Palms on wall — 46
  16. Turning the palms — 47
  17. Stabilizing the arms: Belt around elbows — 48
  18. Stabilizing the arms: Elbows on blocks or inverted chair — 49

Moving On with the Pose — 50
  19. Moving the shoulder blades in: Starting with forearms on the floor — 50
  20. Moving the middle back in: Starting with the head low — 51

Restorative Adho Mukha Svanasana — 52
  21. Relaxing the brain: Head support — 52
  22. Passive extension of the spine: Wall rope around front groins — 53

Uttanasana — 55

About Uttanasana — 55

Legs and Pelvis — 56
  1. Checking the symmetry: Buttocks against the wall — 56
  2. Increasing the thighs action: Back of legs against the wall — 57
  3. Stabilizing the legs: Leaning over the backrest of a chair — 58
  4. Extending the calves: Standing on a slanted surface — 59
  5. Stand high; bend low: Standing on a raised platform — 60
  6. Compact legs: Belt around feet and pelvis — 61
  7. Folding deeply into the pose: Belt around back and legs — 62

Opening the Shoulders — 63
  8. Creating movement in the shoulders: Holding a block behind the back — 63

Restorative Uttanasana — 65
  9. Resting in half-inverted pose: Back against the wall — 65
  10. Relaxing the brain: Top of the Head on block — 66

Utthita Trikonasana — 67

About Utthita Trikonasana — 67

Aligning the Feet — 68
  1. Correct alignment of the legs: Using a reference line — 68

Activating the Back Leg — 69
  2. Anchoring the back foot: Outer foot against the wall — 69
  3. Activating the back leg: Foot on belt — 70
  4. Activating the back leg: Pulling the leg with belt — 71
  5. Lifting the inner groin: Partner pulls the back leg — 72

Turning the Legs Out — 73
  6. Turning the legs: Two belts on the upper thighs — 73
  7. Turning the front leg out: Foot turned more than 90° — 74
  8. Knee turned out; buttock turned in: Entering from Utthita Parsvakonasana — 75

Activating the Front Leg — 76
  9. Activating the front leg: Lifting the toe mounds — 76
  10a. Activating the front leg: Heel on block — 77
  10b. Stretching the front leg: Sole against the wall — 78

Opening the Pelvis — 79
  11. Opening the groins: Diagonal alignment — 79
  12. Ensuring lateral alignment: Back against the wall — 81
  13. Broadening the trunk and relaxing the eyes: Facing the wall — 83

Maintaining Length Along the Sides of the Trunk — 84
  14. Extending the sides of the trunk: Front hand on wall — 85
  15a. Bending from the hips: Partner pulls the front hip — 86
  15b. Pulling the front groin while stabilizing the back leg — 87

Correcting Hyper-extended Knees — 88
  16. Active work for hyper-extended knee: Pressing the foot against the wall — 88
  17. Stabilizing hyper-extended knee: Supporting the calf with block — 89, 90
  18. Turning the chest: Upper hand holds weight — 90
  19. Turning the chest: Hands holding a chair from behind — 91
  20. Rolling the shoulders back: Bottom palm on block — 92
  21. Moving the shoulders back: Arms behind the back — 93

Stretching the Top Arm	94
22: Stretching the top arm: Holding a rope	94

Virabhadrasana II — 95

Bending the Knee to Form a Square — 95
1. Squaring the front leg: Belt from knee to back leg	96
2. Squaring the front leg: Supporting the knee with a block	97
3. Reducing muscular effort: Resting the buttock on a chair	98

Stretching the Back Arm — 99
4a. Activating the back arm: Back palm against the wall	99
4b. Aligning the chest above the pelvis: Back hand holds a wall rope	100
5. Aligning the chest above the pelvis: Partner holds the back arm	101

Lifting and Opening the Chest — 102
6. Lifting the chest: Holding a block	102

Virabhadrasana I — 103

About Virabhadrasana I — 103

Turning Sideways — 103
1a. Learning the sideways orientation: Entering by stepping back	104
1b. Turning sideways: Entering from Vimanasana	105
2. Opening the chest: Belt attached to the back leg	106
3. Arching back: Hands against the wall	107
4. Activating the back leg: Supporting the heel	108
5. Reducing muscular effort: Front thigh rests on chair	109
6. Moving the tailbone in: Pubic bone against a wall corner	110
7. Experiencing lightness: Helpers lift the groins	111

Upper Body — 112
8. Activating the arms: Belt around the elbows	112
9. Activating the arms: Holding a block	113
10. Stretching upward: Holding a ceiling rope	114
11. Moving the thoracic vertebrae in: Arms behind the back	115

Virabhadrasana III — 116
1. Learning to balance: Supporting the hands	117
2. Horizontal alignment: Supporting the pelvis with a chair	119
3. Aligning the back (lifted) leg: Hands on blocks	120
4. Compacting the standing leg: Belt from foot to pelvis	122
5. Learning to stretch horizontally: Entering from Urdhva Hastasana	123
6. Opening the chest: Arms behind the back	124
7. Stabilizing the pose: Belt on back leg	125
8. Floating in Virabhadra III: Holding wall ropes	126
9. Restorative Virabhadra III: Hands on wall, back leg on stool	127

Parsvottanasana — 128
1. Shifting weight to the back leg: Hands on wall	129
2. Pelvis alignment: Supporting the front groins on a chair	131
3. Anchoring the back leg: Foot against the wall	132
4. Intensified forward bend: Hands catching the back knee	133
5. Stabilizing the pelvis: Pulling the front groins with belt	134
6. Opening the shoulders: Hands in Gomukhasana	135

Prasarita Padottanasana — 136
1. Insuring symmetry: Using floor lines	136
2. Activating the thighs: Buttocks against the wall	137
3. Activating the legs: Bracing the outer ankles with a belt	138
4. Activating the legs: Pressing outer feet against wall/block	139
5. When the head does not reach the floor: Tilting the pelvis forward	140
6. Creating space in the pelvis: Pulling the inner groins	141
7. Intensifying the downward stretch: Standing on blocks	142

Introduction

Yoga was revealed by the ancient sages as a way of spiritual realization and transformation; it was transmitted to us by a succession of sages (rishis) and Gurus. Texts like The *Yoga Sutras of Patanjali*, the *Bhagavad Gita* and the *Shiva Samhita* define and describe the essence of yoga, the yogic state, and yogic conduct. Many interpretations of these ancient texts have evolved over the years, including several books by my own teacher, Yogacharya B.K.S. Iyengar.

Yoga is not just a theory; it is a practical philosophy, a path to be travelled with intention, action, sensitivity and dedication. Only by putting the *sutras* into practice in our own lives can their full meaning and significance be revealed to us. Mere theoretical study of the texts will not lead to transformation and liberation. Iyengar's brilliant contribution has been to formulate ways in which the practice of asana and pranayama can be used to transform our bodies and minds through self-reflection, seeking to achieve the yogic state of knowing the eternal soul within.

Asanas are not mere exercises; they enable us to study our bodies and minds and to get acquainted with our limitations, tendencies and potentialities. Iyengar had developed the practice of asanas to a level of art and science. In his book *The Tree of Yoga*, he writes:

"Mahatma Gandhi did not practice all the aspects of yoga. He only followed two of its principles – non-violence and truth, yet through these two aspects of yoga, he mastered his own nature and gained independence for India. If part of yama could make Mahatma Gandhi so great, so pure, so honest and so divine, should it not be possible to take another limb of yoga – asana – and through it reach the highest level of spiritual development? Many of you may say that performing asana is a physical discipline, but if you speak in this way without knowing the depth of asana, you have already fallen from the grace of yoga." [2]

In this book, he shows how all eight limbs of *Ashtanga Yoga* can be expressed and practiced through a deep study of the third and fourth limbs (asana and pranayama). Of course, practicing asanas as physical exercises has its own merit; it may keep your body flexible, healthy and light, but if you do not accompany your practice by observing and studying your mind, you will miss the opportunity to develop your intelligence and uplift your consciousness (By 'intelligence' I do not refer merely to one's IQ level but rather to one's ability to

[2] *The Tree of Yoga* in the chapter: The depth of asana

perceive one's self and one's surroundings without biases, and to act skillfully in the pursuit of good according to one's own values and sense of truth).

An examination of the role of props in the asana practice of B.K.S. Iyengar helps us to understand his method. The wide range of props serves as a tool to make the practice accessible to people of all age groups and health conditions. Together with B.K.S. Iyengar's detailed instructions and thorough interpretations of ancient yogic texts, the props have enabled millions to realize his vision that "Yoga is for All."

About the Use of Props

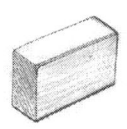

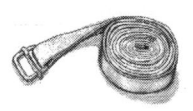

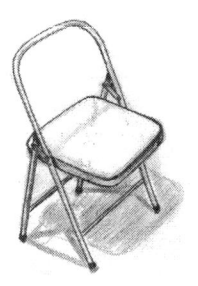

This is how Iyengar explains why he introduced props into his practice and teaching:

"I was preoccupied trying various ways to improve and perfect my own practice. I used to pick up stones and bricks lying on the roads and used them as 'supports' and 'weight bearers' to make progress in my mastery of asana…

Props help to perform the asanas with ease… The student understands and learns asana faster on props as the brain remains passive. Through passive brain one learns to be alert in body and mind. **Props are guides to self-learning**[3]*. They help accurately without mistakes."* (In 70 Glorious years of Yogacharya B.K.S.. Iyengar, page 391)

Christian Pisano adds to that:

"Props thus allow us to unfold the space of an asana and acquaint us with certain asanas that may otherwise be too difficult to practice. Props create understanding of the correct gesture (mudra) and attitude (bhava) of asana. Props let us stay longer in an asana, thus permitting deeper penetration of unexplored bodily regions." [4]

[3] Highlighted by present author
[4] The Hero's Contemplation

While props are an important characteristic of Iyengar Yoga, they should not be confused with its essence. Props are a means for achieving an end - such as alignment, stability, precision, and prolonged stays in asanas.

The usage of props covered here is intended to direct awareness to different aspects of the asanas and to different parts of the body, in order to deepen and enhance the understanding of the asanas. At the same time, practitioners should be careful not to develop dependency on props; rather, props should be employed intelligently in pursuit of a mature and mindful practice of asanas.

Iyengar continues his description:

"Now, talking of the pros and cons of using props, one of the criticisms leveled against props is that one becomes habituated and lacks the will to attempt doing independently. Is this the fault of props? Certainly not! Props are to feel the asana. But I never say that they should be used on a permanent basis. Props give the sense of direction. When sense of direction sets in, I want my pupils to do the asanas independently sooner or later… The props are meant to give a sense of direction, alignment and understanding of the asana."[1]

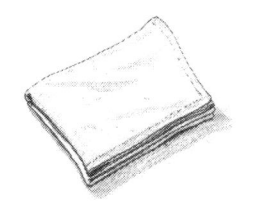

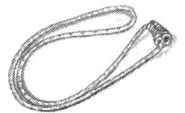

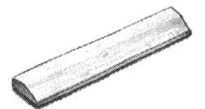

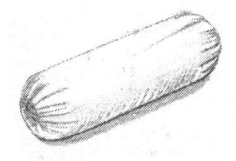

Ultimately the body and mind are also external props to help 'the seer to dwell in his own true splendor' (*Yoga Sutras of Patanjali*, I.3), or as Pisano expresses it: *"… Props can be regarded as an outer weave that points to the very essence of the asana, in a purely subjective way. There will therefore always be some swaying between using an external prop and using the body itself as a prop. Ultimately, the body-mind is itself only an external prop."*[2]

To sum it up, props make it possible for every person to enhance his/her *Sadhana* (study and discipline of yoga), regardless of physical limitations. By using props adequately one can:

- Perform asanas which are difficult to perform independently
- Achieve and maintain correct alignment during the practice
- Stay longer and relax in challenging asanas, thus attaining their full benefit
- Study and investigate asanas on a deeper level
- Continue practice and improve one's condition despite illness, injury, or chronic condition

[1] *Ibid.*
[2] *Ibid.*

About this Guide

This guide is the fruit of my 35 years of *Yoga Sadhana*. It has evolved from a continuous journey of practice and study, in my home practice; at RIMYI under B.K.S., Geeta, and Prashant Iyengar; in countless workshops that I took or offered in Israel and around the world; and from daily work with teachers and students in my own Iyengar Yoga Center in Israel.

Often, when preparing a class or a workshop, I search for new ways of highlighting the principles of asana practice using props. I believe that many of my colleagues share a similar need. *Props for Yoga* is my modest attempt to address this need.

Since the original publication of *Light on Yoga*, the book which laid the foundation of the 'Iyengar Method', many books have been written in an attempt to elaborate and explain the wealth of knowledge embedded in that fundamental and by now classic text. The most prominent one is the beautiful book by B.K.S. Iyengar himself: *Yoga – the Path to Holistic Health*. Geeta's book: *A Gem for Women* and her booklets: *Yoga in Action, Preliminary and Intermediate-I courses* are important additions to that body of knowledge. Other books like *Yoga the Iyengar Way* by Silva, Mira & Shyam Mehta further clarify and specify the method. Most of these books, however, are intended for the general public, and cover mostly the basic usage of props. There are also several books showing the use of props specifically for Yoga Therapy. This guide is intended primarily for teachers and experienced practitioners of the Iyengar method. It presents and **explains more thoroughly how to use props to learn and achieve basic actions required in the classical asanas**. While some of the variations may be well known, many others are new and innovative ways that have not yet been documented.

My previous book, *A Chair for Yoga*, focused on the use of a single prop in the practice of a large number of asanas. In contrast, this book deals with a much smaller set of asanas but utilizes a variety of props. I limit the discussion to the simple, commonly available props such as blocks, belts, blankets, walls, bolsters, ropes, etc.

The present volume of the guide is the first in a series. It covers standing asanas and includes one practice sequense. Future volumes will focus on other families of asanas. Each will include practice sequences of various lengths and levels. These sequences will demonstrate how to use specific props for a complete practice session. The sequence included with this volume (See Appendix 1) demonstrates usage of blocks for standing poses, inversions and back bends.

The Structure of the Guide

This volume of the guide contains one chapter: Standing Asanas. The chapter begins with a short introduction followed by a number of representative asanas. For each asana a number of variations with different props are offered. Each variation is presented in the following order:

   a. Props in use
   b. Short introduction
   c. Step-by-Step Instructions
   d. Effects of practicing this variation
   e. Tips – special points to observe in this variation
   f. Applicability – in what other asanas the prop can be used in this way

The **Step-by-Step Instructions** (part c), illustrated by many photos, provide the technical information needed in order to position the body and use the props. The **Effects** section explains why the specific variation is given. It tells what we can learn from using the prop in the specified manner or how it might help us avoid common mistakes in alignment. The **Tips** section gives some clues regarding physical as well as mental actions you should do while staying in the asana in order to get the desired effect.

Note: *Asana practice works on many levels. Our presentation refers mostly to the seen and explicit level, the anamaya kośa (the structural, anatomic body). However asanas have deep effects on the more internal kośas including the organic-physiological sheath (pranamaya kośa) and the psychological sheath (monomaya kośa). This text, being a practical guide, focuses on the technical aspects of the practice. This does not mean that the deeper effects of the practice are less important. We leave it for you – the reader - to pursue and experiment on your own these internal effects.*

How to Use this Guide

Keep the following in mind when using this guide:

- This guide is not a substitute for learning with a certified Iyengar Yoga teacher. The subtleties of the instructions in the Iyengar method cannot adequately be captured in a book. So, while it can help you study and explore the asanas, please remember that no guide can observe you and correct the mistakes you may perform while doing a variation.

- Work by comparison and analysis: Do the pose several times with and without the props. Observe your sensations when doing the pose with the prop and then try to recreate those sensations without the prop. Do not use the props habitually, but rather use them for learning in a creative and innovative way; study and compare the effects to enhance your understanding. Do not develop dependency on props; rather, employ them mindfully. Always remain fresh and alert!

- The possibilities are virtually endless; use your imagination and creativity to find new ways of using props.

You should also note the following:

1. For the sake of clarity, each variation we present focuses on the use of a single prop, or on one specific way to work on an asana. However, some of the variations can be practiced in combination or in sequence. To avoid confusion, we do not show such combinations, but rather encourage you to try it on your own.

2. To facilitate quick access to the material in the guide use the detailed *Index* and the *Table of Contents*. The *Index* contains references to the variations according to the prop used and the asana taken – this is helpful if you wish to see all the variations that use a certain prop.

3. When working in pairs, it is recommended to work with a partner of the same gender and, as much as possible, of the same size and flexibility. Always be watchful and prudent when helping other people.

4. Certain variations refer to plates in *Light on Yoga*. Those are marked by the symbol LOY followed by the plate number. For example "LOY Pl. 100" refers to plate number 100 in *Light on Yoga*.

5. The guide shows only a sample of what can be done with props. In particular, the number of variations using a chair is limited. For extensive use of chairs in Iyengar Yoga practice, please refer to *A Chair for Yoga – A complete guide to Iyengar Yoga practice with a chair*, by the same author.

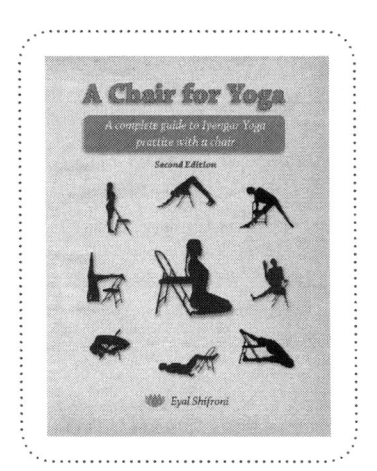

CAUTION Users of this guide must have a solid foundation in yoga practice, preferably obtained through regular classes with a certified Iyengar Yoga teacher. Some of the variations shown in this guide are advanced and should not be attempted without guidance and supervision. The author takes no responsibility for any injury or damage that may occur due to improper use of the material presented.

Enjoy your practice!
....

If you have any comments or feedback…I'd love to hear it.
Please write to me at:
eyal@theiyengaryoga.com

Chapter 1
Understanding the Standing Asanas

About Standing Asanas

Standing poses (asanas) are the basis for Iyengar Yoga practice. These poses open and strengthen the body, develop flexibility and build the muscle actions required for more advanced asanas. Beginners learn how to use the legs for activating the lower torso and how to use the arms for activating the upper torso. By extending the muscles of the legs and groins, one attains free movement at the hips. This allows the spine to extend freely and in the long run will prevent back pain. By creating movement in the shoulder girdle, the shoulders retain their flexibility and the chest is broadened. This improves breathing and circulation and keeps the body agile and light and the mind fresh.

Standing postures are a good starting point for learning yoga asanas. In a classroom environment, the standing postures allow students and teacher to see each other most easily. They involve more external action, and demand less mentally. Their challenges and rewards are also more immediate than those of other classes of postures.

Standing poses are ideal for introducing the principles of alignment. When standing, our field of vision is broad and we are more aware of the space around us. It is here that we learn to align ourselves by orienting our body in reference to the floor and wall planes and correct the alignment of our limbs accordingly. In this sense, standing poses can lead us from *Vikalpa* (fantasy, delusion) and *Viparyaya* (wrong knowledge, illusion) to *Pramana* (valid knowledge).

Standing poses teach us to activate and integrate all of our elements: we get rooting and grounding from our feet (earth); we sense flow and movement within us (water); we generate and release energy and enthusiasm (fire); we open the chest and relax our skin to enable continuous, uninterrupted breathing and bring lightness (air); and we develop awareness of our inner organs and the space within us (ether).

Standing poses are challenging and rewarding. They develop will power, strength, endurance and stamina – all of which are fundamental elements of Yoga. Even if you are an advanced practitioner, do not discard these poses from your practice routine. Always return to the basics!

Tadasana

About Tadasana

Tadasana is a pose that every beginner learns, and we always come back to it. The more you practice it, the more you learn to appreciate its subtleties. The pose creates balance and stability, height and extension, compactness from outside as well as expansion from inside. In general, the variations listed below are applicable to other straight-standing poses, such as Urdhva Hastasana, Urdhva Namskarasana and Urdhva Baddhanguliyasana.

Tadasana is also called *Samasthiti*. In Sanskrit, *Tad* means mountain and *Sama* means stable, even and *sthiti* means state or condition. This pose combines the height and solidity of a mountain with balance and evenness. One of the meanings of *Samasthiti* is 'standing upright without moving'. When you join your legs and stand upright, note how the weight of your body tends to shift from one foot to the other. This becomes more apparent when closing the eyes: vision and balance are strongly connected.

With open eyes, but unfocused gaze, look forward at eye level and mentally observe the shoulder blades. Relax any movement or hardness in the eyeballs. When your eyes become quiet and soft, lower the inner gaze down as if to observe the heels. Check if your weight is distributed evenly on your two heels. Can you maintain an even and stable (*sama*) pose without letting the weight shift from one heel to the other? Observing this will give you a different experience of this seemingly simple pose! It can become a meditative pose!

Occasionally, hold the pose for five minutes or more. Physically that is not difficult; but mentally it presents an interesting challenge!

Tips

- Do the pose with open eyes but without looking at any specific object. Imagine you are looking far forward to the horizon, where the sea meets the sky.

- Broaden your field of vision and soften your eyes, as if looking from the ears; observe the body's internal state and actions.

- Relax the eardrums and allow them to recede toward the back of the skull.

- Let the top of the brain recede into the base of the brain, and then let the brain recede down into the heart center.

⚠ CAUTIONS

People with scoliosis should rest the spine against a wall edge (see Variation 14 of this pose).

If you are prone to dizziness do the pose with your back against a wall.

Feet and Legs

We start Tadasana with attention to the base. The feet, legs and pelvic girdle enable the grounding of the pose, embodying its earth element.

Tadasana Variation 1

Activating the feet: Block between feet

Props
Block

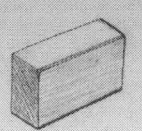

→ Stand with the legs slightly apart. Place a flat block in between and in contact with the inner sides of the feet.

› Lift the toe mounds of the right foot, bend and use your fingers to open and spread the skin of the mounds. Spread the toes and place them such that the big toes touch each other and the small toes are spread outward.

› Press the big toe mounds and the inner heels down to the floor and lift the inner ankles.

› Press the 'neck' of the toes down to the floor.

› Lift the right heel, extend it back, away from the arch and place it so that the outer heel is pressed down, the heel bone is wide and both sides of the ankle are vertical.

› Now stand straight. Compare the different sensations in your right and the left legs.

› Repeat the same work on the left foot.

› Press from the outer feet against the block.

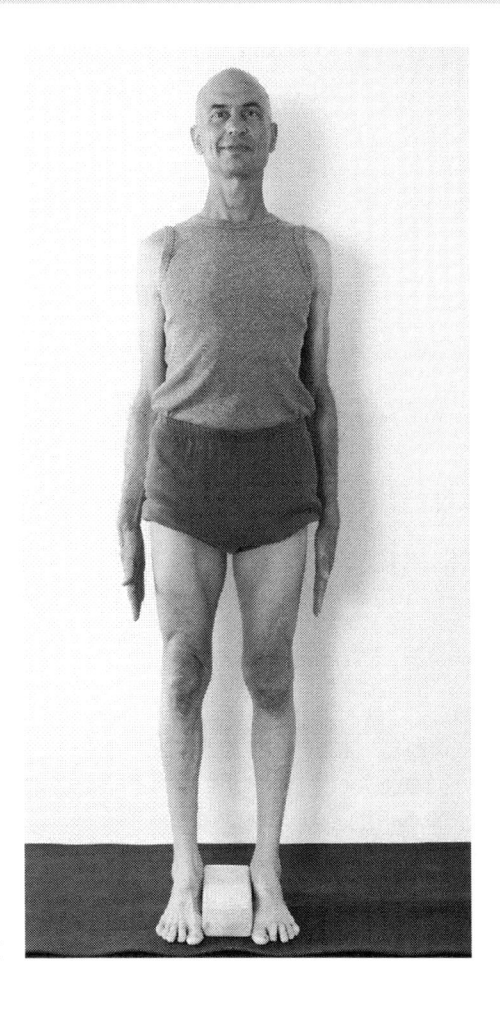

Effects

Improves the sensitivity and action of the feet and develops balance and stability. The resistance of the block activates the feet and ankles; this improves the work of the entire leg and teaches to lift the arches of the feet. After adjusting the first foot you will observe a remarkable difference between the legs. This will teach you the correct feeling of the base of Tadasana.

Tips

✓ Check that the outer heel is performing a 'little Tadasana', i.e., it is upright and vertical. Then check if the inner arches and inner ankles of both feet are lifted.

✓ Do not press the tips of the toes to the floor, as this will bend the toes. Energetically move the metatarsal bones back toward the heels while extending the toes forward.

✓ Spread the skin of the soles of the feet as if you want to touch 'Mother Earth' with every cell of the sole.

✓ Observe the shape of both feet and legs – are both legs symmetrical?

✓ Identify which foot carries more weight, then check in which eye the vision is sharper – is there any connection between feet and eyes?

Tadasana
Variation 2

Activating the knees: Block between knees

Props
block
1 or 2 belts

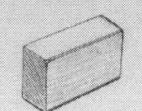

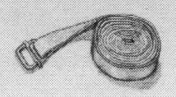

→ Hold a block between the knees.

› Move the outer knees backward and press the inner knees against the block. Now move also the inner knees backward without letting the outer knees move forward.

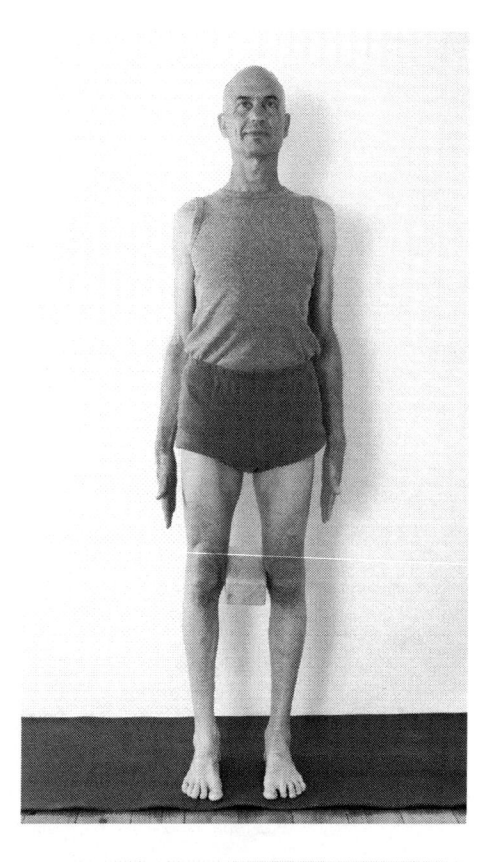

› A belt around the middle of the shins is useful for people with rounded shins (O shape). Another belt can be placed in the middle of the thighs.

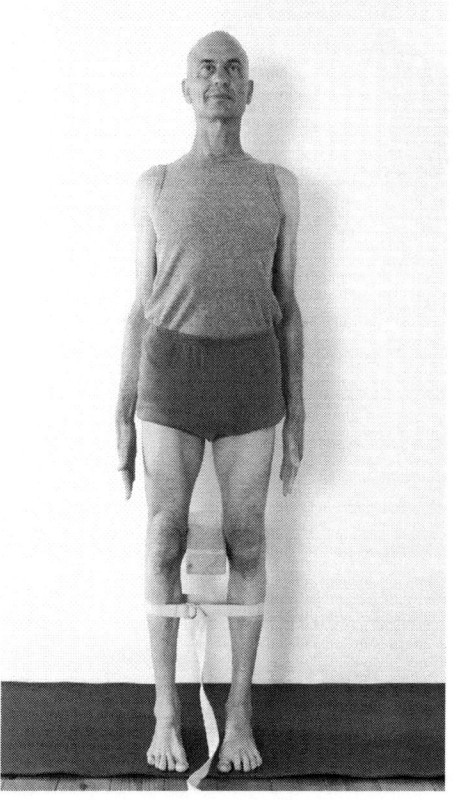

Effects
The resistance of the block activates the knees and sharpens the awareness in the thighs. Gradually, "o"-shape and "x"-shape legs will become more parallel.

Tips
✓ Learn to move the outer ligaments of the knees backwards, in order to balance the inward rotation of the upper thighs and to correct 'knocked knees'.

✓ After lifting the kneecaps, move them back into the knees and open the back of the knees.

6 Props for Yoga / Chapter 1 / Tadasana

Tadasana
Variation 3

Activating the thighs: Block between thighs

Props
block

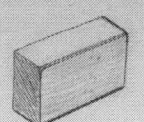

→ Stand with your legs slightly spread, place a block vertically between the thighs and press the legs against it. Move the feet closer to each other, until the pressure of the block on the thighs is equal all along its contact surface.

> Roll the upper thighs inward, as if you are trying to move the block backward.

> Simultaneously, extend the buttock muscles down, move the tailbone in and toward the block, as if you try to move the block forward.

> Move the front thighs backward.

> You can also keep the block in between the thighs as above, and tighten a belt around the thighs.

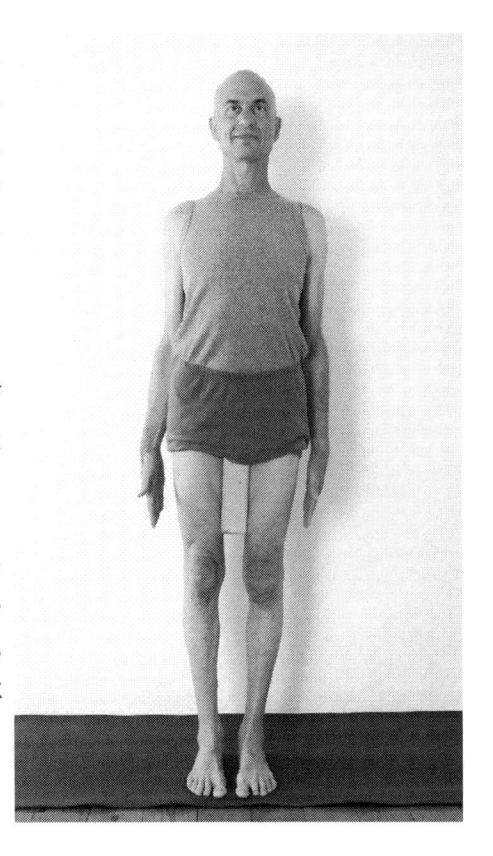

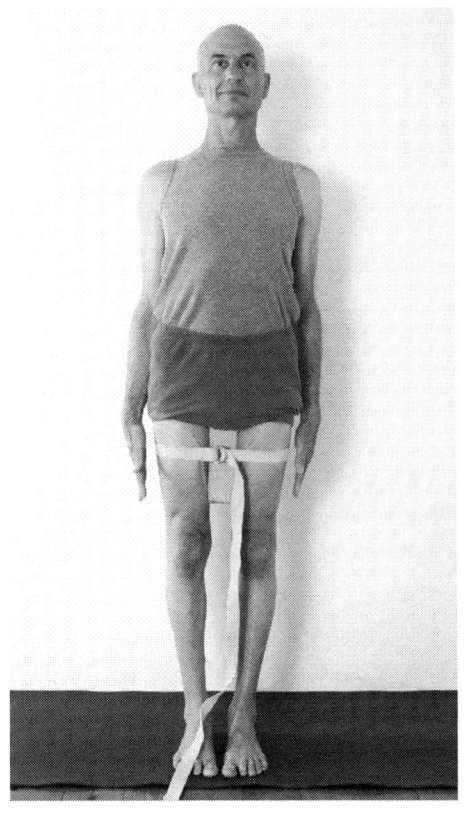

Effects
Helps to learn the inward rotation of the thighs. Pressing against the block creates compactness in the legs without shrinking the inner space; this has a deep organic effect in the lower abdomen.

Tips

✓ Turn the thighs until the inner front thighs touch the block and the outer front thighs face forward.

✓ The shape of the thighs should resemble a block – i.e. the front thigh should face the wall in front, the sides should face the walls at the sides, and the back of the thigh should face the wall behind.

✓ Imagine you are standing on a pointed-heels shoes (not recommended to do, but you can imagine…) and tuck these pointed heels down into the ground. Observe the effect on the thighs.

Applicability
Any pose in which the legs are together and straight; e.g. *Sirsasana, Sarvangasana & Setu Bandha Sarvangasana* (LOY Pl. 259) and *Dandasana*.

Props for Yoga / Chapter 1 / Tadasana 7

Tadasana
Variation 4

Props
2 belts

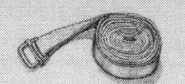

Turning the upper thighs in: Belt on each groin

→ Wrap two belts, one around the upper thigh of each leg, just below the groins.

> Tighten each belt with the buckle at the inner groin and pass the loose ends between your legs to the back.

> Catch both belts from behind your thighs and pull backwards.

> Observe how the skin of the buttocks and the top back thighs is moving from inside out and the sacral band is widened.

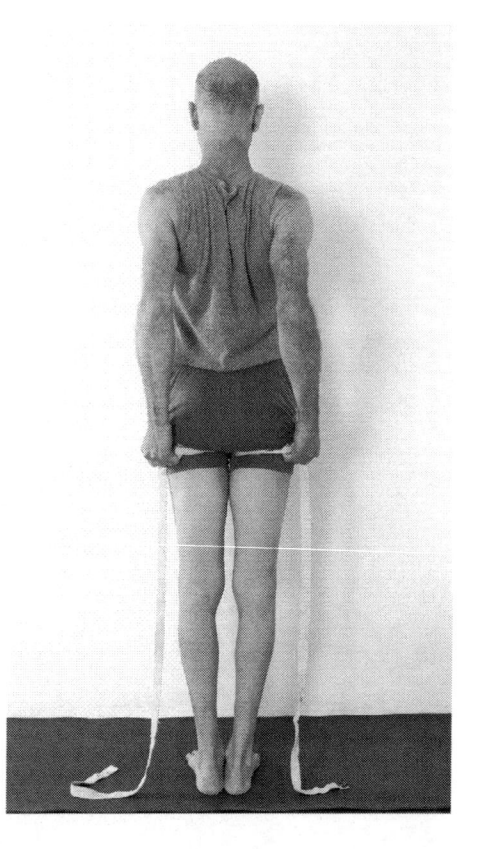

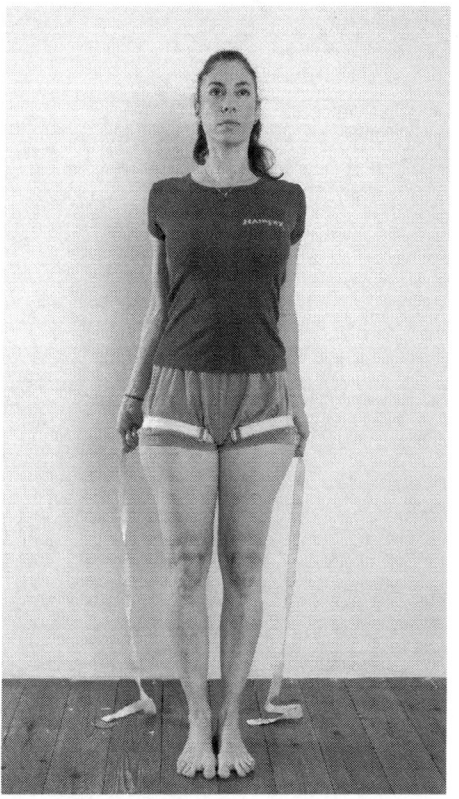

Effects
Pulling the belts clarifies the turning action that should be done in the thighs and its effects on the pelvic area.

Tips

✓ Pull the belts to learn how much the upper thighs can turn in.

✓ Observe the effect of this turning on the sacral band, the lumbar, the lower abdomen and its internal organs.

✓ When doing without the belts you can use your two hands to turn the upper thighs one at a time.

Applicability
This technique may be used for any pose which requires turning the thighs in, e.g. *Parsvottanasana* and *Virabhadrasana I*.

Tadasana
Variation 5

Stabilizing the pelvis: Belt around pelvis

Props
1-2 belts

→ Place a belt around the middle of the pelvis. Tighten it so that it presses against the greater trochanters (the two boney bulges on the sides of the pelvis) and touches the middle of the pubic bone. Bend the knees slightly and tighten the belt.

› Use both hands so that the belt is tightened evenly on both sides of the pelvis.

› If one hip joint feels weaker than the other, tighten the belt from that 'weaker' side towards the 'good' side.

› For best results use two belts, tightened in opposite directions.

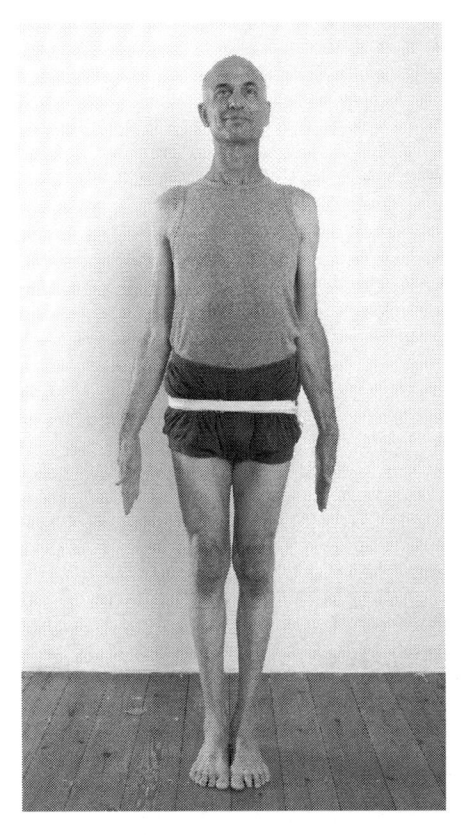

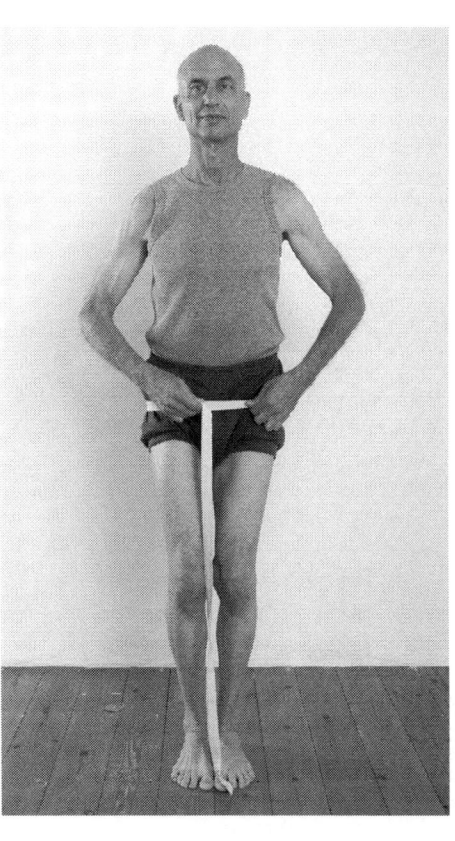

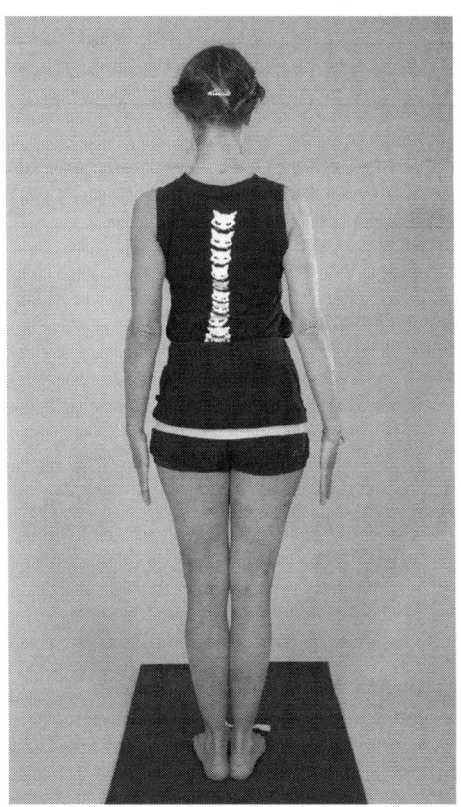

Effects
The belt presses against the femur heads and stabilizes the balls of the joints in their sockets. This is very healthy for the hip joints.

Tips

✓ Observe the touch of the skin with the belt; where is it more pronounced: at the back or at the front?

✓ Move the base of the pelvis forward to touch the belt with your pubis while tightening the mid-buttocks in, away from the belt.

Applicability
People suffering from hip joint problems will benefit from wearing the belts around the pelvis during regular practice.

Props for Yoga / Chapter 1 / Tadasana 9

Tadasana Variation 6

Moving the sacrum in: Block between sacrum and wall

Props
block

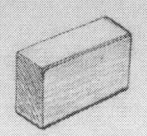

→ Stand with your back to the wall. The distance from the wall should match the length of the block you are using.

› Insert the block between the sacro-lumbar area and the wall. Bend your knees ❶.

› Slowly straighten the knees while dragging the sacral skin down ❷.

› Move the front thighs back to press the block with the sacrum.

› Roll the shoulders back and stand straight in Tadasana.

› You can also take the arms up to Urdhva Hastasana or Urdhva Baddhanguliyasana. Resist the tendency of the thighs to move forward when you lift the arms.

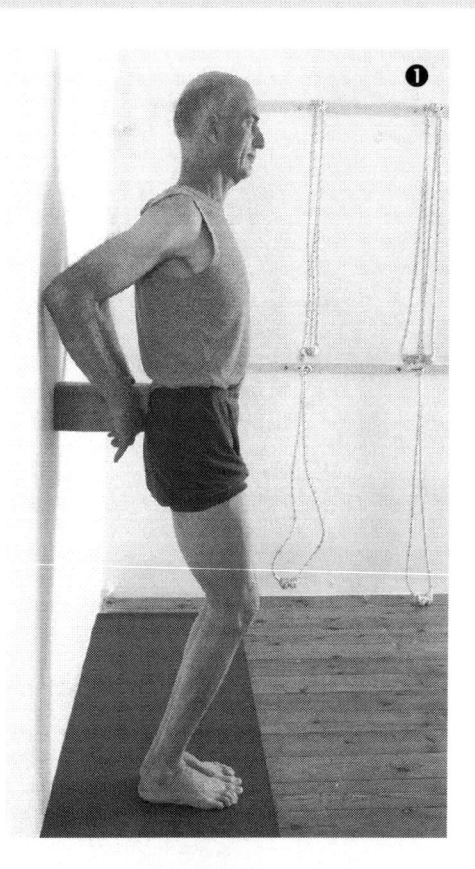

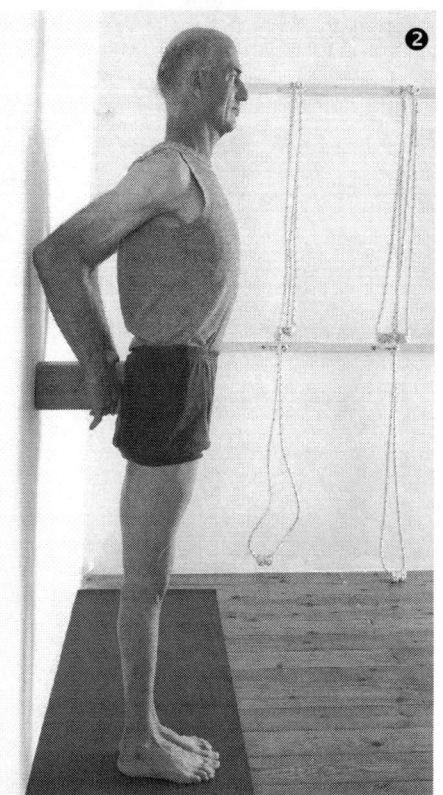

Effects

The block helps to hold the sacrum inside the pelvis, which in turn allows the whole spine to extend freely. This induces widening and relaxation of the lower abdomen. The pressure against the block clarifies the instruction: 'Move the tailbone in'.

Tips

✓ Observe: is the content of the front thighs more pronounced than that of the back thighs? Imagine you move the content of the front thighs back, to fill the back of the thighs.

Tadasana
Variation 7

Thighs back, buttocks in: Two opposite pulls

Props
2 ropes
2 helpers

This variation produces a similar effect to the previous one but with a different method.

⟹ Stand in Tadasana and have one helper stand behind and the other in front of you.

> The front helper wraps a belt around the middle of your buttocks; the rear helper wraps a belt around your frontal upper thighs.

> Then the rear helper pulls the front thighs backward, while the front helper pulls the mid buttocks forward.

> These two opposite pulls should be balanced.

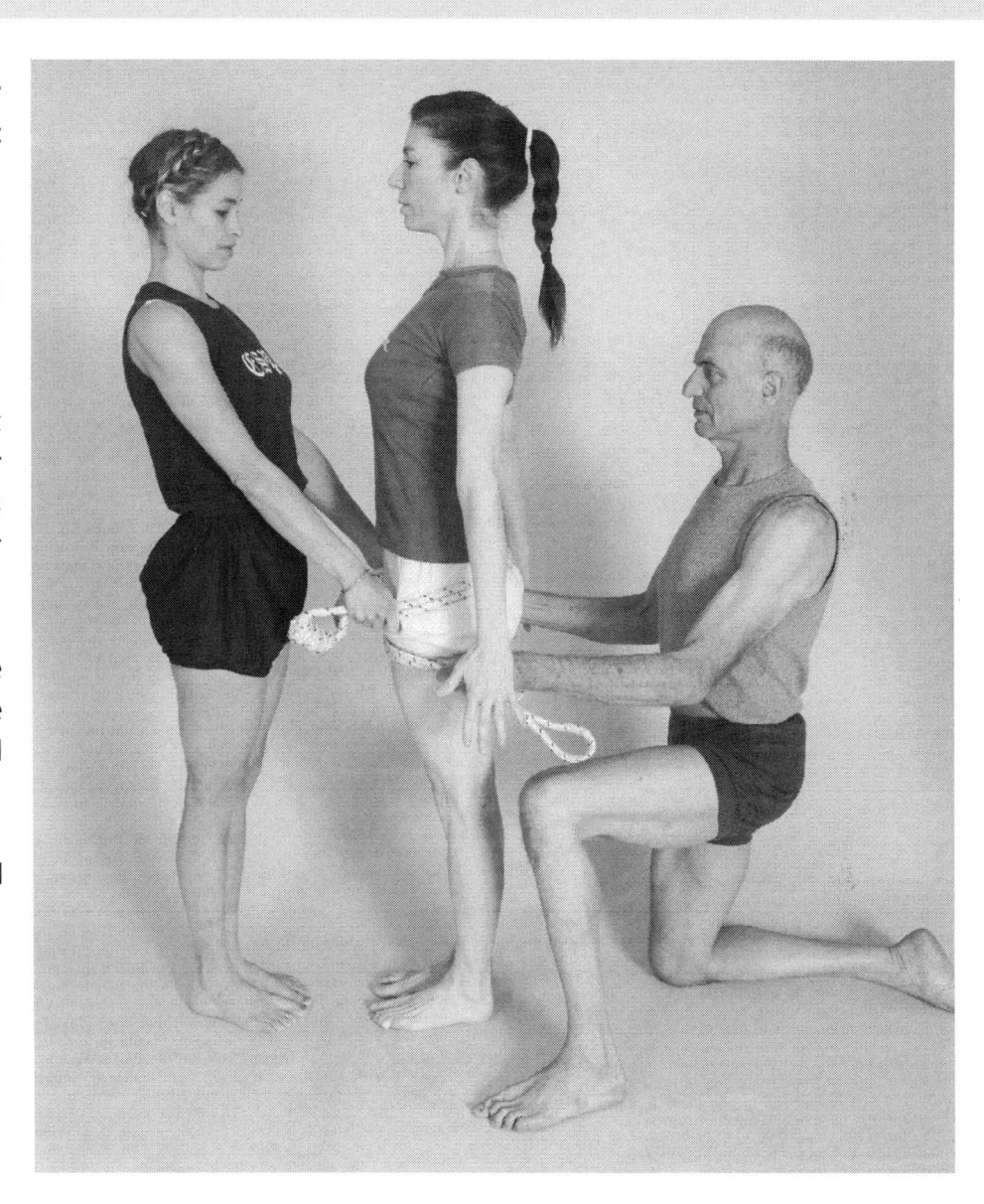

Tips

- Extend the skin of the soles from the arches toward the heels and stamp the heels down.

- Lift the front thigh muscles and move them back, closer to the bone.

- Looking from the side, the hip joint should be just above the ankle joint.

- Lift the lower ribs high above the abdomen and broaden the chest.

- Experience the effect of these actions with helpers and then try to recreate it on your own.

Effects

The pull of the two ropes clarifies the simultaneous actions of the upper legs and the pelvis. When the pelvis finds its correct vertical alignment and is held stable, the abdomen is drawn towards the spine without tension in the abdomen muscles. The pose immediately feels taller, lighter and effortless.

Tadasana
Variation 8

Sensing the bones of the legs: Standing on two blocks

Props
block

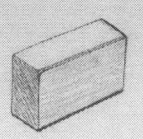

→ Stand on two blocks with toes extending beyond the front edge of the blocks.

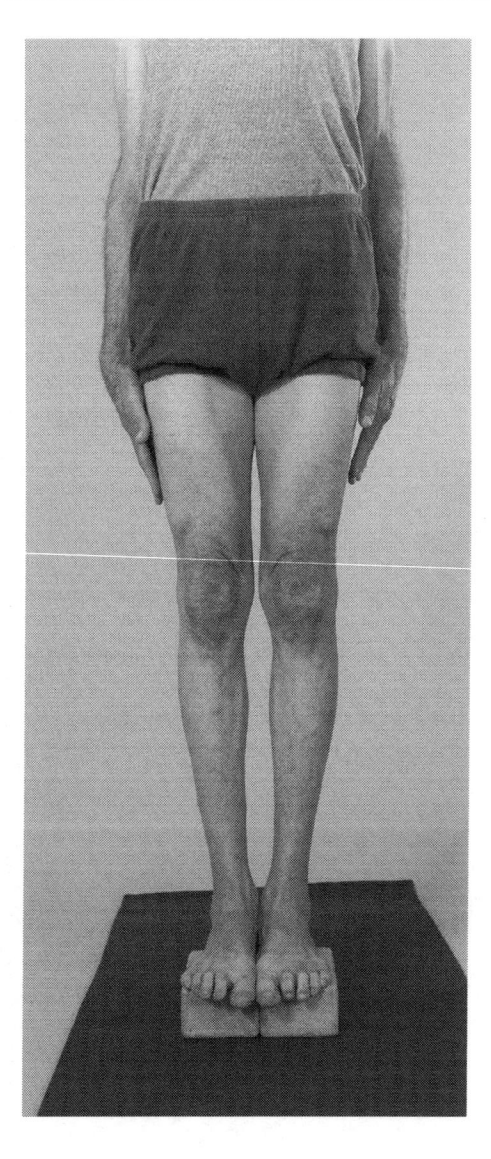

Effects
The resistance of the blocks creates a more tangible lengthening and density in the bones of the legs. You not only feel higher, but also taller, lighter- almost floating. Releasing the toes over the edges of the blocks teaches to release undue tension in the toes.

Tips
✓ Release the toes over the edges of the blocks.

Applicability
Vrksasana, Uttanasana, Prasarita Padottanasana.

Tadasana
Variation 9

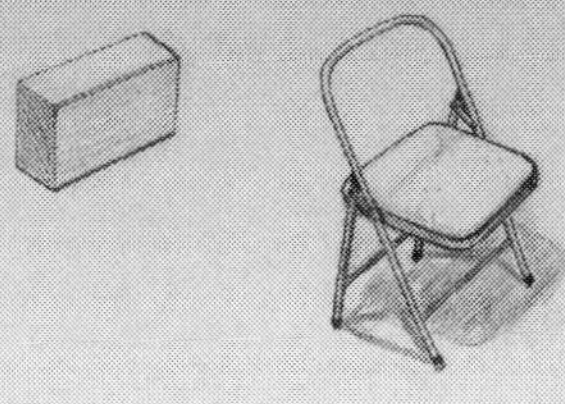

Extending the calves: Standing on a slant

Props
block or chair

→ We show two ways to stand on a slanting surface.

1. Using a block:

> Stand with the toe mounds lifted on a block ❶.

> Move your front thighs back and the tailbone inward.

> You can also stretch the arms up to Urdhva Hastasana or Urdhva Baddhanguliyasana ❷.

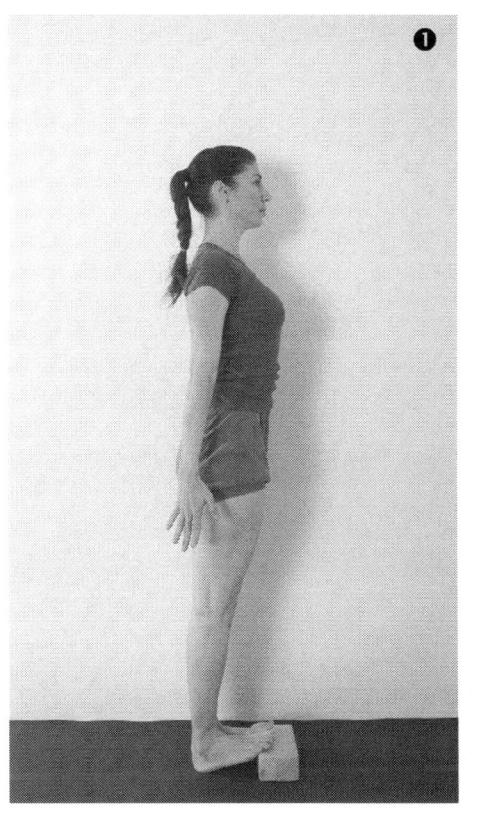

2. On inverted chair:

> Stand on the back side of the seat of an inverted chair.

> To prevent the body from falling back pull a rope attached to a wall ❸, or hold a firm and stable object.

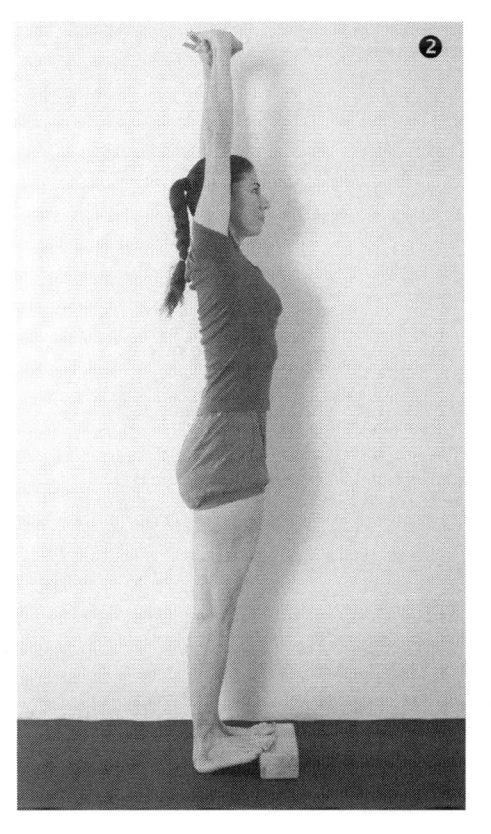

Effects

Beginners often find it hard to lift the knee caps and hold them in place. In this variation the quadriceps (front thigh muscles) are automatically activated and the knee caps are lifted and pulled back. It also stretches the calf (gastrocnemius) muscles and the Achilles tendons.

Applicability

Uttanasana.

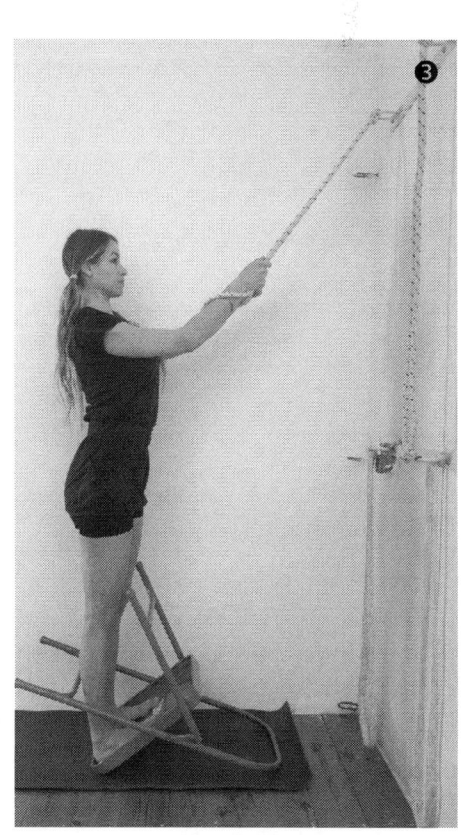

Props for Yoga / Chapter 1 / Tadasana 13

Arms and Chest

The legs are the base of Tadasana, but in order to open the chest, the arms and the shoulders should work as well. Following are several variations that help to develop the actions of the arms, shoulders and shoulder blades.

Tadasana Variation 10

Props
Belt

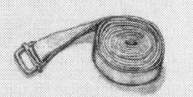

Activating the arms: Belt around forearms

→ Wrap a belt around your forearms to keep them at shoulder-width.

› Lift the side chest up and stretch the arms down.

› Move them sideways, as if to stretch the belt.

› Extend the palms and fingers down in line with the arms.

> **Note:** People who find it hard to straighten the elbows can wrap the belt around the bones of the outer elbows; this will help them to move these bones in.

› Another option is to interlock the fingers behind the back (Paschima Baddhanguliyasana) and stretch the arms initially back and then down (while lifting the side chest up).

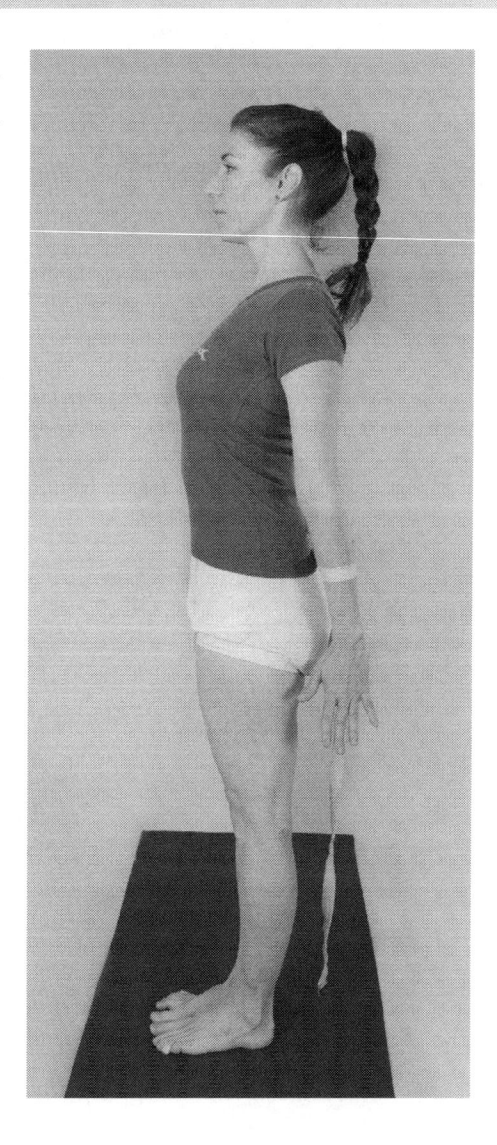

Effects

Activating the arms against the belt moves the shoulders back and the shoulder blades in, which in turn opens the chest. The arms action becomes much clearer when working against resistance.

Tips

✓ Work the arms against the belt to move the shoulder blades in while rolling the top shoulders downward and the outer shoulders backward.

✓ Move the shoulders down, and at the same time lift the bones of the upper arms (humerus) into the shoulders.

Tadasana Variation 11

Moving the trapezius down: Shoulder traction

Props
a rope
and a belt
(or 2 belts)

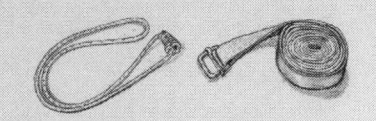

→ Wrap a rope (or a belt) around your shoulder blades and under the armpits. Hold the rope with its knot in front of you ❶.

> Throw the knot over your head to the back so that the rope is placed on top of your shoulders near the neck.

> Now catch the knot behind your back and pull down, while lifting the chest up ❷.

You can use a belt to intensify the stretching (and to free the arms):

> Loop a belt through the rope (or first belt) and tie it around your heels.

Note: For tall people, this belt must be a long one!

A general remark: **If you do not have a long belt you can form one by connecting two regular belts.**

> Bend the knees slightly and tighten the belt ❸. Make sure the rope is placed symmetrically near the neck (on the inner trapezius) Then straighten the legs against the pull of the belt ❹.

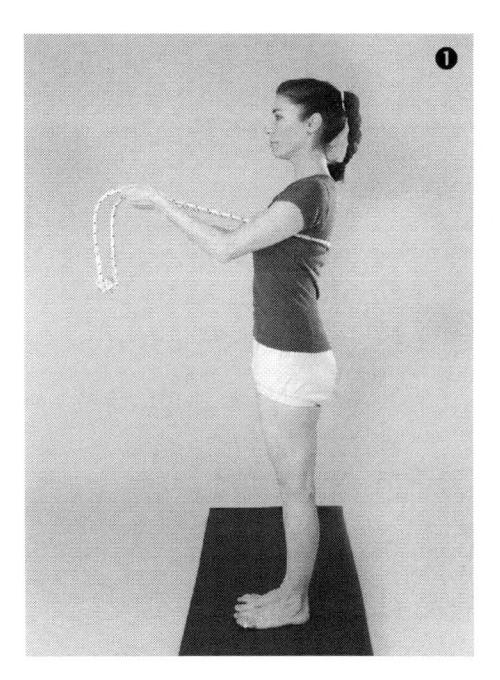

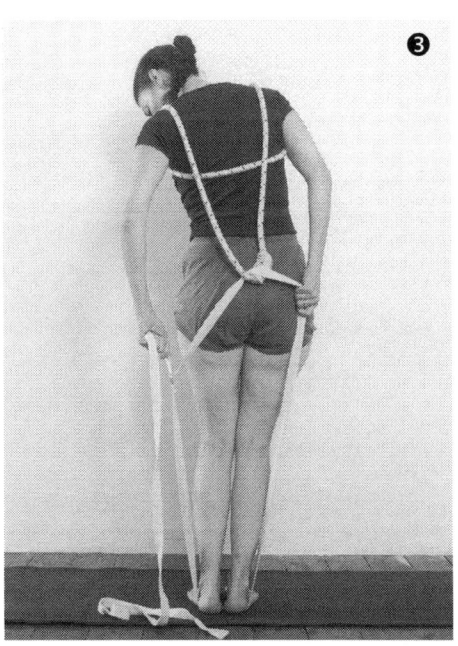

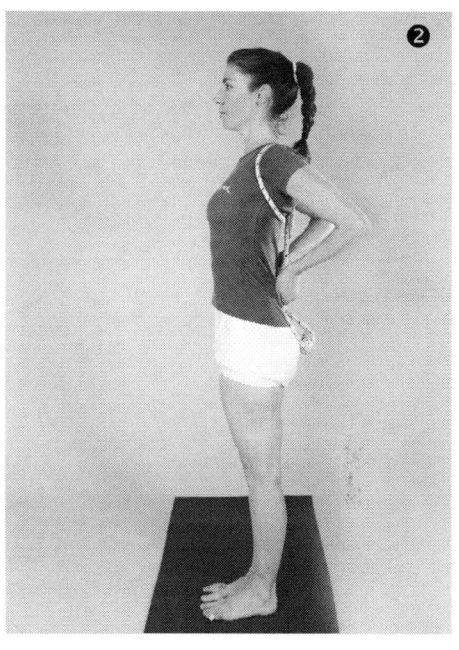

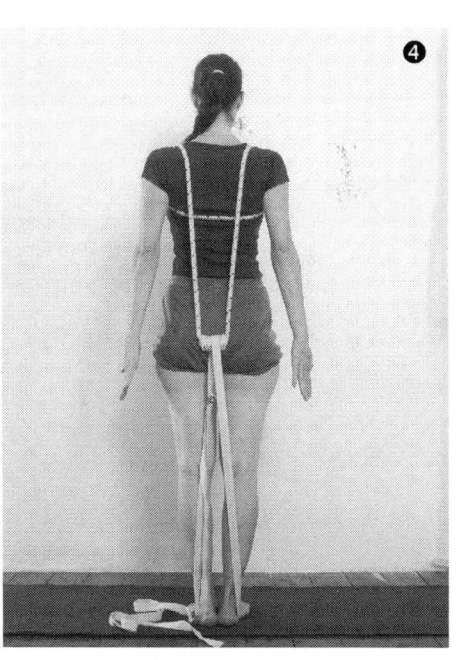

Tips

✓ Once freedom in the neck is felt, learn to get this effect without the belt. Remind yourself during your daily activities to soften the trapezius and move it down.

Effects

Placing the belt on the heels pulls the shoulders back and down without employing the hands. This enables doing other asanas while maintaining this shoulder traction.

Tadasana
Variation 11 (cont.)

Moving the trapezius down: Shoulder traction

⟶ There is another, slightly better way to place the rope, but this requires the help of another person. Photos ❺, ❻ and ❼ demonstrate how this is done.

▷ Once the rope is set, you can catch the knot and pull down.

▷ Using a belt, like in ❹ you can free the arms and use your heels to stretch the belt. Then you can lift the arms up to Urdhva Hastasana ❽ or Urdhva Baddhanguliyasana.

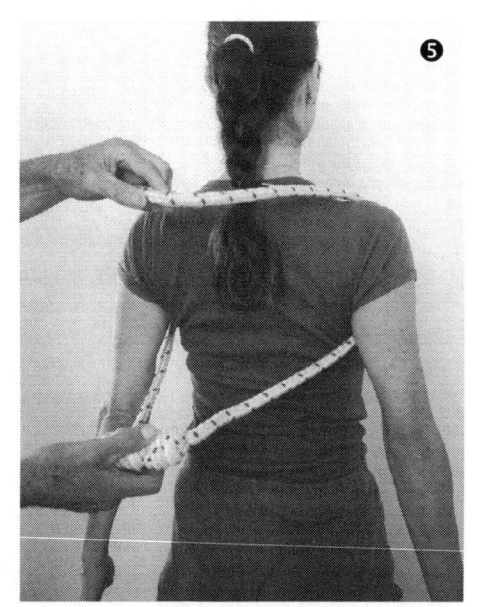

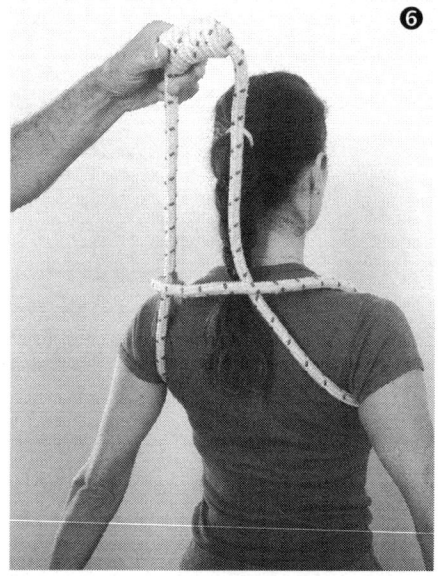

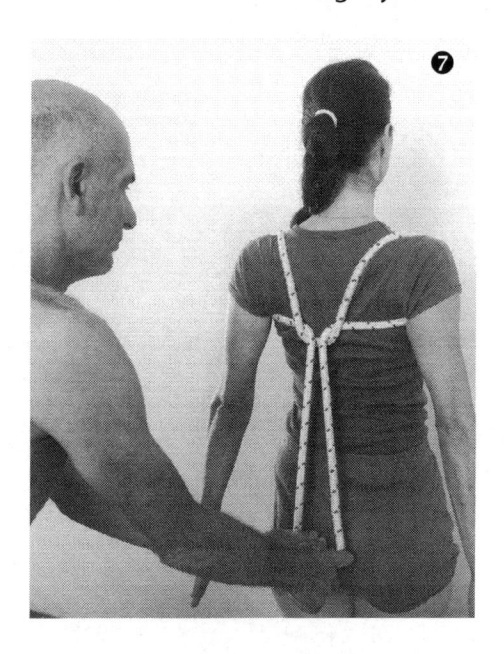

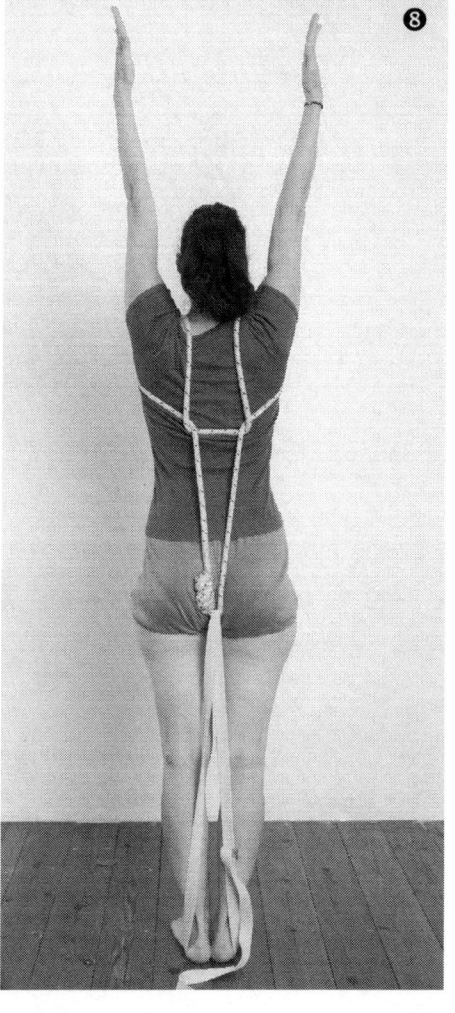

Effects

Tension in the trapezius muscle is a common trigger for neck pain and headache. The trapezius tends to harden and bulge upward, thus limiting the movement of the neck. Pulling the trapezius muscle down helps to soften it and thus release tension accumulated in this area. It also helps to roll the shoulders back and down.

Applicability

In a similar fashion, the partner can pull the rope while you do other asanas, like: Utthita Trikonasana and Adho Mukha Svanasana (see page 43).

Tadasana
Variation 12

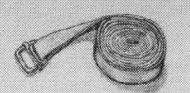

Sensitizing the top chest: Belt around chest

Props
belt

→ Loop a belt around the top chest and fasten it; then stand in Tadasana. ❶

> *Note:* If a partner is available, he or she can help you by tucking the shoulder blades under the belt and tightening it from the back. This way the belt can be adjusted more precisely. ❷

➢ You can also lift the arms to Urdhva Hastasana.

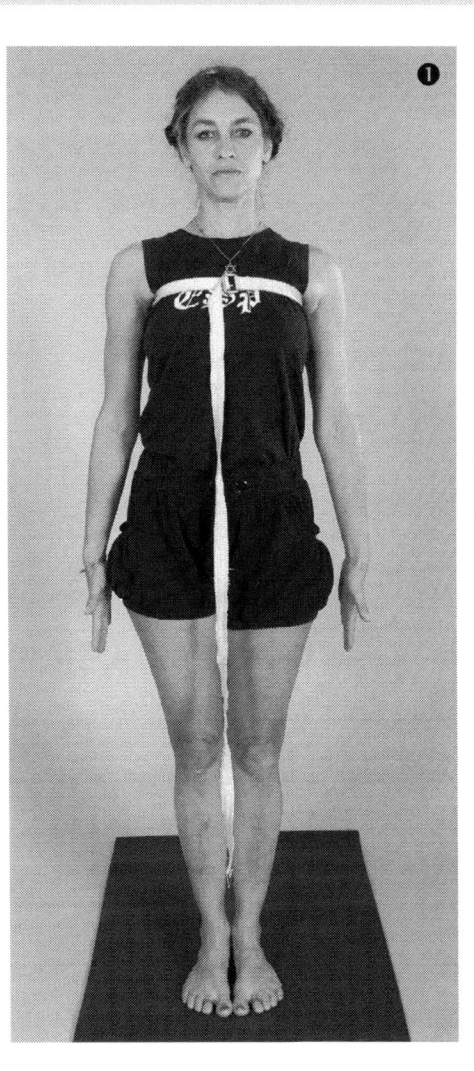

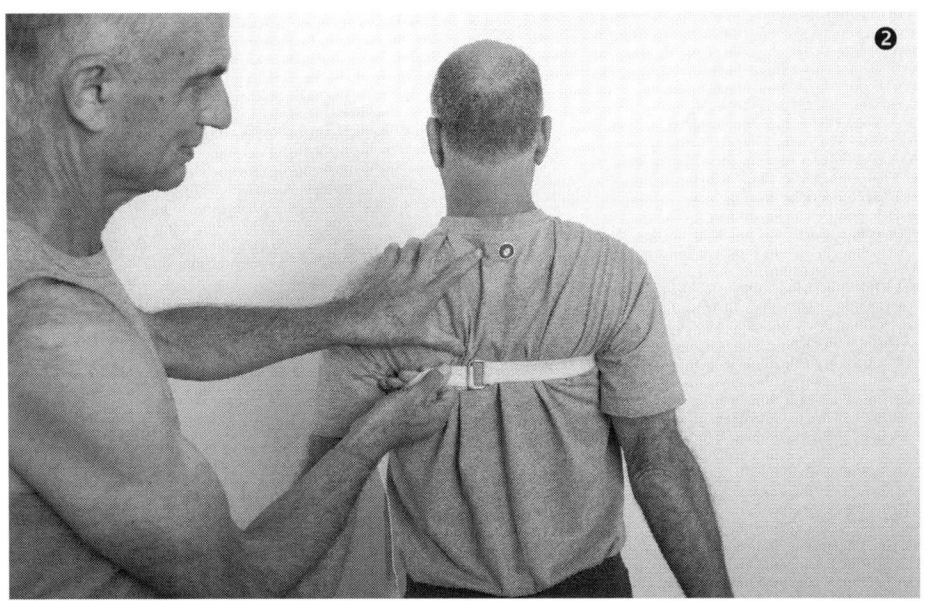

Effects
The touch of the belt brings awareness to the top chest and shoulder blades. It helps to keep the shoulder blades in place and activates the entire top chest.

Tips
✓ In some cases, the shoulder blades stick out of the body ('winged' shoulder blades); this is not a healthy condition. To correct it, move the lower part of the shoulder blades toward the spine. The sensation of the belt will help you learn this action.

Applicability
The belt may be used in this way for the entire practice session, but it is especially useful for: *Adho Mukha Svanasana, Sirsasana, Adho Mukha Vrksasana* and standing poses like *Utthita Trikonasana, Virabhadrasana* and so on.

Props for Yoga / Chapter 1 / Tadasana 17

Tadasana
Variation 13

Aligning the spine: Spine on a wall edge

→ Stand with the middle of your back against the corner of a rectangular column (or the protruding edge of two adjoining walls).

› Using the vertical edge as the centerline, place your heels around its bottom; then position your tailbone and the middle of the occiput (the rear bone of the skull) against it. Now align the spine vertically, vertebra after vertebra, along the same vertical line.

> *Note:* The lumbar vertebrae should not touch the protruding edge (there should be a healthy lumbar lordosis).

› Place your hands on the pelvis, bend the knees slightly and move the buttock muscles (gluteus) down and the tailbone in. ❶

› Slowly straighten the knees while moving the front thighs backward. ❷

› You can lift the arms up and check their position relative to the walls behind you. ❸

> *Note:* If a wall corner is not available, you can use the narrow side of an open door.

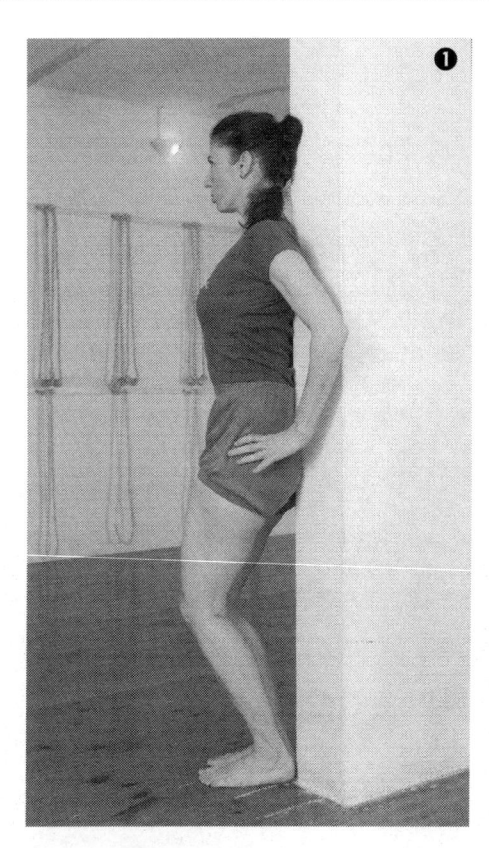

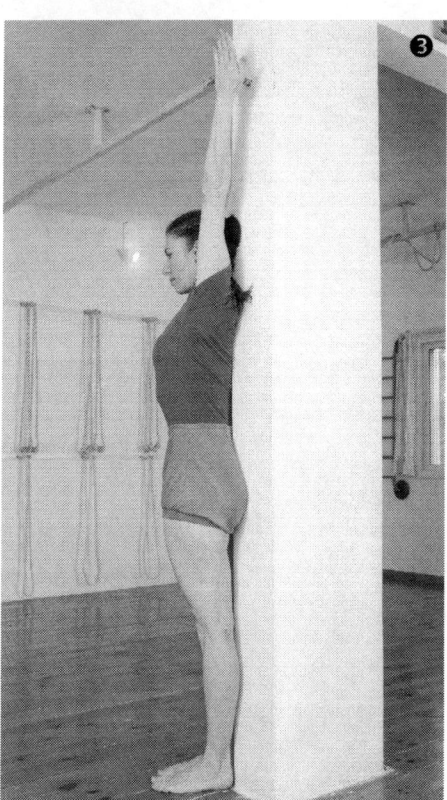

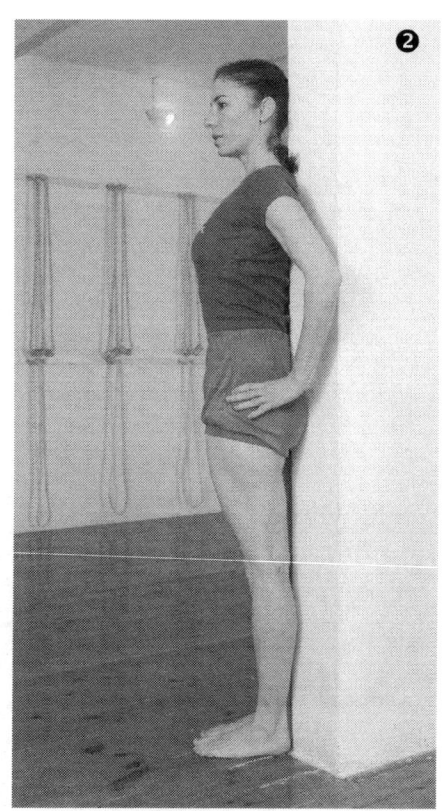

Effects

The vertical line of the corner enables you to check that your spine is straight. When standing in the middle of the room, the spine may tilt, lean or turn to one side. This becomes habitual and one may not even be aware of it. The corner line brings awareness to the spine's curvatures and allows one to check if the lumbar curve (lordosis) is excessive. This variation is a must for people with scoliosis.

Tips

✓ If the distance between your lumbar and the vertical edge is excessive when the legs are straight, work more on pushing the tailbone in.

Urdhva Hastasana

Many of the variations shown above for Tadasana are applicable also for Urdhva Hastasana. Here we add a few variations for learning the upward extension of the arms.

> **⚠ CAUTIONS**
>
> Do not stretch the arms up more than 30 seconds if you have high blood pressure or a cardiac condition. If you are prone to dizziness, practice with your back against a wall.

Urdhva Hastasana
Variation 1

Stretching the sides: One arm stretches the other

⟶ Lift the arms up and with the left hand hold the right wrist and pull it up; extend up the whole right side of the trunk. ❶

› Catch the upper arm and turn it inward (the triceps muscle turns in). ❷

› Release and then stretch both arms upward at shoulder width.

✓ Compare the feeling in the sides of the trunk: which side feels more extended? More alive?

› Now use the right hand to extend the left arm and side.

› Then stay in Urdhva Hastasana and observe the stretch of both sides.

› Take the arms down and then repeat Urdhva Hastasana. Try to achieve even stretch when lifting both arms at the same time.

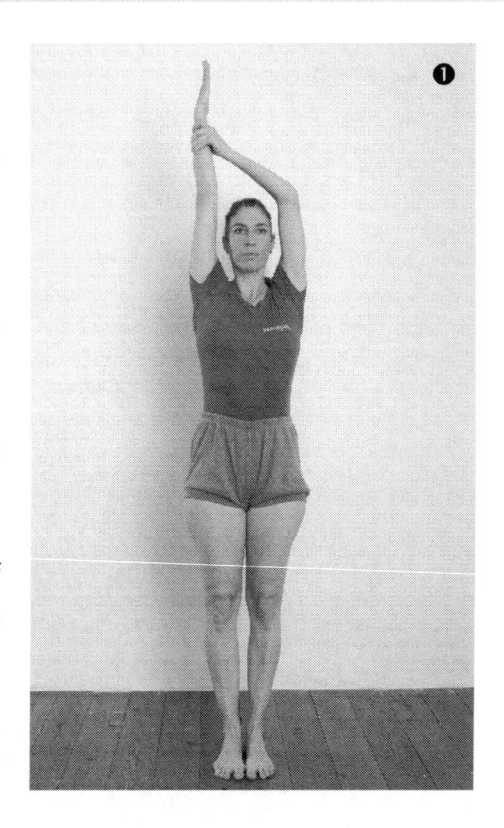

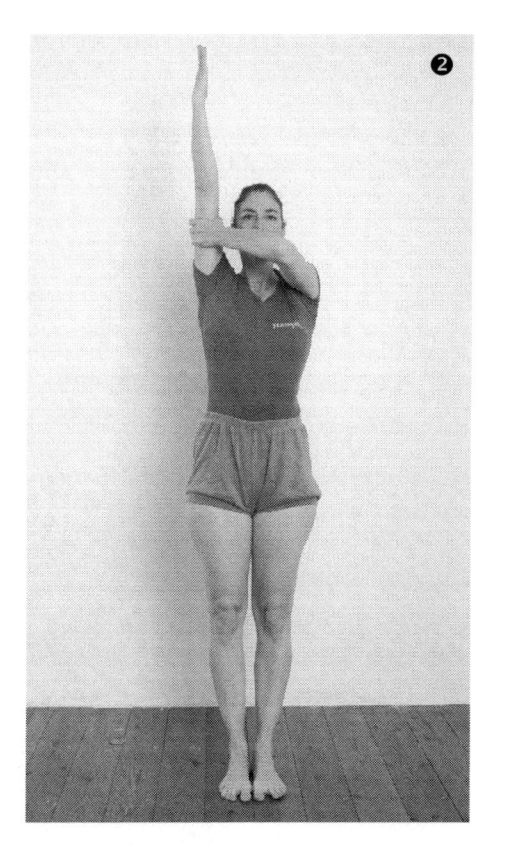

Effects

Stretching each side separately clarifies the role of the arms in lifting and extending the sides of the body.

Urdhva Hastasana
Variation 2

Activating the arms: Belt around forearms, block between palms

Props
belt
block

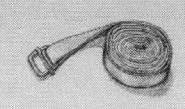

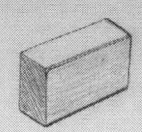

→ Place a belt around the mid-forearms or the elbows, tighten it to shoulder width and then hold a block between the palms.

Press on the blocks and stretch the arms up. ❶

Effects: the combination of the block and belt helps to strengthen and stabilize the arms. The belt is especially useful for people who find it hard to straighten the elbows.

Now, try to do the same without a belt:

> Balance a block on the crown of your head and take your hands down to Tadasana. ❷

> Carefully extend your spine, so as to push the block up with your head.

Note: Be alert to catch the block in case it falls (or use a rubber block).

> Now, hold the block between the bases of the palms and stretch the arms up to Urdhva Hastasana. Keep pressing the palms against the block. ❸

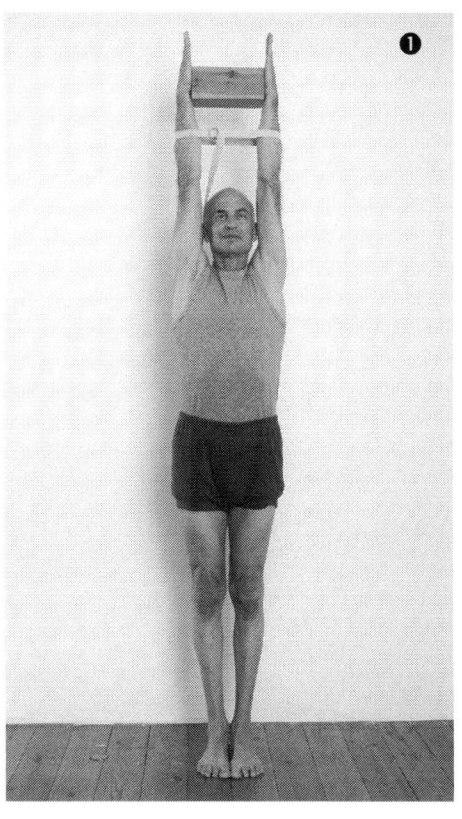

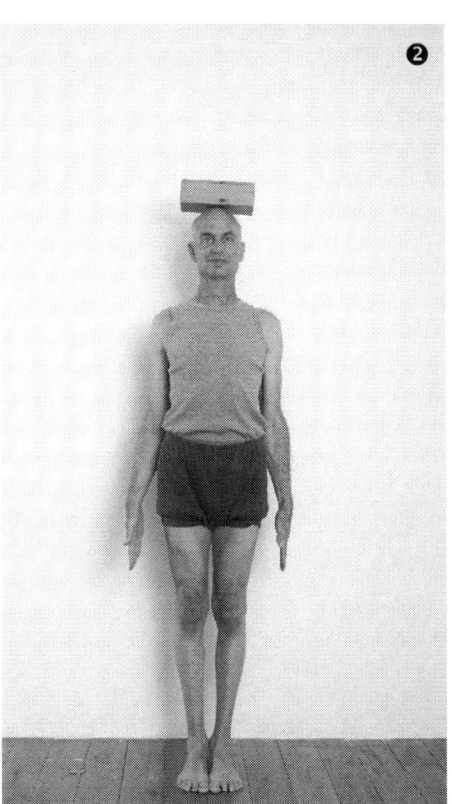

Effects
pressing the palms against the block (without grasping it) activates and strengthens the arms.

Tips

✓ If pressing the block at the base of the palms is too difficult, bend your fingers and grasp it firmly.

✓ Move the wrists back and at the same time extend the thumbs up.

✓ The joints of the ankles, hips, shoulders and wrists should all be on one vertical line.

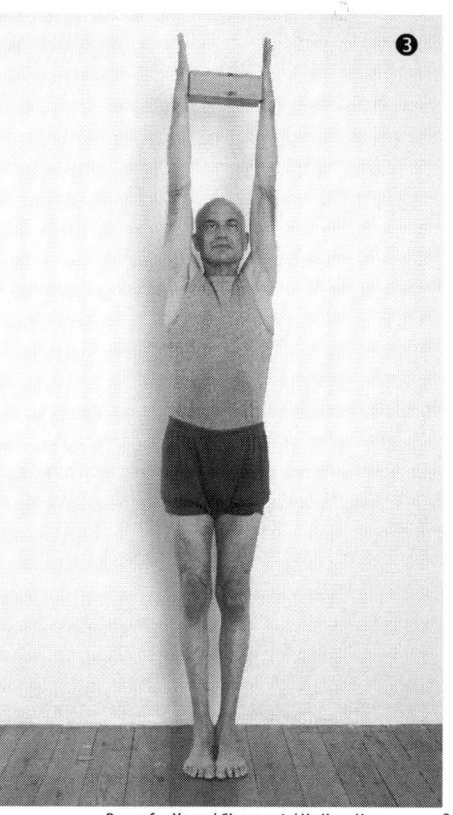

Urdhva Hastasana
Variation 3

Extending the armpits: Facing the wall, palms on blocks

Props
wall
2 blocks

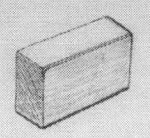

⟶ Face the wall standing about 50 cm (20 inches) away from it. Lift the arms holding two blocks and press the blocks against the wall.

▷ Slide the blocks up while moving the chest and head forward toward the wall.

▷ Move the shoulder blades in and lean the forehead on the wall. Keep the tailbone in.

▷ Extend your arms up from the armpits. Press the blocks evenly.

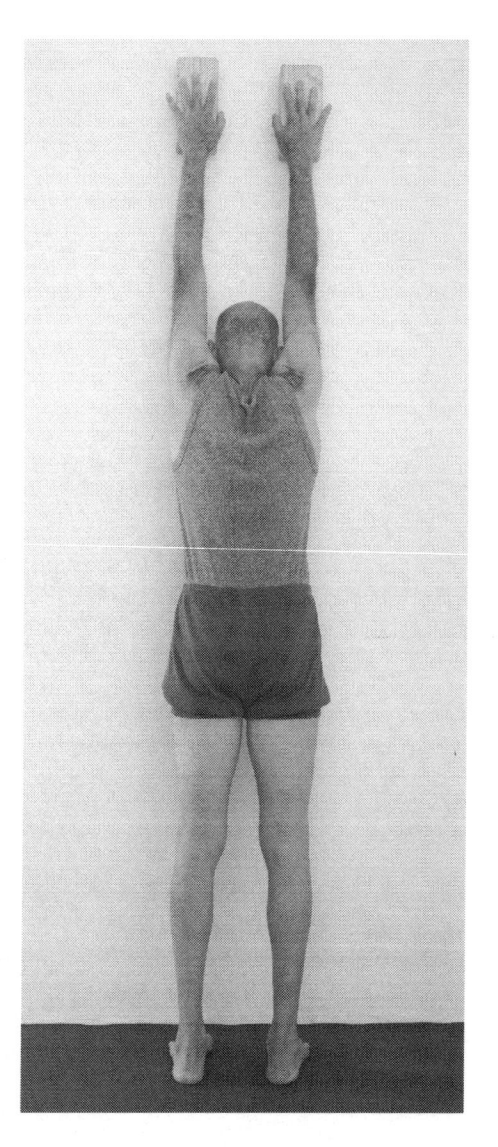

Effects
The resistance of the blocks helps to open and extend the armpits.

Tips

✓ Slide the blocks upward on the wall.

✓ Learn to activate the shoulders without shortening the armpits.

Urdhva Hastasana
Variation 4

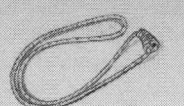

Extending the entire body upward: Holding a ceiling rope

Props
ceiling rope

→ Stand in Tadasana directly below a rope attached to a ceiling anchor.

› Lift the arms up to Urdhva Hastasana. Slightly lift the heels off the floor and catch the rope high up.

› Now, without releasing the grip of the hands, lower the heels down to the floor.

› Keep holding the rope for a while, sensing your increased tallness. Breathe into the extended chest.

› Now release the rope; try to maintain the upward extension achieved with the rope.

Note: Although ceiling ropes are not very common, they are not difficult to install and can be very helpful in many asanas.

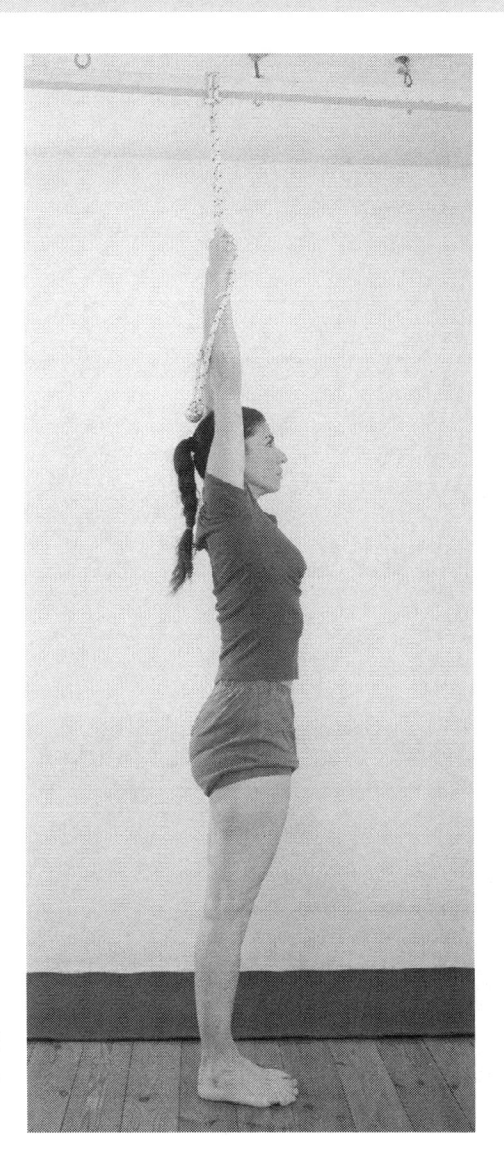

Effects
The rope creates length in the spine and upper body; when releasing the rope one can feel the drop of the spine and learns the action required to prevent it.

Applicability
Ceiling ropes can be used for many standing asanas as well as for other groups of asanas. See for example variation 4 of Vrksasana and Variation 22 of Utthita Trikonasana.

Vrksasana

Vrksasana is usually the first balancing pose one learns. It combines the arm action of Urdhva Namaskarasana with balancing on one leg. If joining the palms is too difficult – keep the hands separated, as in Urdhva Hastasana.

Tips

- In Tadasana you learn the firmness and stability of a mountain; in Vrksasana you learn the delicate and flexible balance of a tree!

⚠ CAUTIONS

Do not stretch the arms up more than 30 seconds if you have high blood pressure or a cardiac condition. If you are prone to dizziness, practice with your back against a wall.

Opening the Pelvis

Vrksasana is also where some basic actions of the lateral standing poses are learnt. It is the first pose to work on broadening the pelvis. This is done by moving the buttock of the lifted leg in and extending the inner thigh, while keeping the Tadasana action of the standing leg and the tailbone.

Vrksaasana
Variation 1

Moving the femur head in: Bent leg against the wall

The hip joint is a ball-and socket joint that connects the femur bones to the pelvis. Wear and tear in this joint is a common complaint in old age; many people need to go through a hip joint replacement surgery. Displacement of the femur head is one of the factors contributing to this problem. This variation (and similar others) helps to maintain the health of the hip joints by keeping the femur head of the bent leg deep in the socket of the ilium bone (acetabulum) of the pelvis.

⟶ To do the pose with right leg lifted:

> Stand approximately half a meter (1.5 feet) from the wall with your right side to the wall.

> Bending the right leg, use your right hand to lift the foot and place the heel against the inner groin of the left leg.

> Keep the left (standing) leg strong as you press the right sole against the inner left thigh.

> Move the left front thigh back (as in Tadasana).

> Lower the right knee as much as possible and place it against the wall. If needed, adjust your distance from the wall.

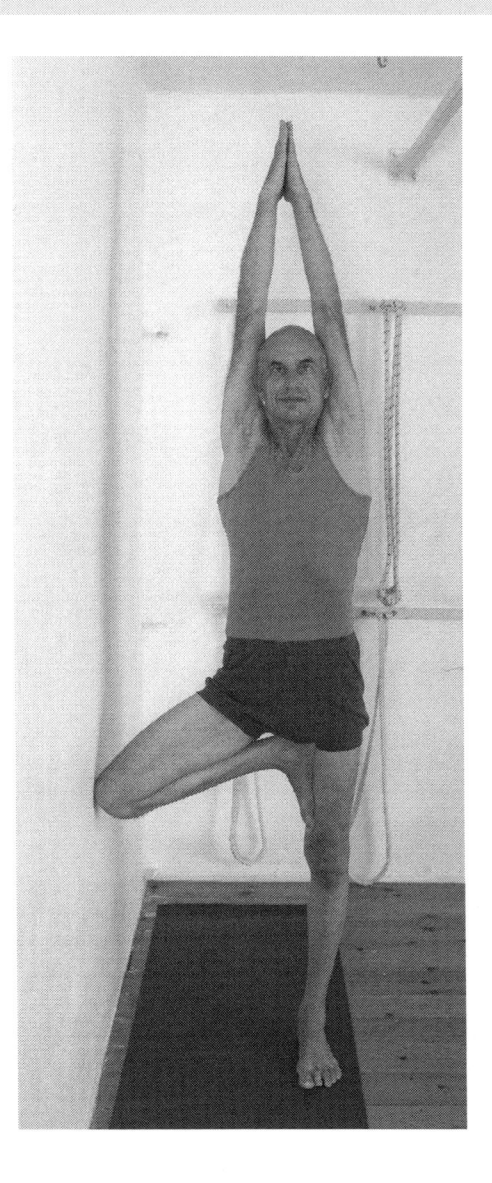

Effects

The resistance of the wall prevents the right foot from sliding down due to insufficient strength in the standing leg. The femur head is held firmly in its socket, creating an effective pivot for the outward rotation of the bent leg.

Tips

✓ Lift the leg and fold it until there is no space between the thigh and the shin and the heel touches the perineum.

✓ Extend the buttock of the lifted leg down and take it in (forward) resisting its tendency to bulge backwards.

✓ Maintain the internal sensation of Tadasana in the trunk.

Vrksaasana
Variation 2

Increasing the movement of the hip joint: Back against the wall

⟶ To do the pose with right leg lifted:

› Stand in Tadasana with your back against the wall.

› Lift the right leg and fold it to Vrksasana. Sensing the touch of the buttocks on the wall, verify the alignment and leveling of the pelvis girdle

› With hands lifted, keep the front thigh of the standing (left) leg pressed firmly backwards towards the wall.

› Without letting the left thigh move forward, tuck the right buttock in, extend the right thigh from the inner groin to the inner knee and roll the knee out. Using your right hand, push the knee back toward the wall, while keeping the even touch of both buttocks on the wall.

› When feeling stable, move slightly away from the wall to practice the free-standing pose.

Note: A helper can stabilize the left side of the pelvis and gently push the right knee to the wall.

Effects
The wall helps to maintain the balance and detect misalignment in the pelvic area: you will immediately feel any tilt, turn or unevenness. It also clarifies the action of lengthening the adductor muscles of the inner thigh.

Applicability
All lateral standing poses.

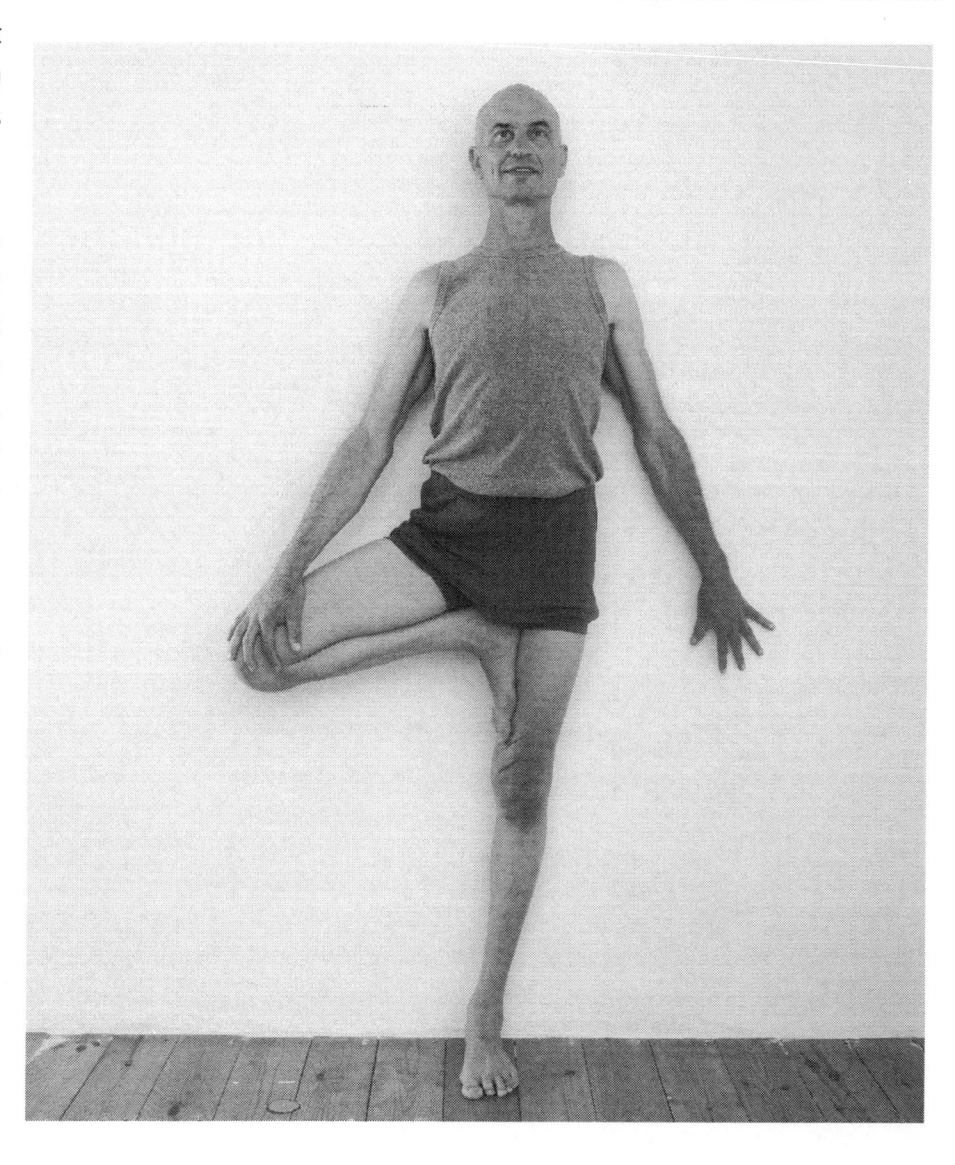

Vrksasana Variation 3

Widening the pelvis: Facing the wall

Props
2 foam blocks

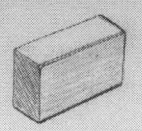

⟶ To do the pose with right leg lifted:

> Stand in Tadasana facing the wall.

> Place one block between your upper left thigh and the wall and hold the other block.

> Lift the right leg to Vrksasana and place the foam block between your right inner knee and the wall.

> Now move the right buttock toward the wall.

Note: Wooden blocks are not recommended due to safety reasons. Would not want one of those heavy blocks falling on your toes!

Note: A helper can gently push the right buttock down and in toward the wall.

Effects

The first block prevents the forward movement of the left thigh. The second block provides a fulcrum for the movement of the right buttock. This variation is more effective when a partner helps to move the buttock in.

Applicability

All lateral standing poses.

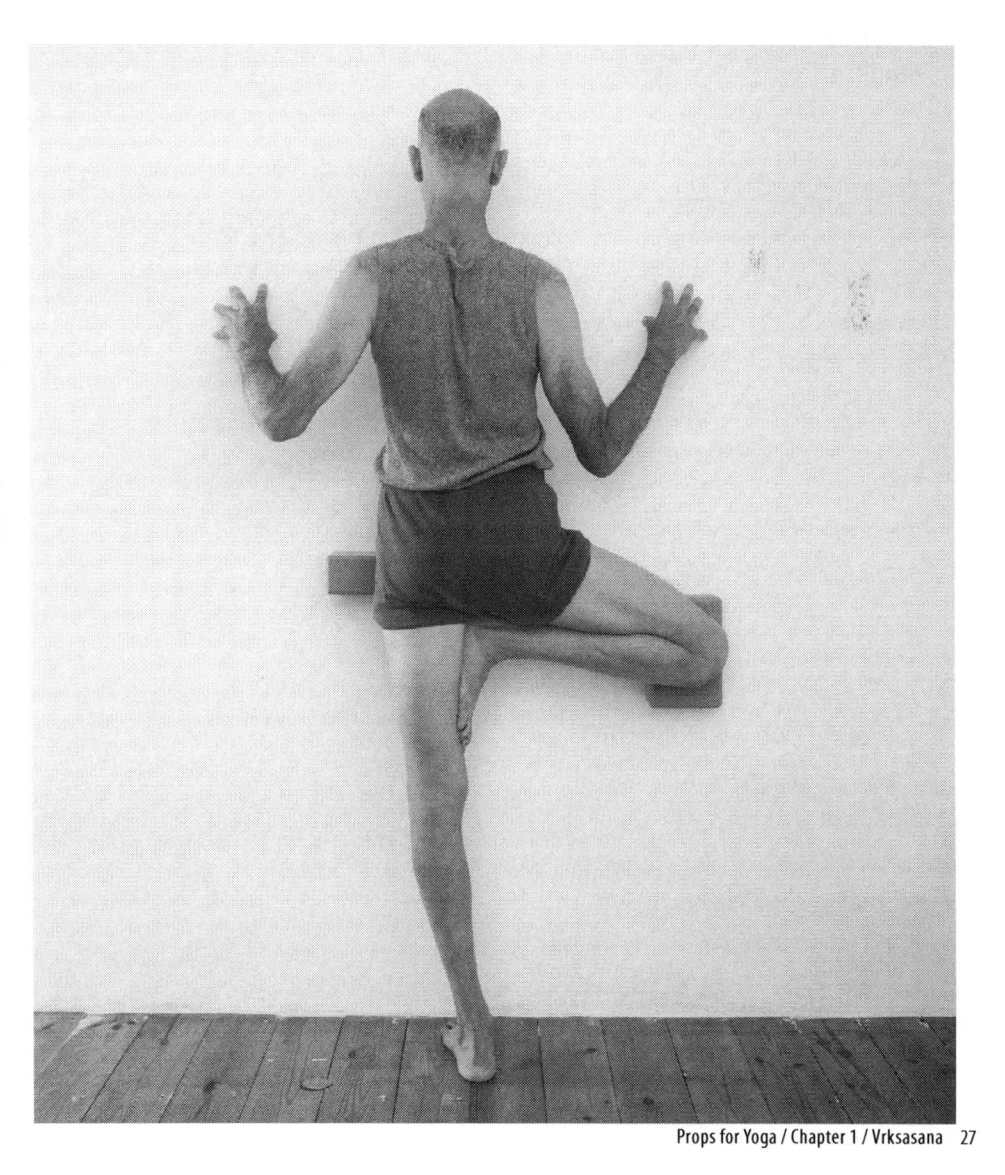

Stretching Up

In addition to balancing you should stretch up in this pose and be as tall as a cypress tree. Here is a variation that teaches this.

Vrksaasana Variation 4

Extending the body upward: Holding a ceiling rope

Props
ceiling rope

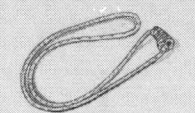

This variation is similar to the variation 4 of Urdhva Hastasana (page 23).

→ To do the pose with the right leg lifted:

- Stand in Tadasana directly below a rope attached to a ceiling anchor.

- Lift the right leg to Vrksasana and extend the arms up. Slightly lift the left heel off the floor and catch the ceiling rope higher up.

- Now, without releasing the hand grip, lower the heel down to the floor.

- Keep holding the rope for a while, experiencing your increased tallness. Breathe into the extended chest.

- Now release the rope; try to maintain the same upward extension achieved when using the rope.

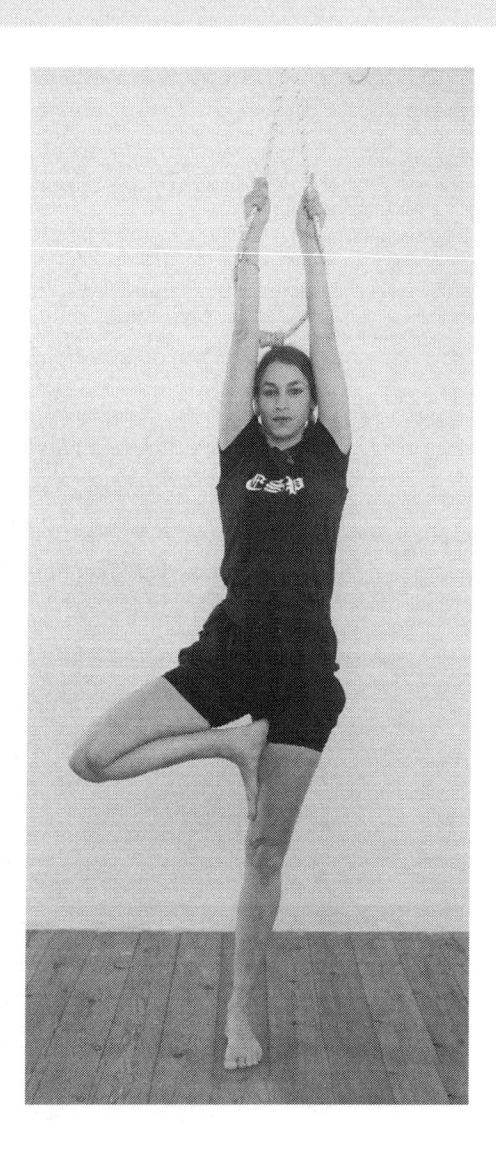

Effects
The rope helps to extend the body upward and to keep it in balance.

Tips
✓ Learn to maintain balance and internal extension without the prop.

Applicability
Ceiling ropes are helpful in many standing poses (and also in sitting poses). We shall show some examples of their usage in subsequent variations.

Adho Mukha Svanasana

About *Adho Mukha Svanasana*

I love those yoga T-shirts that say: "Another Day, Another Dog Pose"; and I do practice this pose every day. It has a unique combination of forward extension with concave back action. It charges the entire body; activating all the four principal organs of action (karmendriyas) – the arms and the legs and fits well into many types of sequences.

The final position of Adho Mukha Svanasana –"downward facing dog pose" in Sanskrit - is not easy to attain. However, beginners can perform its preparatory stages and benefit from it tremendously, especially with the help of props or a partner. It is often practiced as a warm up for other asanas.

The general shape of the pose is triangular. B.K.S. Iyengar once said that in this pose, the awareness should embrace the buttocks like snow covering the peaks of the Himalayas. The energy of the body moves from the palms back and up to the buttocks area. The photo in *Light on Yoga* (LOY, Pl. 75) shows the pose with the head resting on the floor and hence, many people try to bring their head to the floor prematurely. If you are a beginner, work first on lifting the buttocks, moving the weight of the body back and pressing the heels down. Only after this has been achieved, start working on concaving the back. In some future day, your head may indeed reach the floor but don't get over-ambitious about it! If you wish to experience the effect of resting the head on the floor but are not ready for the full pose, use a block or a bolster to support the forehead (see below).

General Structure of the Pose

In Adho Mukha Svanasana there should be exact symmetry between the left and the right sides of the body and an even distribution of weight on the palms and the feet. The following variations help to learn the correct structure of the pose.

> *T i p s*
> The general shape of Adho Mukha Svanasana resembles a triangle; the energy of the pose moves from the base (palms and feet) through the body up to its top (the buttocks). In the final pose, the awareness embraces the top of the triangle like snow resting on top of a Himalayan peak.

> ⚠ **CAUTIONS**
> If you have high blood pressure or frequent headaches, support your head with a bolster (see Variation 21 below). If you are prone to dislocation of the shoulders, ensure that your arms do not rotate outward. Practice this asana in advanced pregnancy with a chair or other support for the hands and head.

Adho Mukha Svanasana
Variation 1

Finding the distance between feet and palms

A common question that comes up is: "What is the correct distance between the palms and feet?" The classic way of entering the pose from Chaturanga Dandasana gives a clue for the correct distance. But beginners often enter the pose from Uttanasana and need to get a feel for the right distance. For that you can try the following:

⟶ First, enter the pose with an intentionally short span between palms and feet ❶. Note the stretch of the spine and the legs. Step forward to Uttanasana.

> Enter the pose a second time, now with an intentionally excessive span between the palms and feet❷. Note how the excessive span limits your ability to shift weight to the legs. Step forward to Uttanasana.

> Enter the pose for the third time. Now adjust the distance such that the weight is distributed evenly between the legs and the arms. Make sure you are able to activate and stretch the legs without compromising the spine's extension.

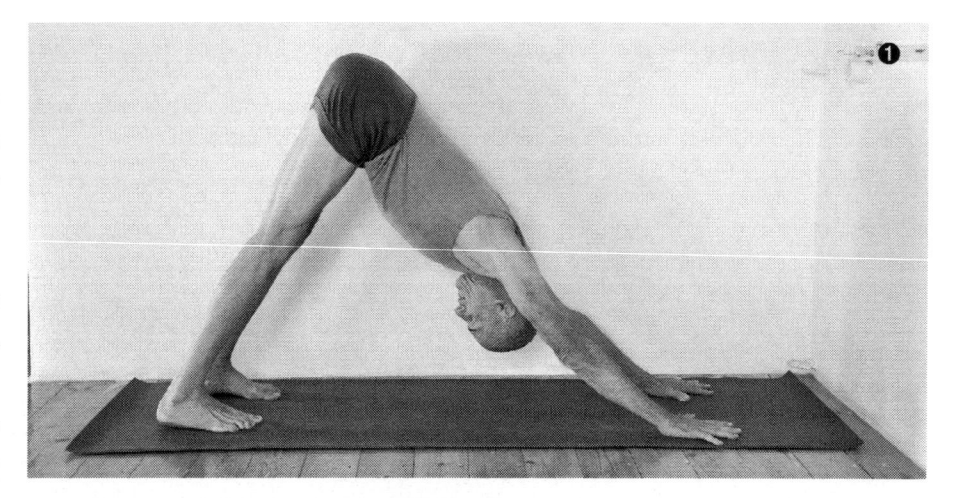

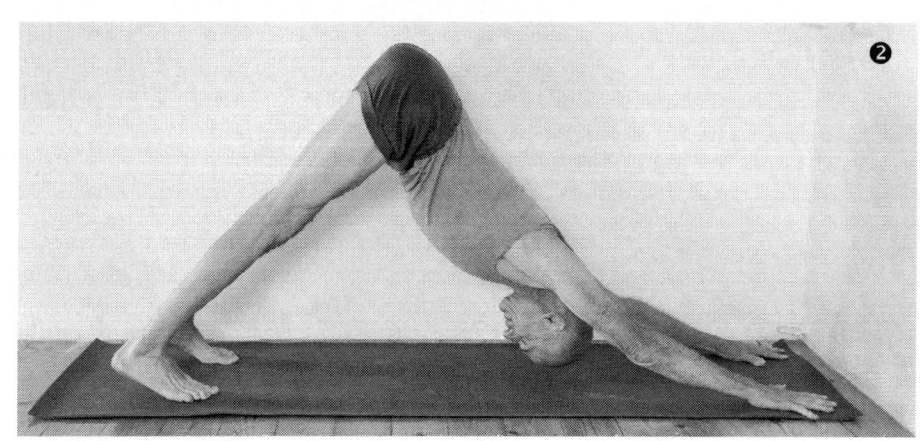

While the above provides a general guideline, be sensitive to your specific body condition. Moreover, the palm-feet distance may vary with the specific purpose of your practice. For example: when I do the dog pose before back bends, I often increase the distance to allow more space in the shoulder girdle and to help concave the spine. This prepares for the actions of the arms and shoulder blades required in back bends. However, when I do the pose before forward extensions I often shorten the distance in order to intensify the work of the hamstrings and the stretching of the calf muscles.

Adho Mukha Svanasana Variation 2

Ensuring symmetry: Using a middle line

Props
floor lines or belt

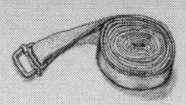

⟶ You can use floor lines to measure the symmetry of the limbs:

> Choose a straight line on the floor. Place the palms symmetrically on each side of it at shoulder width.

> Step back and place the feet symmetrically at hip width.

> Make sure the centerline of the face and the spine are aligned with the floor line ❶.

> If there are no lines on the floor you may create an artificial line using a belt:

> Place the palms and feet at equidistance from the belt ❷.

> Keeping the spine and head above the belt, when moving into the pose ❸.

Tips
✓ Compare the pressure of your left and right palms on the floor – is it equal?

✓ Compare the weight on your left and right feet – is it equal? Can you press both heels equally to the floor?

It is interesting to check if the symmetry can be preserved even when jumping to the pose:

> Stand in Uttanasana with feet equidistance from the middle line.

> Bend your legs, place the palms on the floor, exhale and jump backward to Adho Mukha Svanasana.

> Look at your feet – are they equidistance from the line?

> Now inhale and with an exhalation jump forward to Uttanasana; observe the position of your feet.

> You can jump like this several times, check if you have a repeated tendency and correct it.

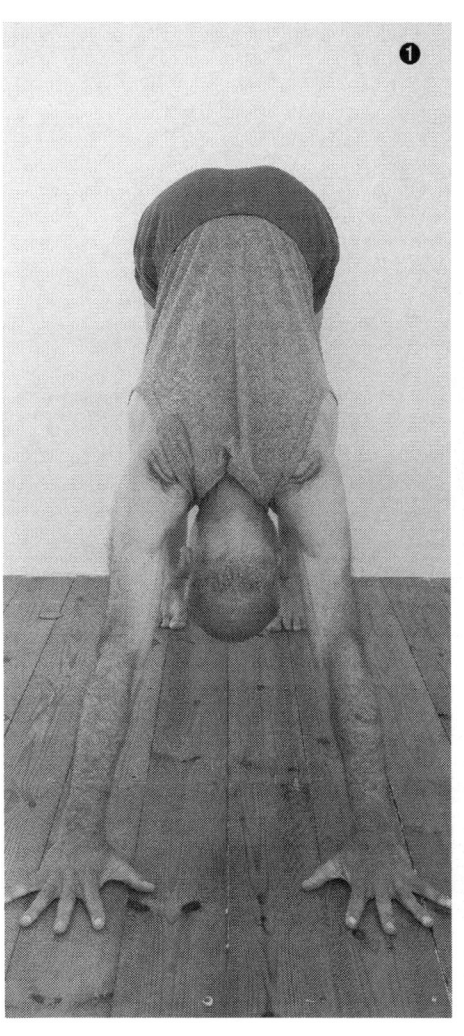

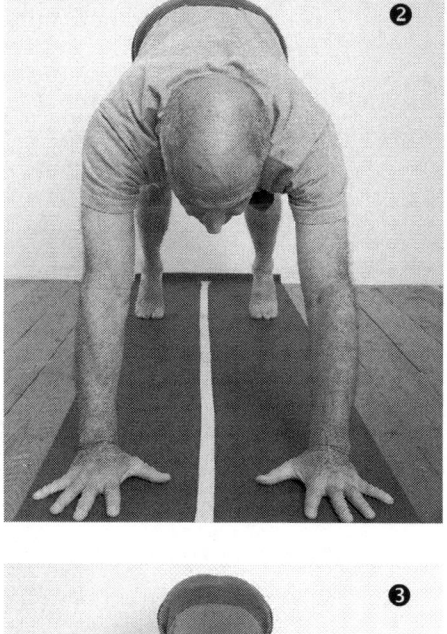

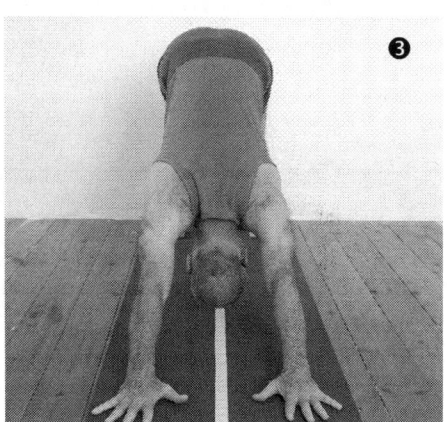

Effects
When perfect left/right symmetry and front/back balance is achieved, the pose assumes a new wholeness. It reminds me of 3D pictures: when both eyes work evenly the two two-dimensional images converge and a third dimension emerges.

Applicability
Floor line can help in many other standing poses. See for example Prasarita Padottanasana (page 136).

Props for Yoga / Chapter 1 / Adho Mukha Svanasana 31

Raising the Palms

The first action one has to learn in this pose is to move the weight from the hands to the feet. For this one needs to activate the legs. This can be learnt by placing the palms on some support. This change in the geometry of the pose reduces the load on the arms and helps to activate the muscles of the front thighs in order to shift weight back. Once the legs become more active, you can challenge them further by lifting the heels or the feet on some support (see below.)

Adho Mukha Svanasana Variation 3

Shifting weight to the legs: Supporting the palms

Props
two blocks
or a chair
wall

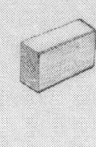

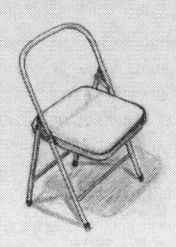

Raising the palms can be done either on a slanted or horizontal support. To use a slanted support:

→ Place two blocks on a mat, slanted and supported by the wall. ❶

› Bend forward and place the palms on the blocks. Spread and stretch the fingers.

› Step backward and enter the pose.

› Push the palms against the blocks, move the front thighs back, lift the heels and lift the buttocks as much as you can.

Now, maintaining the buttocks' height, extend the outer sides of the feet and heels down.

› An inverted chair can be used instead of blocks (see *A Chair for Yoga* for more details). ❷

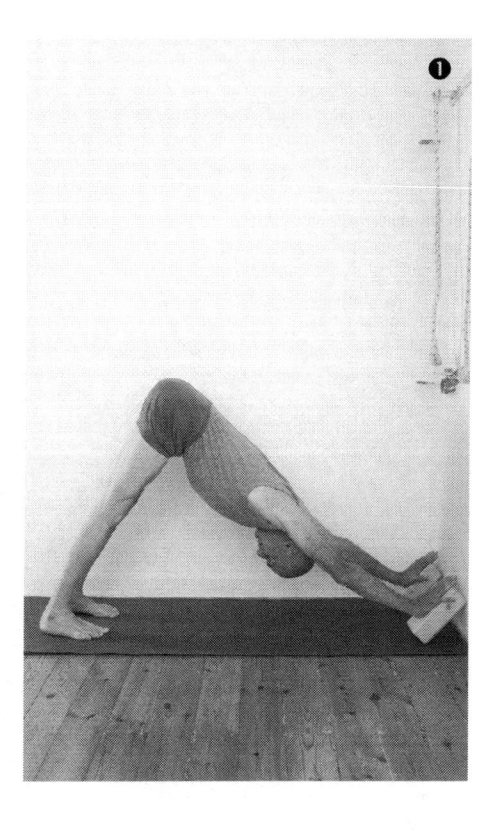

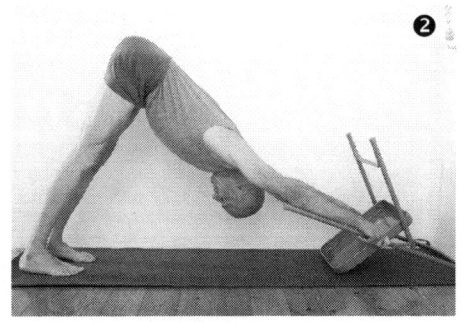

Effects

Raised palm support is a very gentle and nice way to start a practice session as it shifts weight from the hands to the legs. Slanted palm support increases the horizontal vector of the push backward. The heels can reach the floor more easily and form a solid base for the activation of the legs. It helps to move the shoulder blades in and is beneficial for people who suffer from wrist pain in Dog pose.

Tips

✓ The energy should move from the palms, up and back along the arms and trunk all the way to the buttocks. From there it should descend down to the heels.

✓ Lift the heels, extend the skin of the soles back from the arches toward the heels and stamp the heels down.

✓ Learn to cut the outer heels and the outer edges of the feet down. There should be no space left under the outer edges of the feet.

Adho Mukha Svanasana Variation 3 (cont.)

Shifting weight to the legs: Supporting the palms

⟹ To use a flat support for the palms:

> Place two blocks on a mat, flat against the wall.

> Bend and place the palms on the blocks. Step backward and enter the pose. ❶

> Now move forward until the shoulders are above the palms. Lock the elbows, turn the upper arms from inside out (biceps turning out) and extend the inner upper arms to the inner shoulders.

> As you go back to the pose, lift the fingers and palms and press the heel of the palms against the corners of the blocks. Spread and stretch the fingers. ❷

> Stay in the pose for 1-3 minutes, then go to Uttanasana and look at the heel of your palms. The pressure against the blocks leaves a temporary mark. – compare the marks on both palms – this will teach you if you are using the two arms equally.

Depending on the height required for the hand support, you may replace the blocks by a chair or a stool. Place the palms on the seat of the chair ❸ or on the rung (see more in the book *A Chair for Yoga*).

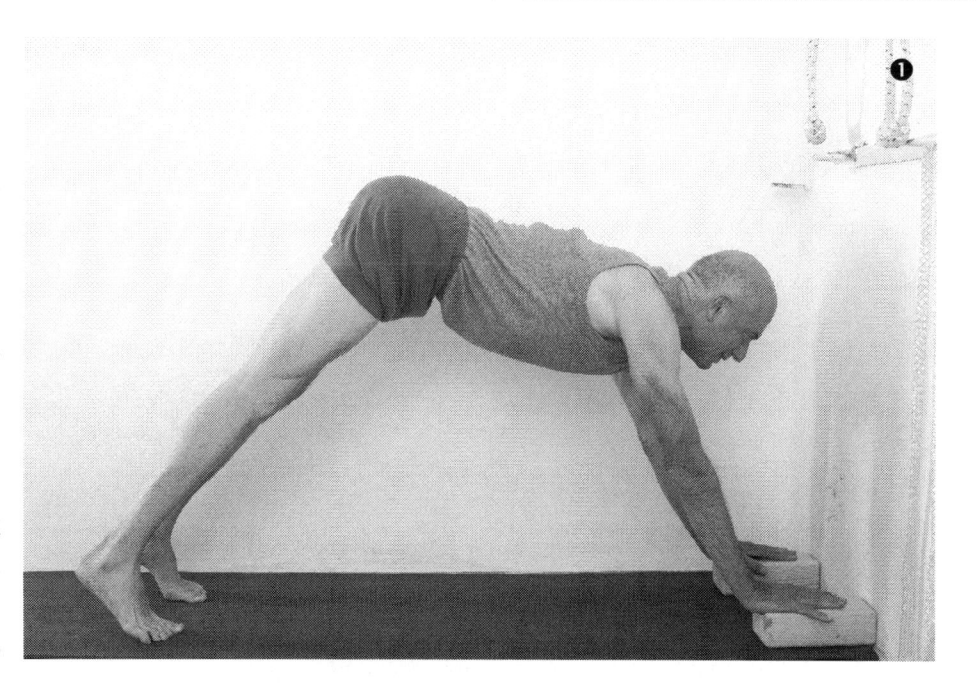

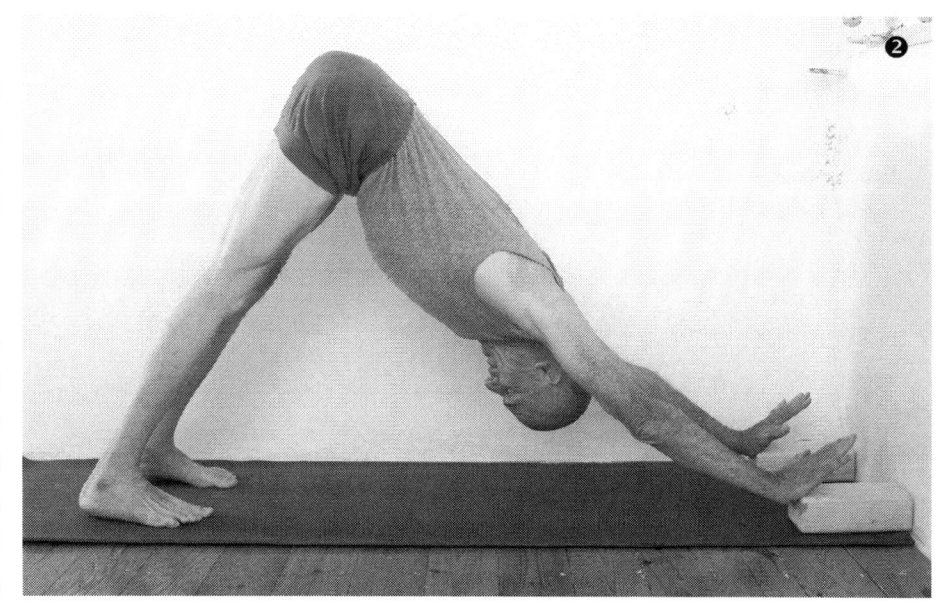

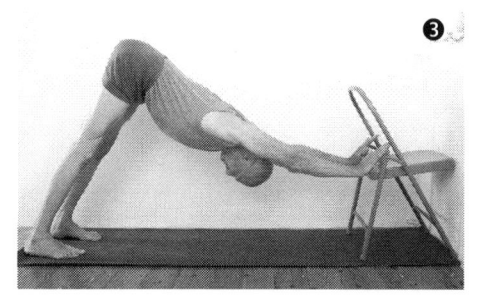

Effects

Lifting the palms on a flat support activates the fingers, palms, arms and shoulder blades. Use this action to concave the back and shift your weight to the legs. For some people this variation helps to lower the heels more than the previous one.

Working with a Partner

The advantage of working with a partner is that the external pull or push gives a sense of how a better pose feels like. This cellular memory will guide you in the future when you perform the pose on your own.

Note: In the following variations with a partner, the instructions are given for the helper, unless otherwise indicated. For convenience's sake, we term the one who does the pose: 'student'.

Adho Mukha Svanasana Variation 4

Stretching back and up: Partner pulls backward with belt

Props
1 belt or
2 belts
a partner

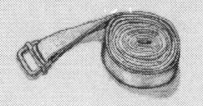

We show three ways in which a partner can help the legs to stretch the torso back and up.

→ Belt around pelvis, partner pulls backward and up:

› After the student enters the pause, place a loose belt around the pelvis.

› Pass the ends of the belt in between the student's legs, from front to rear.

› Hold the loose ends of the belt and pull back and up.

Note: Use your body weight rather than muscle force to pull; keep your back straight and extended.

› Maintain the pull for a while. Remind the student to participate actively in the performance of the pose. Then signal him or her that you are going to release the pull, and do so gradually.

› The student now performs the pose independently for a while.

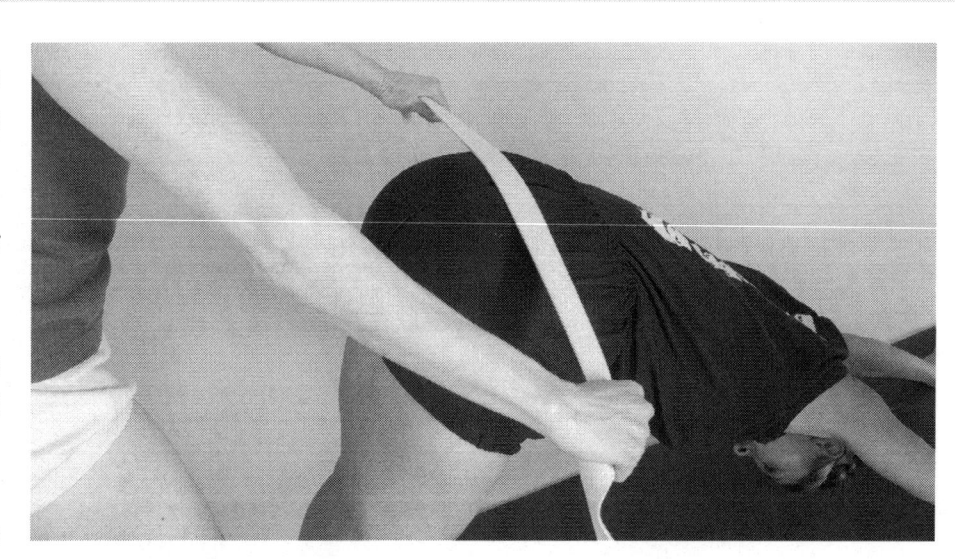

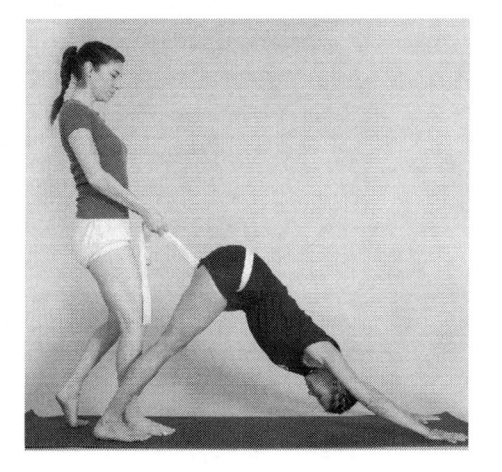

Effects

The pull of the belt helps getting into the pose and activates the muscle action in the correct direction under a reduced load. Once the partner lets go, the student should attempt to retain the same quality of the pose; the partner can continue to guide the student verbally for alignment and symmetry.

Tips

✓ The belt can also be placed simply around the front groins; however, the shown variation has the advantage of creating compactness in the pelvis while moving the inner groins back and turning the thighs inward.

Adho Mukha Svanasana
Variation 4 (cont.)

Stretching back and up: Partner pulls backward with belt

→ Belt around thighs, partner pulls backward:

> Place the belt around the top front thighs and pull it back and up. ❶

Effects
The pull intensifies the widening and expansion of the back of the thighs. The direction of the pull and its intensity clarify the strong thigh action required in this pose.

→ Adjusting the knee with a belt:

> Stand behind the student and place a belt around his/her right leg, just above the knee. ❷

> Observe the movement of the knee. Gently manipulate the pull so as to equalize the motion backward of the two sides of the knee.

> Now, gently release the pull from the right leg while the student maintains the action of the right leg.

> Repeat the same on the left leg.

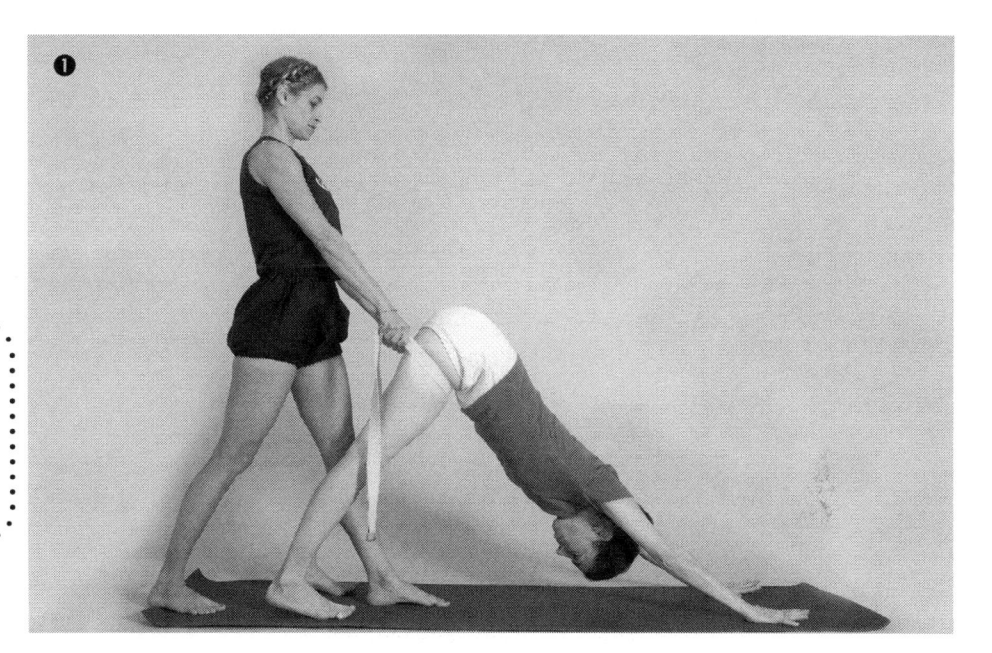

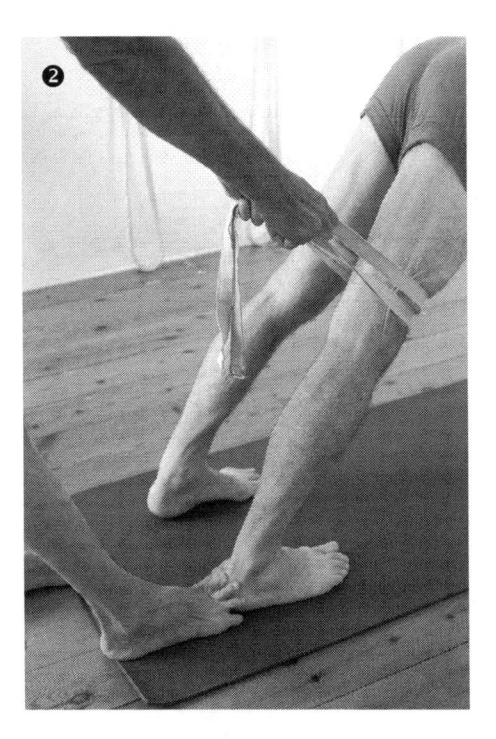

Effects
Pulling the lower thighs helps to realize how much the knees can move back. It opens well the back of the knees. The partner can provide feedback to the student on a part of the body that cannot be regularly seen.

⚠ **Cautions**
Do not place the strap on the kneecap itself.
Skip this variation if the student has hyperextended knees or if there is any sensitivity in the knee.

T i p s

✓ Partner: In most cases, in order to keep the knee aligned, you will need to pull the outer side of the knee stronger than the inner side.

✓ Student: Move the front ankles, the heads of the shins and the top of the thighs backward.

Adho Mukha Svanasana
Variation 5

Rooting the heels: Sitting on the "dog"

Props
wall
partner

In this variation the student is doing the pose while the partner sits on his sacrum.

Note: This variation and the following one can be done only when the student is already capable of stretching the lower back sufficiently to form a triangular pelvis (not a "rounded hill"). The partner should match the student in size and flexibility and preferably be of the same gender.

⟶ After the student has entered the pose with palms against the wall:

> Stand facing the wall, with spread legs, the student's torso between your legs.

> Position your buttocks on the student's sacrum and sit on it gently. Spread your feet on the wall for stability.

> Push the wall with your feet so as to move the student's sacrum away from the wall and his/her heels down to the floor.

Note: In the photo the helper uses a wall rope. This is convenient but not mandatory.

Effects

The partner's push shifts the student's weight towards the legs. The weight on the arms is diminished and the spine gets a good stretch. This variation lengthens the calf muscles and the Achilles' tendons, thus helping to lower the heels to the floor.

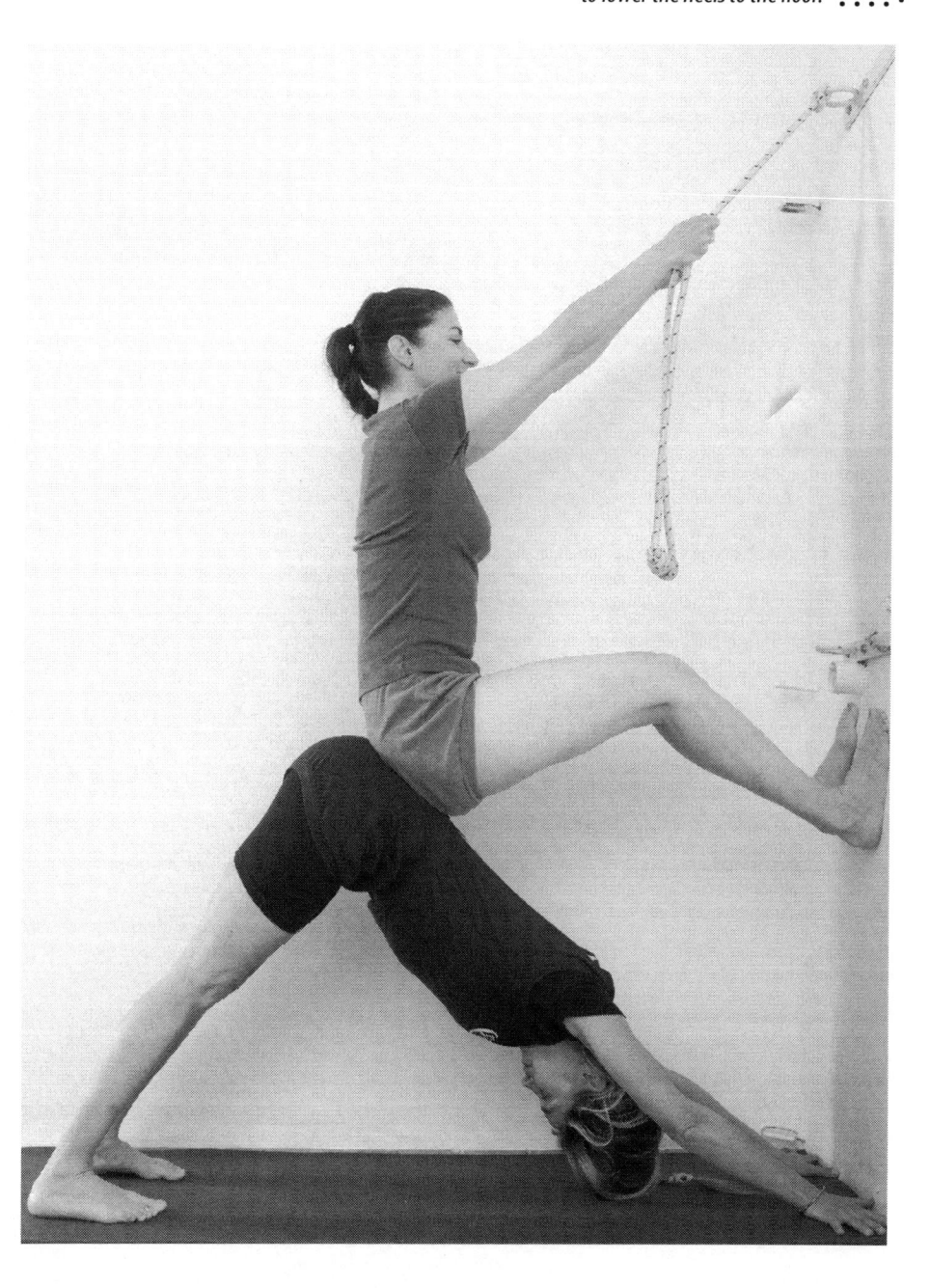

Adho Mukha Svanasana
Variation 6

Moving in the sacrum: "Two dogs"

Props
partner

Here the helper performs a variation of dog pose on top of the student's dog pose.

⟶ After the student has entered the pose:

› Stand about one meter (3 feet) in front of the student's hands, with your back to the student.

› Bend forward and put both hands on the floor; raise one leg at a time and position your feet symmetrically on the student's sacrum.

› Stretch your arms while pushing the student's sacrum back and up; tuck your shoulder blades in and concave your upper back.

Effects

The partner's push helps the student shift weight to the legs, stretch the back, activate the legs and open and lengthen the back of the legs.

The partner is doing a variation of Adho Mukha Svanasana with elevated feet – this is a good way to strengthen and stretch the arms, flex the shoulder girdle and concave the back.

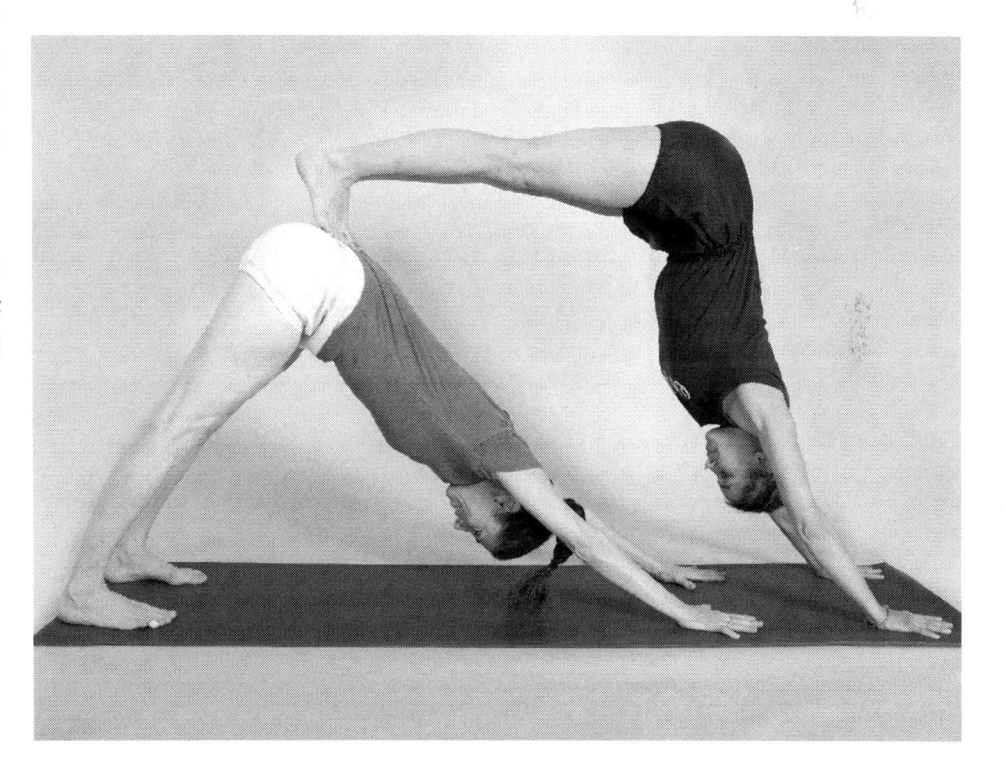

Adho Mukha Svanasana Variation 7

Action and counter-action: Partner pushes against back groins

Props
block
partner

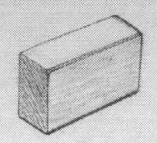

It is easier to push against some resistance rather then to "push the air". In this variation, the partner applies pressure on the student's back groins in order to trigger counter-action in the student.

→ Stand behind the student and place a block against her/his back groins (top of the back of the thighs).

> Push the block forward and down (toward the student's hands) and encourage her/him to push back.

Effects

The pressure of the block triggers the push back. The student learns to adjust the pelvis and mobilize the torso in the correct direction (back and up).

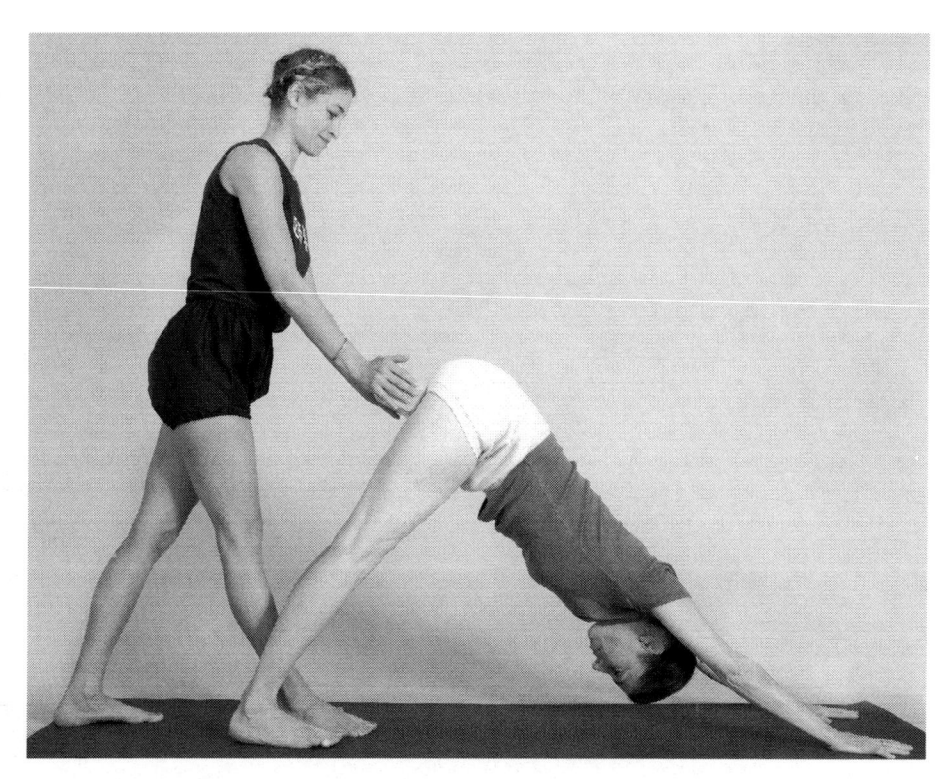

Lifting the Feet

Raising the feet creates length in the lower back and the abdomen.

Adho Mukha Svanasana Variation 8

Sensitizing the buttocks: Elevating the feet

Props
2 or 4 blocks
or a stool

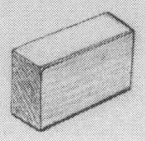

⟹ Place two blocks next to the wall.

› Place the mounds of the toes on blocks and the heels on the wall and do the pose ❶.

✓ *After staying in the pose for a while, move slightly forward, step off the blocks and do the pose with feet on the floor. Observe the feeling in the buttocks and in the pelvic girdle now. Can you re-create the sharp awareness achieved with the raised feet support?*

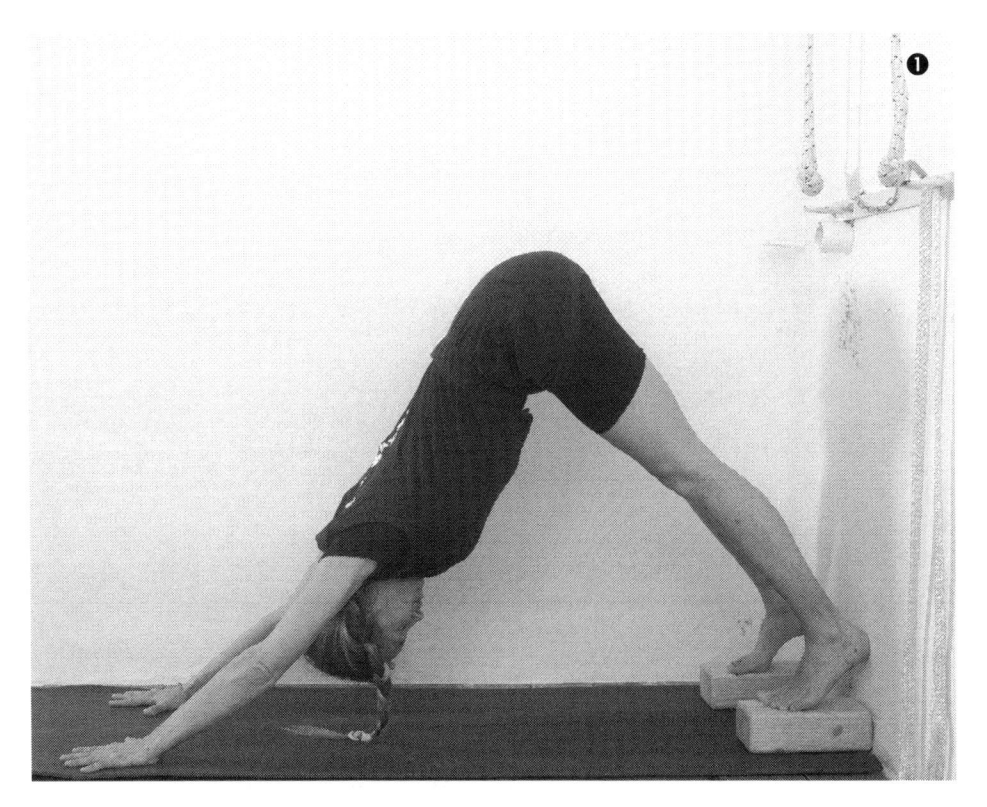

To get a stronger effect you can elevate the feet even higher. For example, you can use four blocks, a low stool ❷ or an inverted chair ❸:

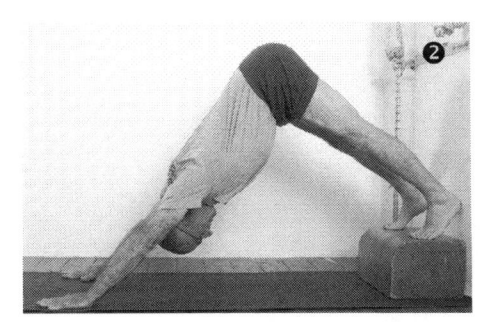

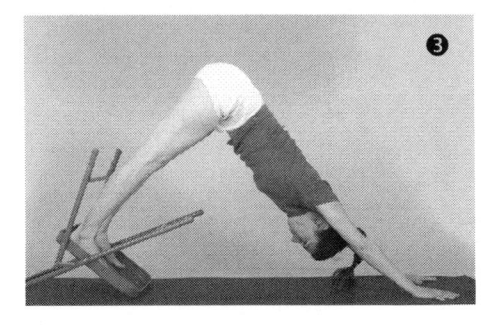

Effects

Raising the feet brings awareness to the top of the pose: the buttocks. It helps one feel what B.K.S. Iyengar meant by giving the image of a snow covering a Himalayan peak. The triangular shape of the pose becomes easier to achieve. The pose becomes more 'inverted', which changes the inner feeling. The lower abdomen is extended and the organs of the pelvis are lifted. This variation is hence beneficial for the reproductive system. It is a recommended practice for post-partum.

Adho Mukha Svanasana
Variation 9

Lifting the entire pose: Feet and palms on blocks

Props
4 blocks

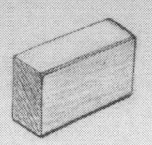

It is interesting to try the pose when both the palms and feet are on blocks:

→ Do the pose and mark the location of your palms and feet on the floor.

> Place four blocks in the marked locations of the palms and the feet.

> Do the pose again, this time elevated by the blocks.

> Stay for a while and record your sensation. Then step off the blocks and do the pose as usual, on the floor.

Effects
The blocks lift both palms and feet so the basic shape of the pose is not changed, still there is a definite effect on the inner feeling of the pose. Although the geometry of the pose is not changed, the pose feels different. The quality of the contact surfaces does make a difference.

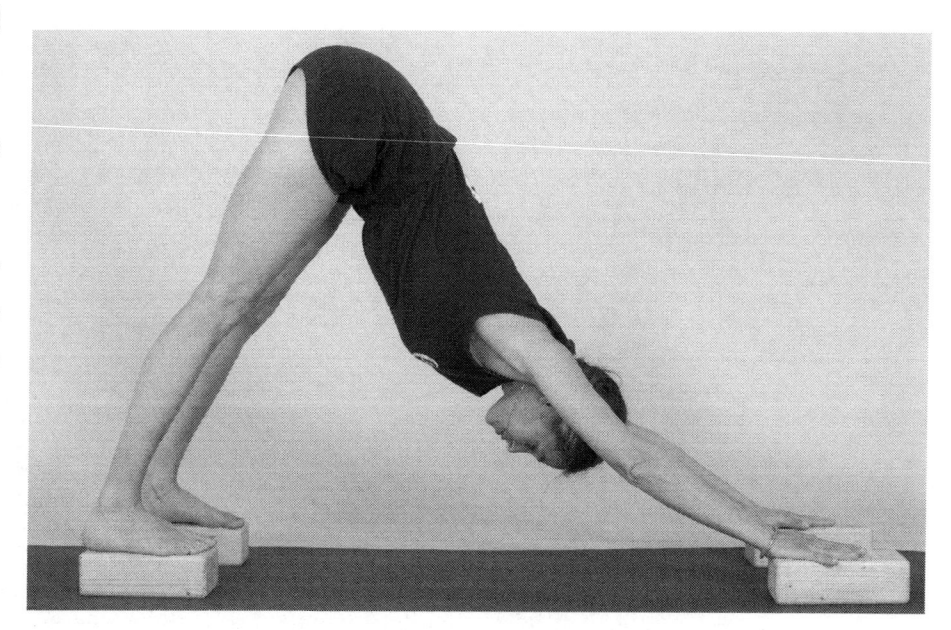

Tips
✓ Compare your feeling when doing on the four blocks with what the feeling of the pose as done usually, on the flat floor. Can you describe this difference and the reason for it? What are the effects of doing on the blocks?

Adho Mukha Svanasana Variation 10

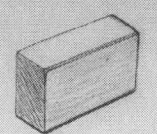

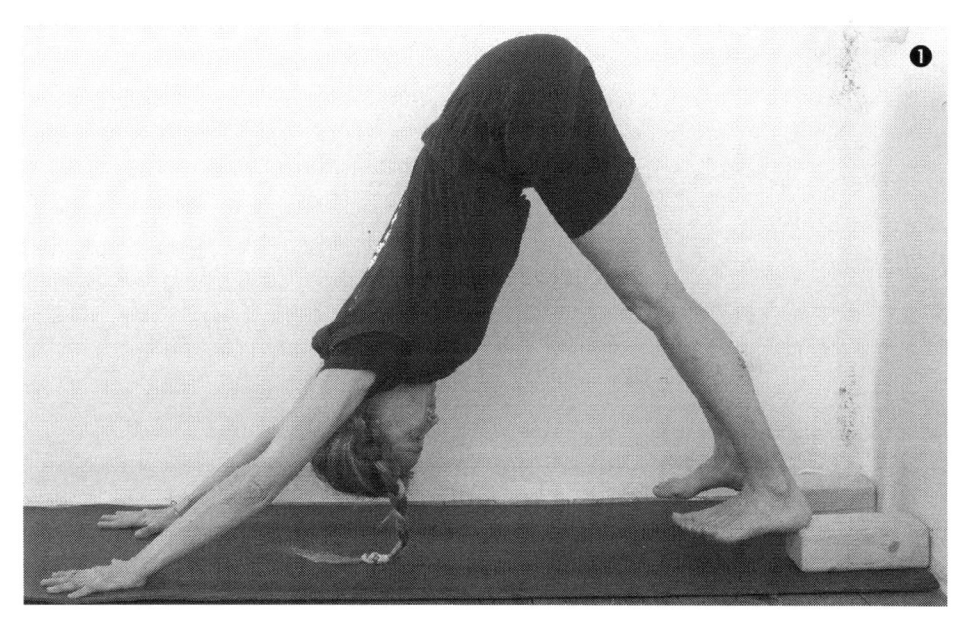

Activating the front thighs: Heels on blocks' edges

Props
2 blocks

Shifting body weight to the legs is the key for achieving full extension of the spine, reducing muscle effort and relaxing in the pose. The following variation strengthens and develops the legs.

⟶ Place two blocks next to the wall. Do the pose on the floor, with the back bones of the heels pushing against the blocks. ❶

› Now place the back edge of each heel on the front edge of the corresponding block.

› Push the heel against the blocks to elevate and spread the toes and soles.

› Move the shin bones and the front thighs back.

› Hold this pose for a while, keeping the backward movement of the legs.

› Now slide the heels down to the floor. ❷

› Press the bottom of the heels down to the floor and the back heel bones against the block.

Effects

Some students find it difficult to activate the quadriceps (frontal thighs muscles) – this variation is for them! It is one of the best ways to activate and strengthen the legs. Observe how the fronts of the legs are moving toward the back of the legs.

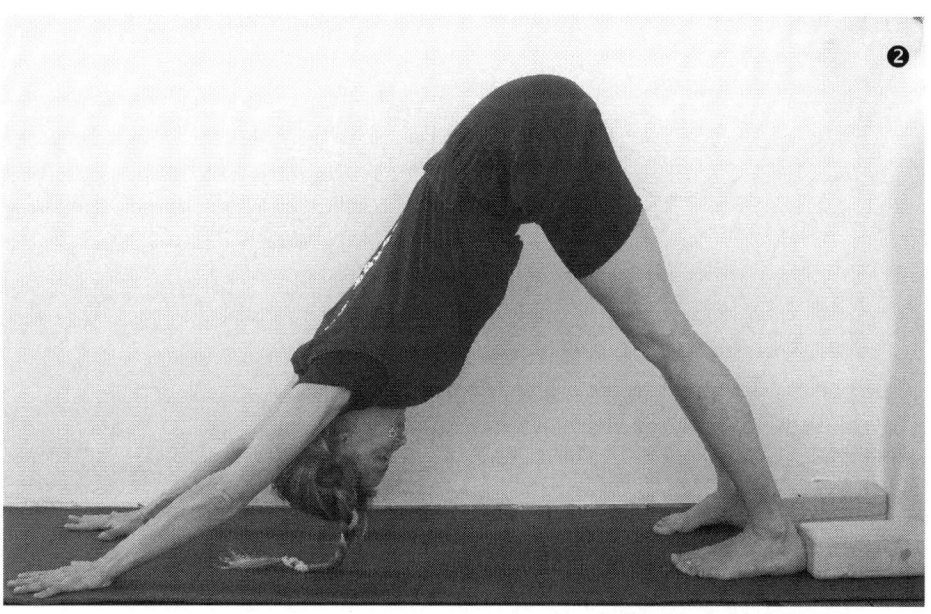

Activating the Arms and Shoulders

Adho Mukha Svanasana is quite a unique pose in that the work of both the arms and the legs is equally important.

✓ You should work the legs like in Tadasana and work the arms like in Adho Mukha Vrksasana (handstand).

Adho Mukha Svanasana Variation 11

Props
partner

Widening the shoulder girdle: Partner helps to turn the arms

The upper arms should rotate so that the biceps muscles are turning outside (away from the center of the body) and the triceps are turning inside (toward the head). It is important to anchor the thumb and the space between the thumb and the index finger, otherwise the turning of the upper arms will lift the inner part of the palms and the base of the pose will weaken.

Working with a partner can clarify this action (instruction for the partner):

⟶ Carefully place your toe mounds on the thumb sides of the palms of the practitioner ❶.

▷ Now hold the arms of the practitioner and gently turn them in the desired direction. (see explanation above) ❷.

▷ Hold for a while and then release and allow the practitioner to do the turning action on his own.

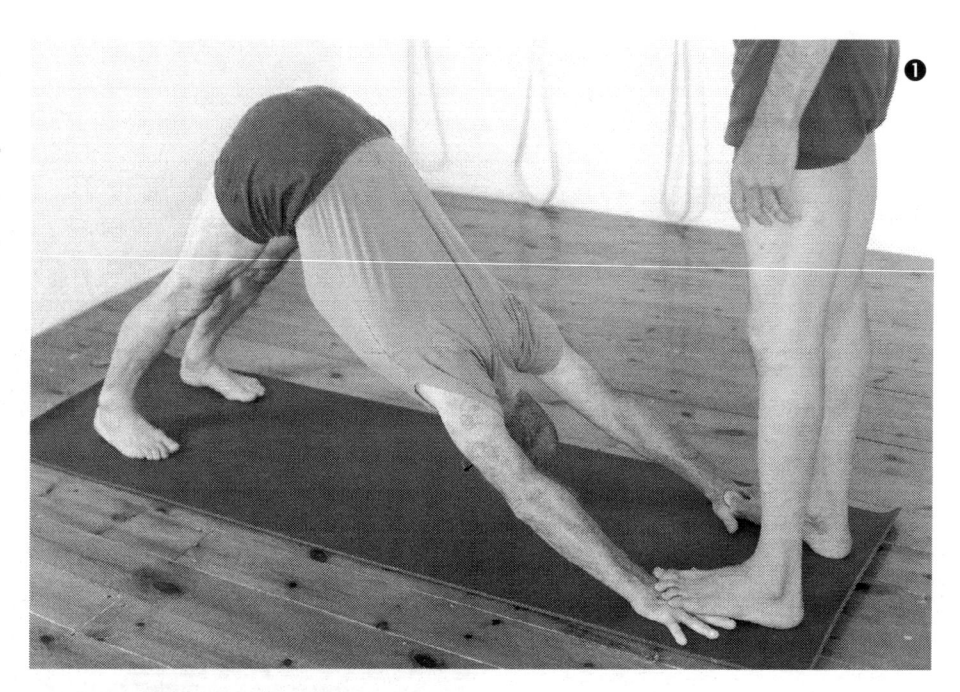

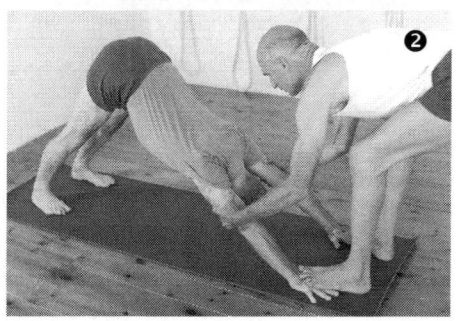

Effects

Turning the upper arms creates width in the shoulder girdle and helps to release the neck. Compare the space between the shoulders in the above two photos. In ❶ there are long wrinkles in the practitioner's shirt; these wrinkles almost disappear in ❷ due to the widening of the shoulder girdle and the upper chest.

Adho Mukha Svanasana
Variation 12

Releasing the neck: Partner pulls the trapezius muscles

Props
belt or rope
partner

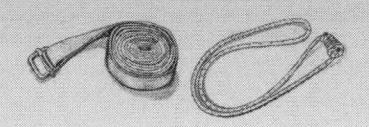

Earlier in this chapter (see Variation 11 of Tadasana on page 17) we explained how to place a rope on the shoulder girdle and hook a belt in order to get trapezius traction. The same can be done in Adho Mukha Svanasana.

→ Arrange the rope (or the belt) as explained in Tadasana.

› Enter the pose and have a partner pull the rope for you ❶.

If no helper is available, it is possible to use a wall hook for this purpose ❷.

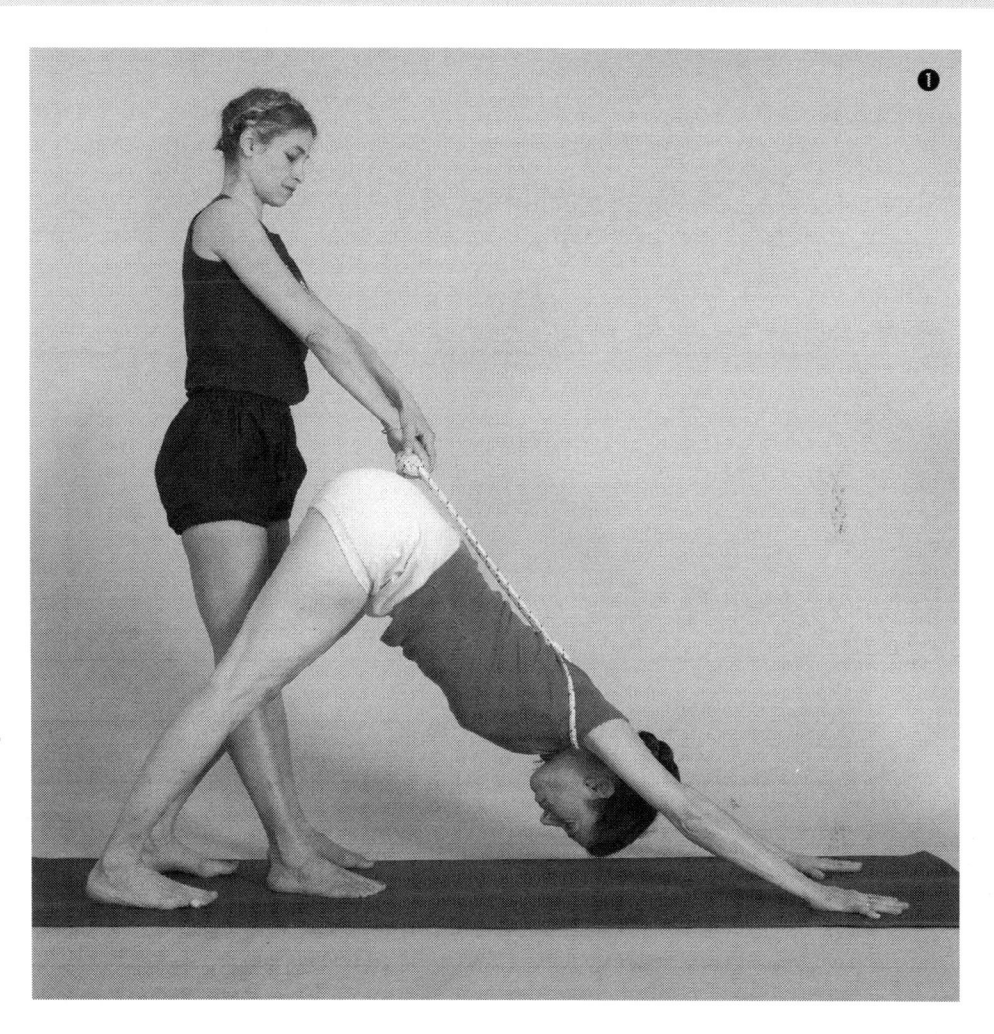

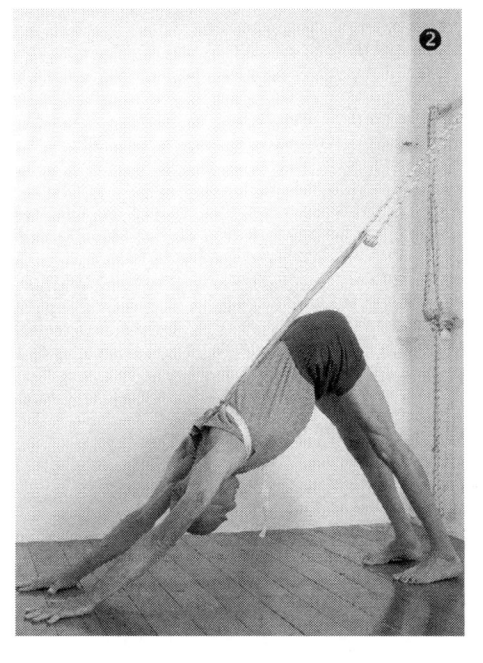

Effects
The trapezius pull releases the neck and creates space in the shoulder area. It also shifts load from the arms to the legs.

Adho Mukha Svanasana
Variation 13

Spreading the fingers: Using wall and blocks

Props
wall
2 blocks

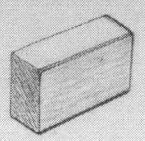

Here are two ways for spreading the fingers and palms:

⟶ Turn the palms slightly sideways and place the tip of the thumbs and the outer sides of the index fingers against the wall.

⟶ Use blocks to spread the thumbs away from the fingers. Use one or two blocks, depending on the length of the block and the width of your shoulders (In the photo, the model uses one flat and one standing block to adjust to her shoulder width).

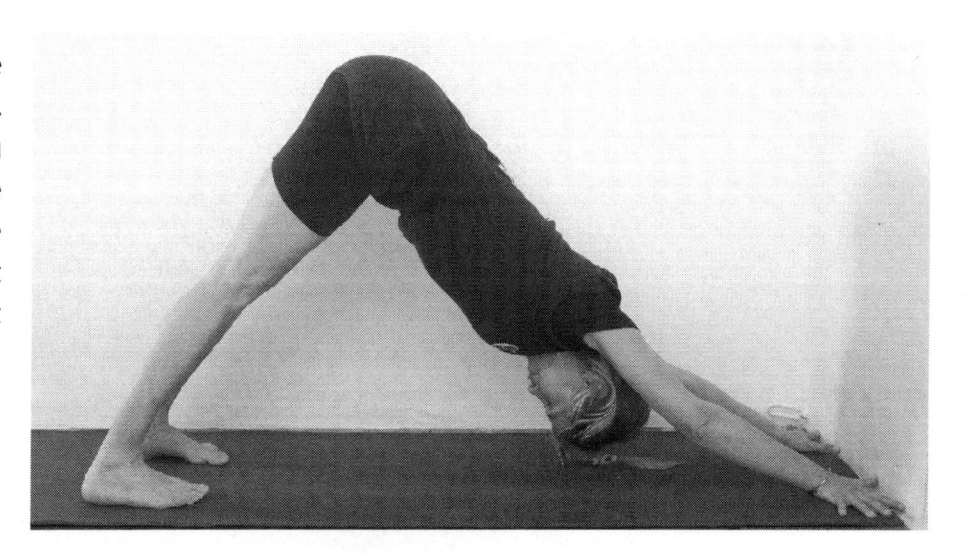

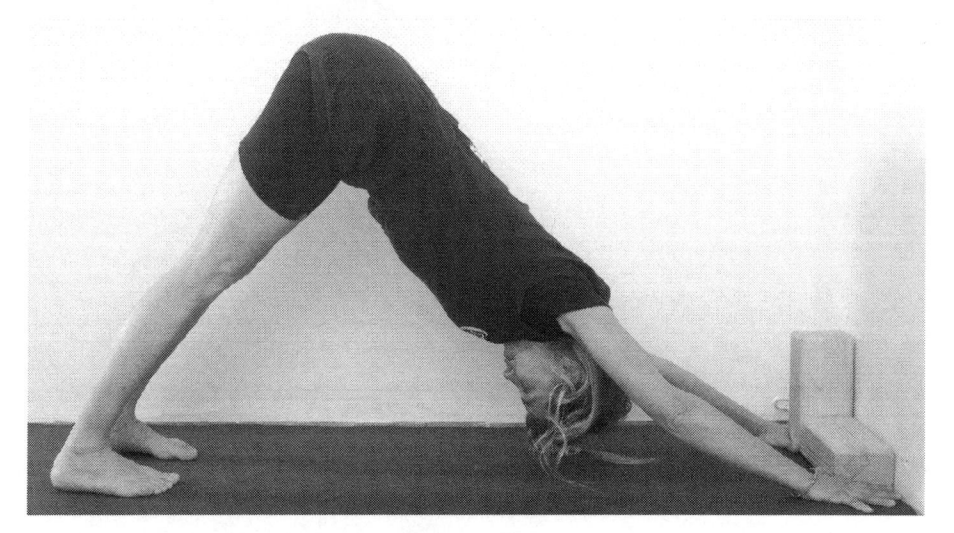

Effects

The grounding of the inner part of the palms is important: it helps to lengthen the inner arms and to rotate the upper arms from inside out. In these variations, the wall and/or blocks help to create space between the index fingers and the thumbs, creating width in the inner part of the palm. This action improves the grounding of the pose in the palms.

Adho Mukha Svanasana Variation 14

Relieving wrist pain: Palms on a slant

Props
Slanted plank ("slant") or a folded mat

Pain in the wrists is quite a common complaint in our era. People suffering from this problem often avoid the dog pose. But in many cases, supporting the carpals ('the heels of the palms') on a raised platform prevents this type of pain.

⟶ Place your carpal bones on a slant ❶, such that the weight is shifted to the finger mounds.

› If no slant is available fold a mat to the required height and place it under your carpals ❷.

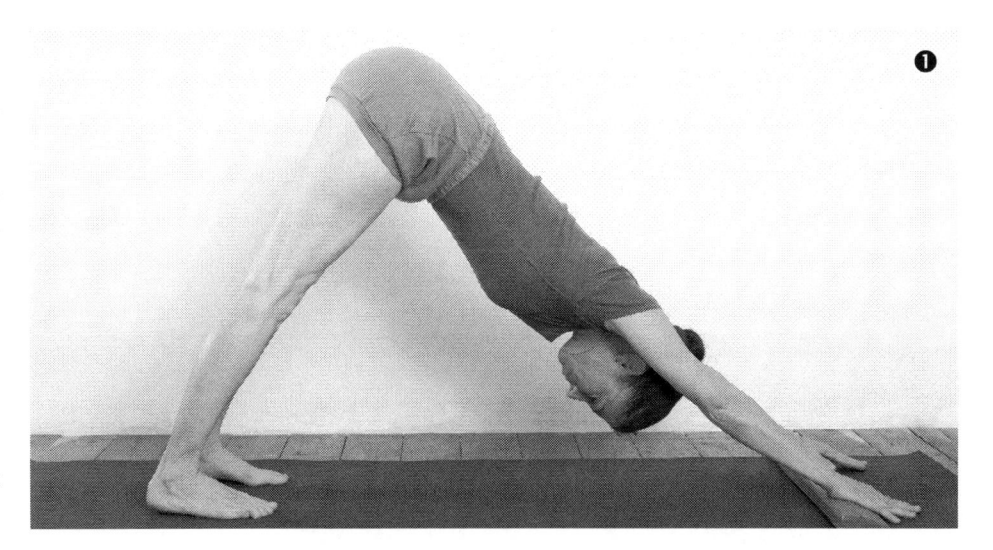

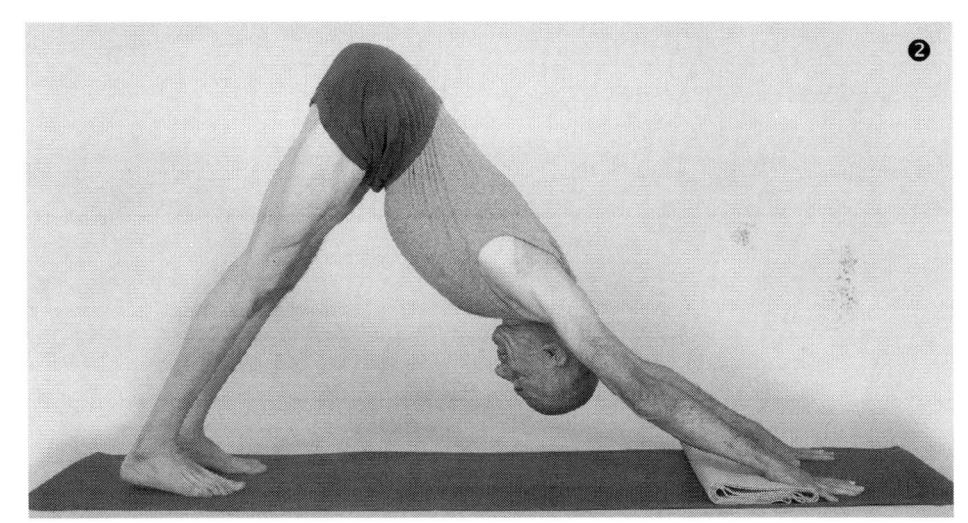

Another useful pose for correcting minor wrist injury is Pada Hastasana: ❸

⟶ Place the palms under the feet. Move them in until the root of each palm is under the toes and press the big toes on the thumb side of the corresponding palm. Lift the lower arms to create space in the wrists.

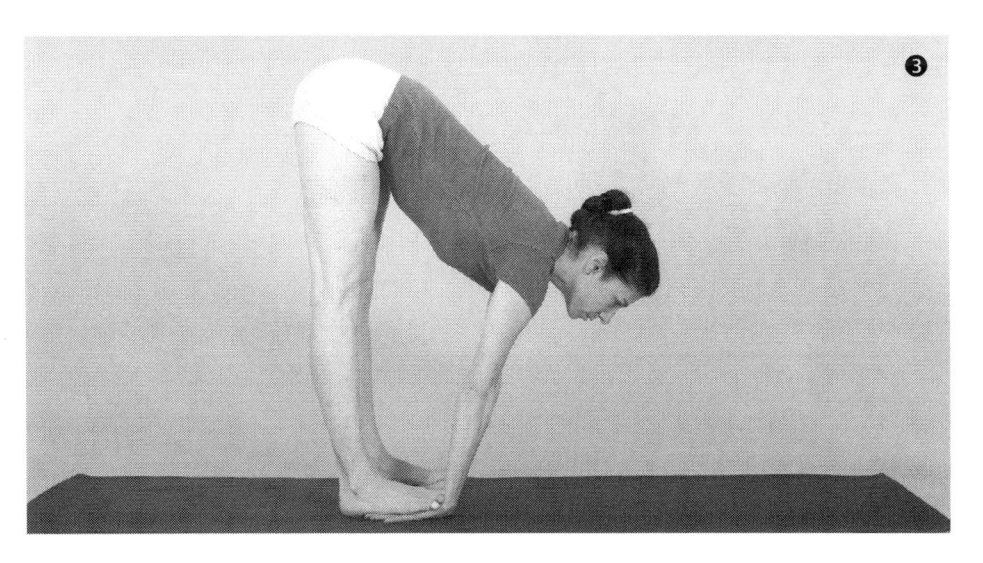

Props for Yoga / Chapter 1 / Adho Mukha Svanasana 45

Adho Mukha Svanasana
Variation 15

Flexing the wrists: Palms on wall

Props
wall

To prevent wrist problems, one needs to make these joints strong and flexible. This variation and the following one, help to achieve this.

→ Kneel and place your palms against the wall, move the root of the palms as close as possible to the wall.

> Now push the wall and straighten your legs to Dog pose.

Note: You can also turn your palms sideways on the wall.

Effects
This variation creates flexibility in the wrists and strengthens the bones of the arms.

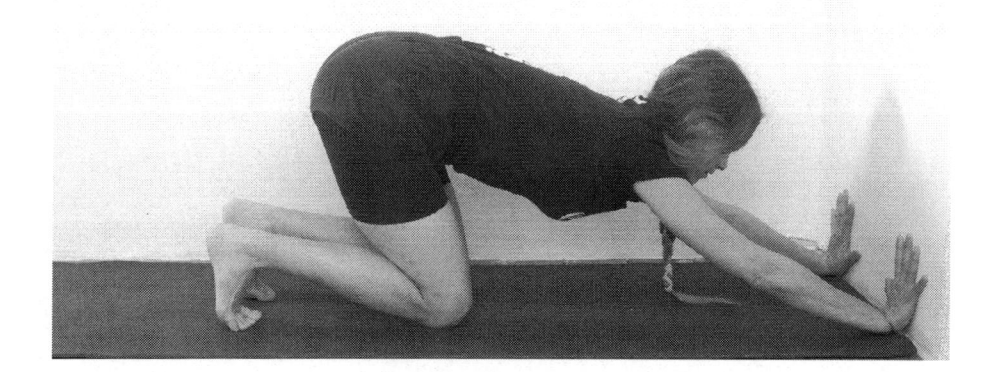

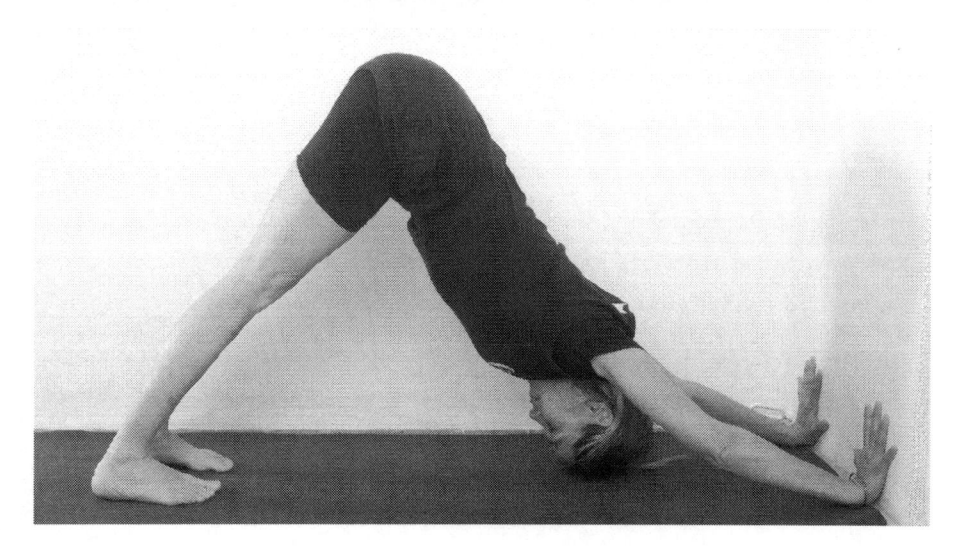

Adho Mukha Svanasana Variation 16

Turning the palms

⟶ Turn the palms outward on the floor and enter the pose.

› Extend the lower arms up and away from the palms.

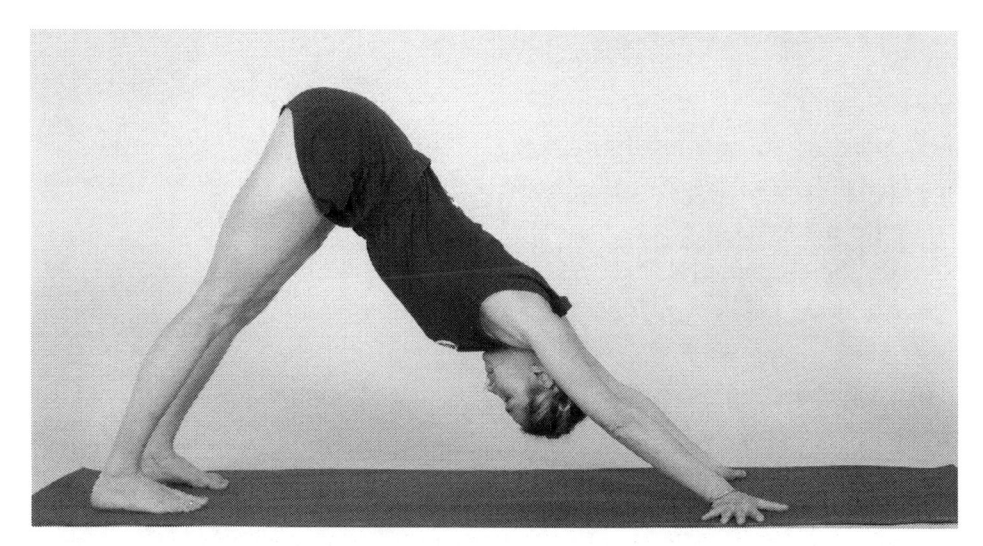

Turning the palms backward:

› Do Urdhva Mukha Svanasana with the palms turned back.

› From there move back to Adho Mukha Svanasana. It is more difficult to move the arms and shoulders back (toward the legs), but the stretch is good for the wrists.

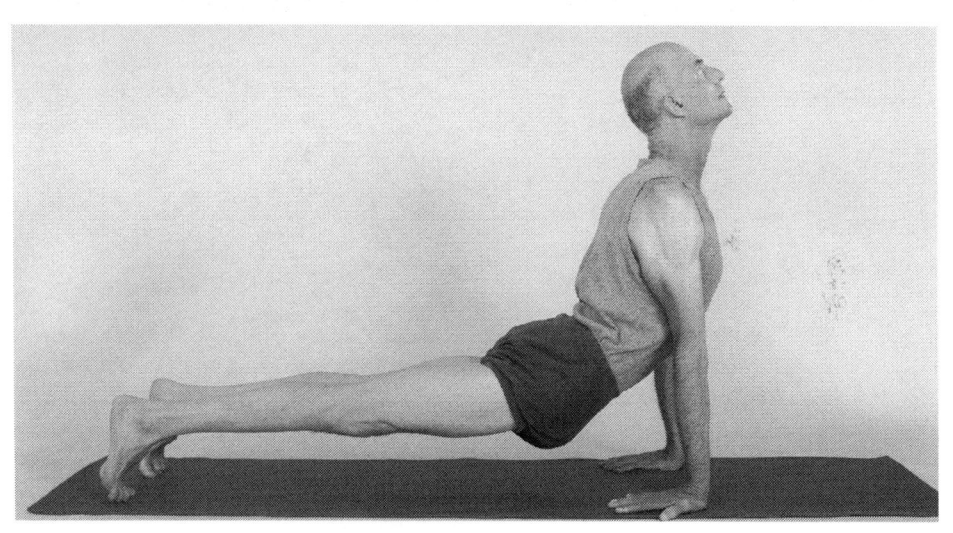

Effects............

Turning the palms and placing a controlled weight on them helps to strengthen the wrists, lengthen the tendons and ligaments of the wrist and make these joints more flexible and healthy. It prepares one for Adho Mukha Vrksasana (full arm balance) with the palms turned back, for Setu Bandha Sarvangasana and for Mayurasana (LOY Pl. 354).

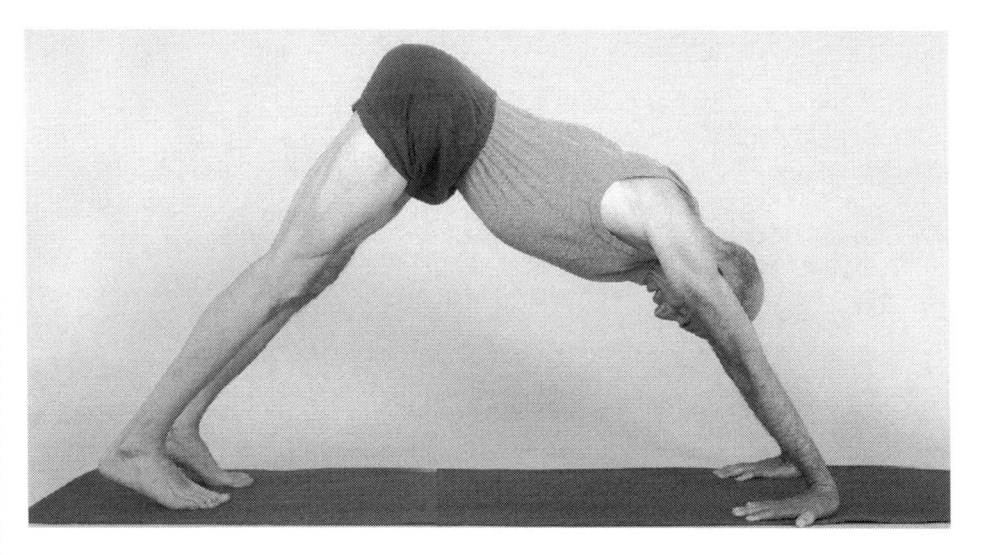

Props for Yoga / Chapter 1 / Adho Mukha Svanasana 47

Adho Mukha Svanasana
Variation 17

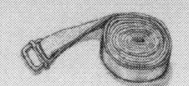

Props
belt

Stabilizing the arms: Belt around elbows.

Elbows can be hyper-extended (i.e., over extended) or hypo-extended (i.e., hard to straighten them). For the hypo type, the outer elbow remains out and the inner arm is short. A belt around the elbows can teach the work one needs to do.

⟶ Loop a belt around the outer elbows and tighten it to shoulder width.

> Do the pose and stretch the inner arms against the resistance of the belt.

Effects
The belt helps to keep the elbows straight; people who have difficulty to do so, will be able to learn this action with the belt.

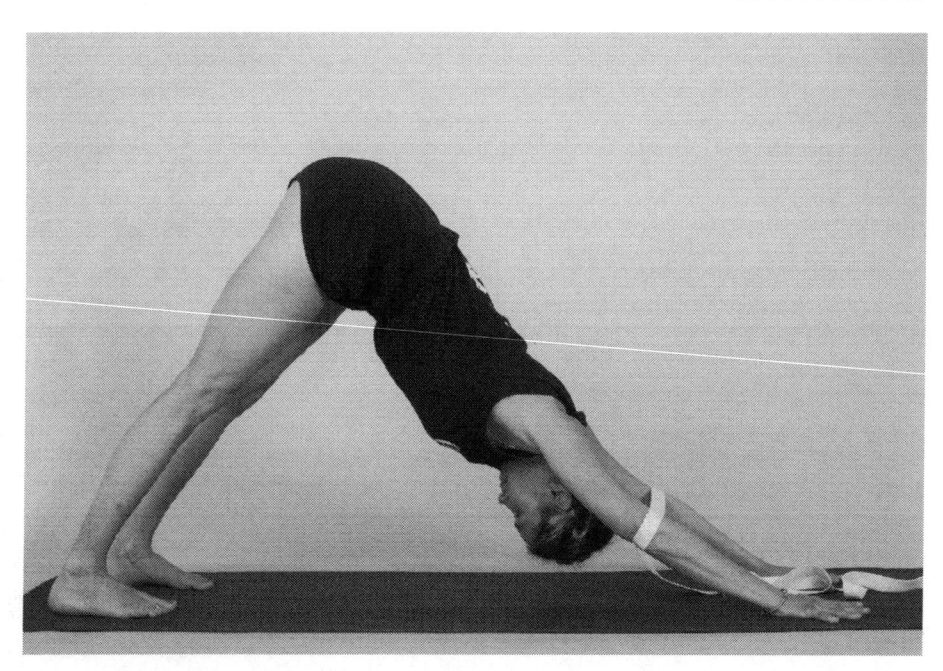

Tips
✓ Use the belt for learning, but do not develop dependency on it. Learn to move the outer elbows in, and to lengthen the inner upper arms up, even without the belt.

Adho Mukha Svanasana
Variation 18

Stabilizing the arms: Elbows on blocks or inverted chair

Props
2 blocks
or a chair

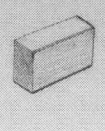

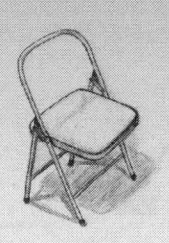

For the hyperextended type, the inner arms become too long. Supporting the forearms helps to limit the excessive extension of the biceps, to balance it with the contraction of the triceps and to register the correct arm sensation in the pose. You can support the elbows with two blocks ❶ or with an inverted chair.

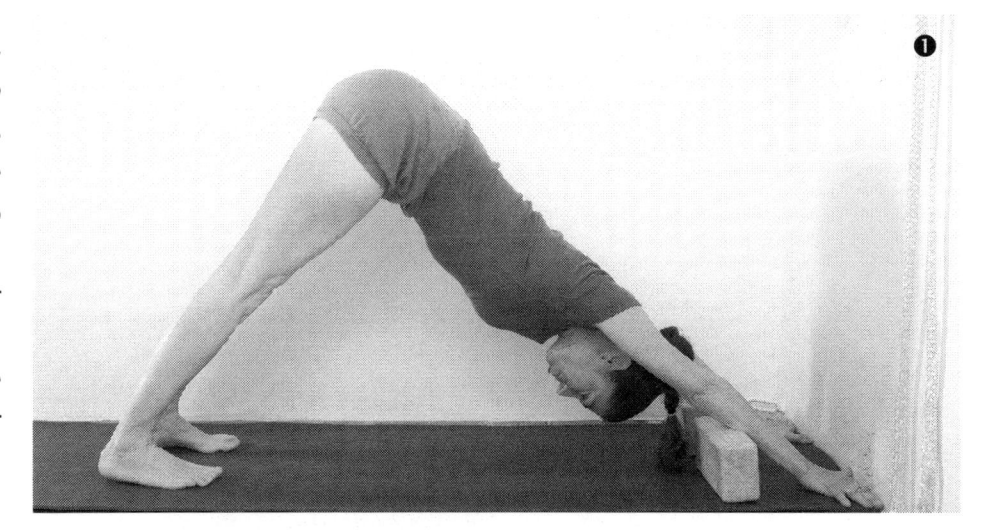

If a partner is available, he or she can tilt the blocks to fit under the lower arms ❷; this improves the support.

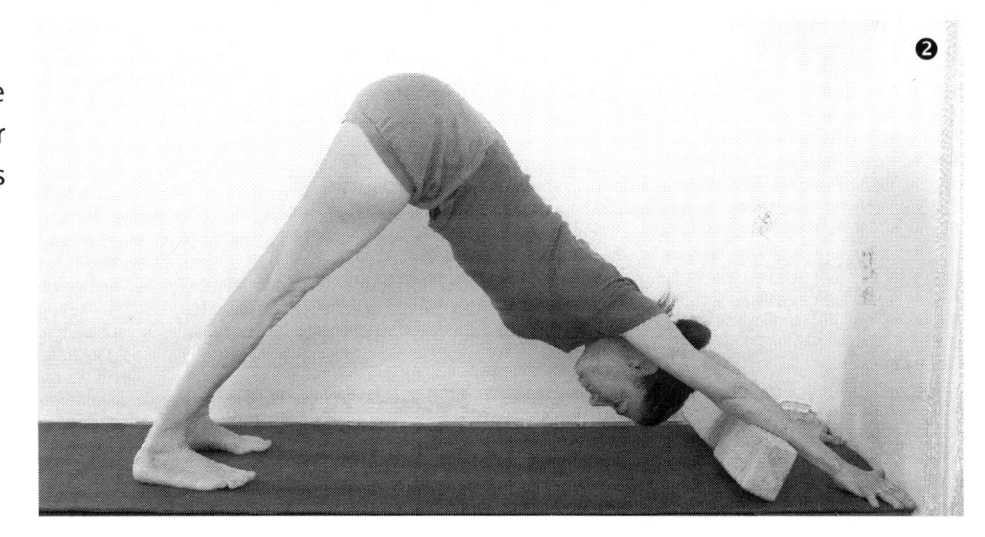

Using an inverted chair for the palms has an additional advantage: the forearms can be supported on the chair's legs ❸.

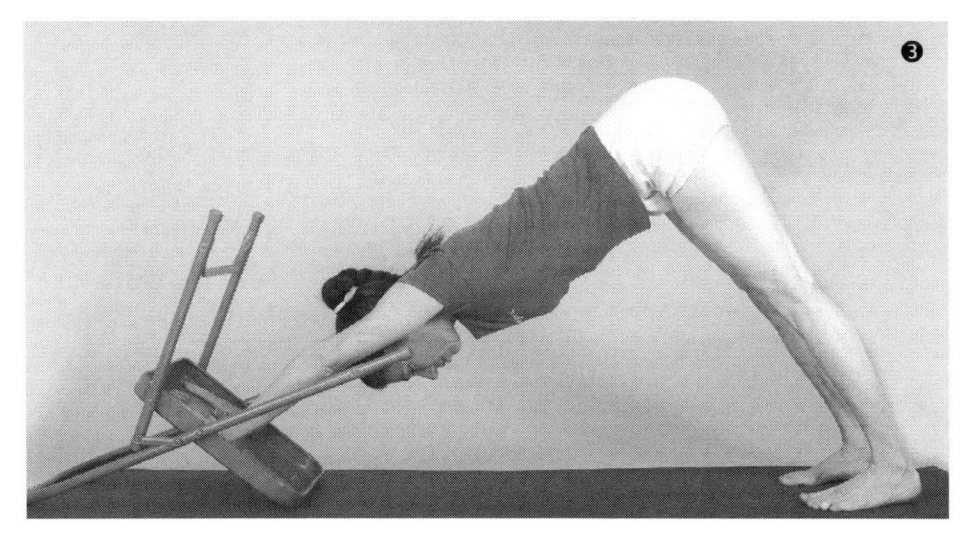

Props for Yoga / Chapter 1 / Adho Mukha Svanasana

Moving On with the Pose

Once the actions of the legs and arms are established, one can work on correct activation of the spine and the shoulders in the pose. The shoulder blades should move deeply into the body and the spine should be concaved toward the legs. Here are two ways to improve the work of the shoulders and shoulder blades.

Adho Mukha Svanasana Variation 19

Props
helper

Moving the shoulder blades in: Starting with forearms on the floor

→ Depending on the width of your shoulders, use a block or two. Separate the thumbs from the index fingers and hold the blocks in between the palms. Make sure the palms are shoulder width apart ❶.

> Place the forearms on floor (like Pincha Mayurasana preparation), concave the back and move the shoulder blades deep in.

> Lift the buttocks up and step in.

> Now, without letting the shoulder blades move out, straighten the arms ❷.

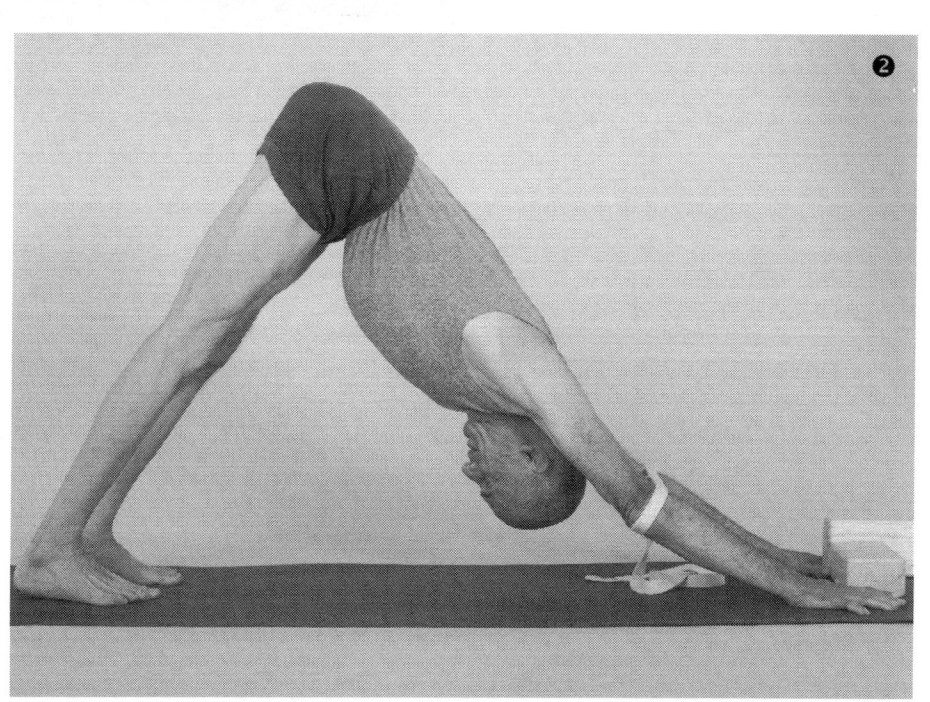

Effects
With the forearms on the floor, it is easier to draw the shoulder blades in; the position of the shoulder blades should then be maintained as one straightens the arms.

Tips
✓ Straighten your arms by moving simultaneously backward and upward (not first up and then back).

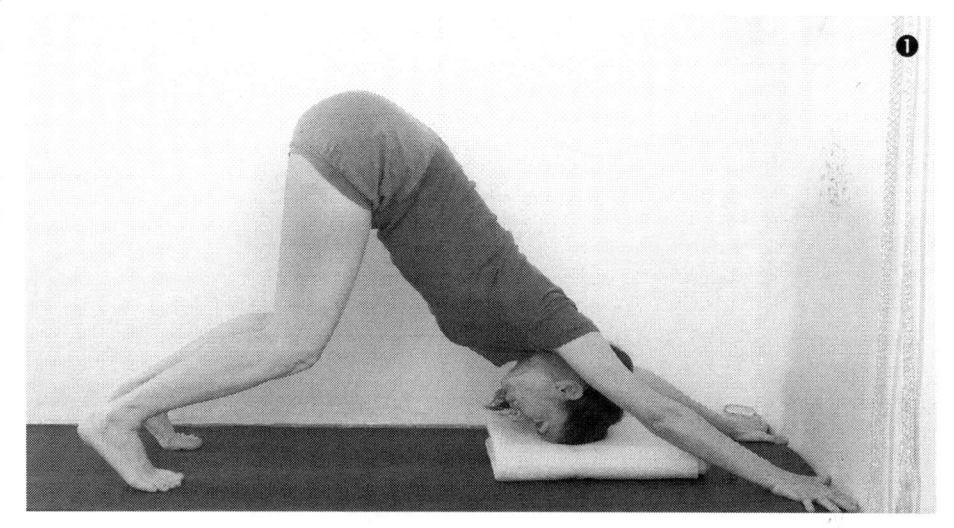

Adho Mukha Svanasana
Variation 20

Moving the middle back in: Starting with the head low

Props
wall
blanket

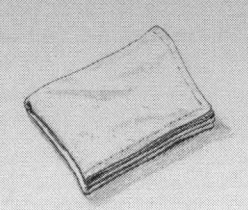

⟶ Kneel on the floor next to the wall; place the fingers against the wall and the head on the floor.

Note: Avoid pushing the shoulders too much in an attempt to put the forehead on the floor; if needed - use a folded blanket to support the head ❶.

▸ Without lifting the head, straighten the knees and press the heels down ❷.

Effects
With the head on the floor, you can draw the shoulder blades in and open the chest; this can be maintained when straightening the legs.

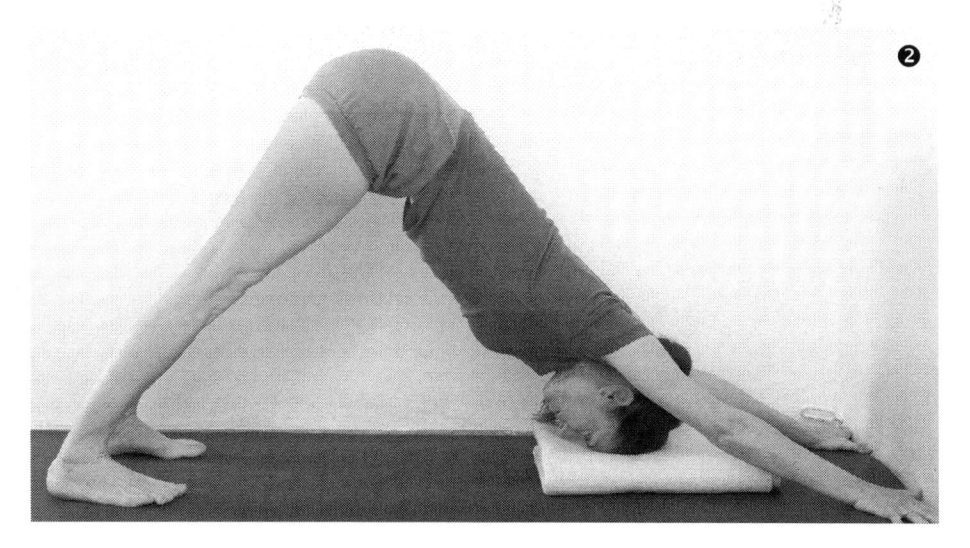

Restorative Adho Mukha Svanasana

B.K.S. Iyengar mentions the following effects of this pose:

"When one is exhausted, a longer stay in this pose removes fatigue and brings back the lost energy." Light on Yoga (see Pl. 75)

"Calms the brain and gently stimulates the nerves; Slows down the heartbeat." Yoga – A Path to Holistic Health, p. 89

Part of this relaxing effect is due to resting the head on the floor. For most people this is relaxing only when using some support for the head. Here are two ways to do the pose with head support for restorative purposes.

Adho Mukha Svanasana Variation 21

Relaxing the brain: Head support

Props
bolster
block
and/or blanket;
wall (optional)

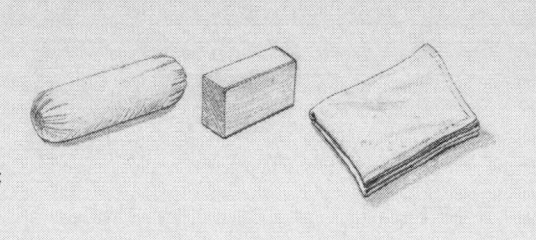

→ Do the pose and hold it comfortably for a while (if the heels do not reach the floor, press them against the wall). Observe the gap between your head and the floor.

› Prepare a support to fill that gap – it can be a block ❶, a bolster, a folded blanket, or any combination thereof.

› Do the pose again with the top part of the forehead (hairline) resting on the support.

› You can also use a slightly higher support and place the entire forehead (hairline to eyebrows) on it ❷.

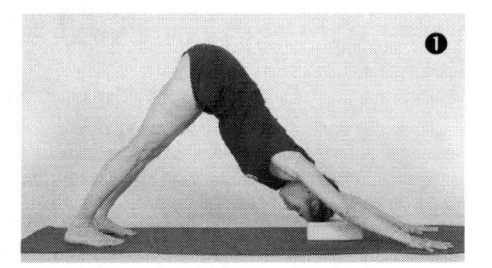

Effects
The support for the head reduces the muscular effort, relaxes the brain and enables a longer stay in the pose with less effort.

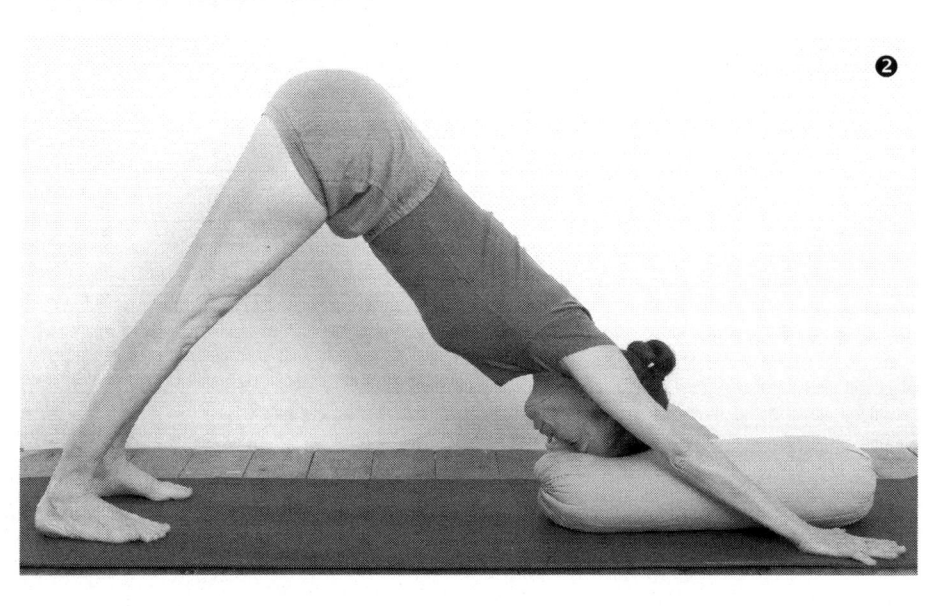

Tips
✓ Compare the difference in your inner feeling between the two head positions.

✓ Breathe rhythmically and observe: what are the effects of staying longer in this pose?

52 Props for Yoga / Chapter 1 / Adho Mukha Svanasana

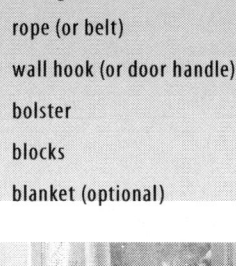

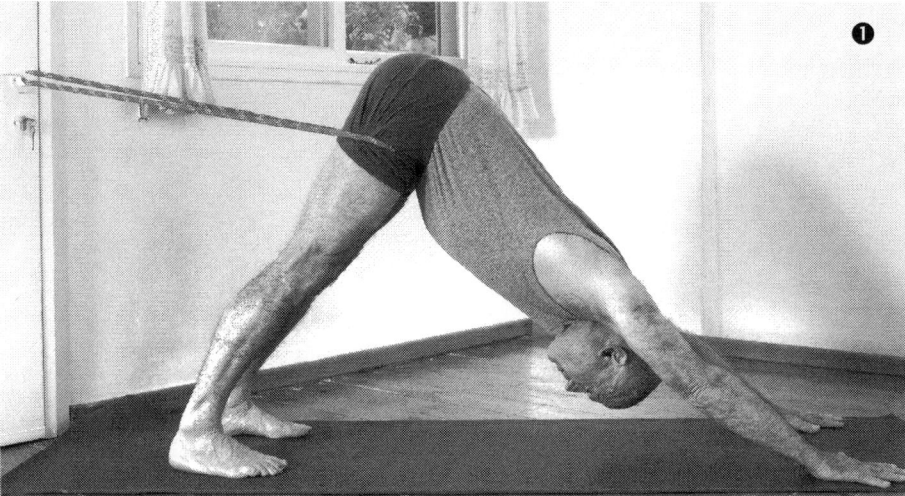

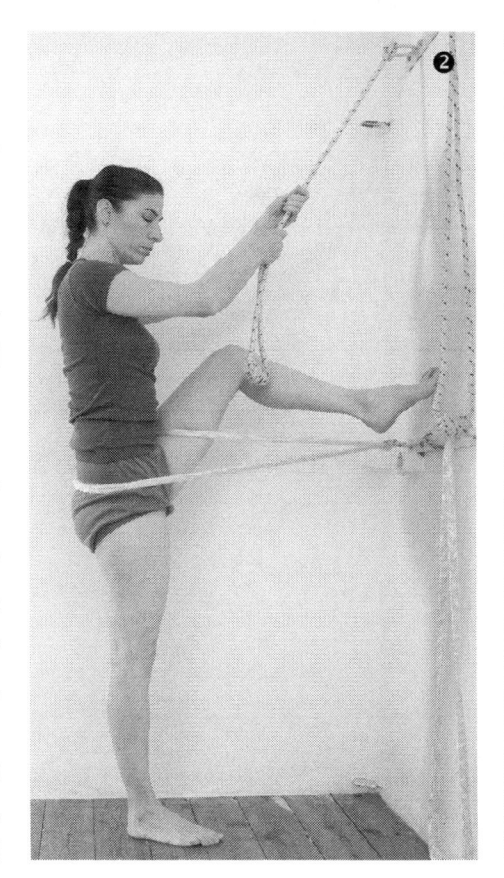

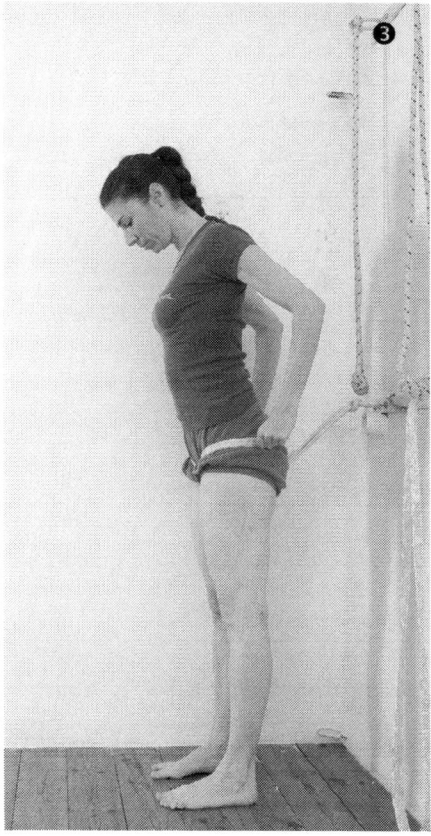

Adho Mukha Svanasana Variation 22

Passive extension of the spine: Wall rope around front groins

Props
rope (or belt)
wall hook (or door handle)
bolster
blocks
blanket (optional)

There are several ways to do the pose with a rope attached to a wall hook. First, we show the 'standard' way.

As can be seen, there is no need for a special hook on the wall; any reliable anchor at an appropriate height may be used for tying the rope. Even a sturdy door handle can do the job ❶.

Another way of entering the pose is my favorite, since it gives more lift and creates more expansion in the pelvis. We show it here using a standard middle wall hook (the pose can also be done with the upper wall hook and a longer rope):

⟶ Stand facing the wall inside the loop of the anchored rope and place it around your pelvis.

▷ Lift one leg from outside the loop ❷.

▷ While turning - move the leg over the two sides of the rope and put the foot on the floor. You are now standing with your back to the wall ❸.

▷ Adjust the rope on your sacrum and groins and bend forward. Place your palms on the floor and step back to touch the wall with your heels.

Note: If the distance to the wall is too far, place blocks to support the heels as in ❹. (see next page)

Adho Mukha Svanasana Variation 22 (cont.)

Passive extension of the spine: Wall rope around front groins

- Now stretch the arms forward and enter the pose.

- Use a folded blanket, block or a bolster to support the forehead, as explained in the previous variation ❹.

    Note: If the palms do not reach the floor easily, place them on blocks or on other suitable support.

- After staying for a few minutes in the pose, step slightly forward and lean your pelvis on the rope to do a forward-slanted Uttanasana ❺.

- Roll the buttocks forward and push the front thighs back. You can also place a block to support the crown of the head.

- To get out of the pose, lift your trunk slowly and gradually. To prevent dizziness, lift the head slowly.

- Release yourself from the rope in reverse: lift one leg and, move it over to the other side, while turning to face the wall.

- Pregnant and menstruating women can do a variation of this pose with two crossed ropes attached to two wall hooks ❻. This creates more width in the lower abdomen.

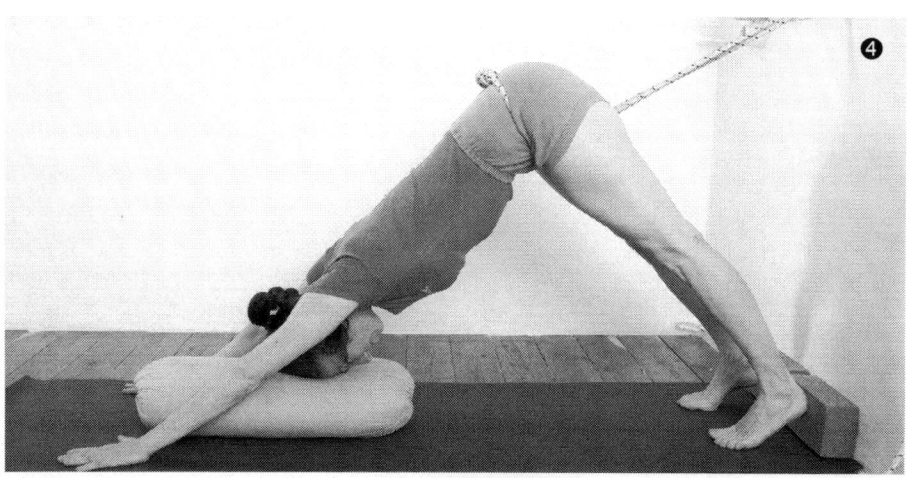

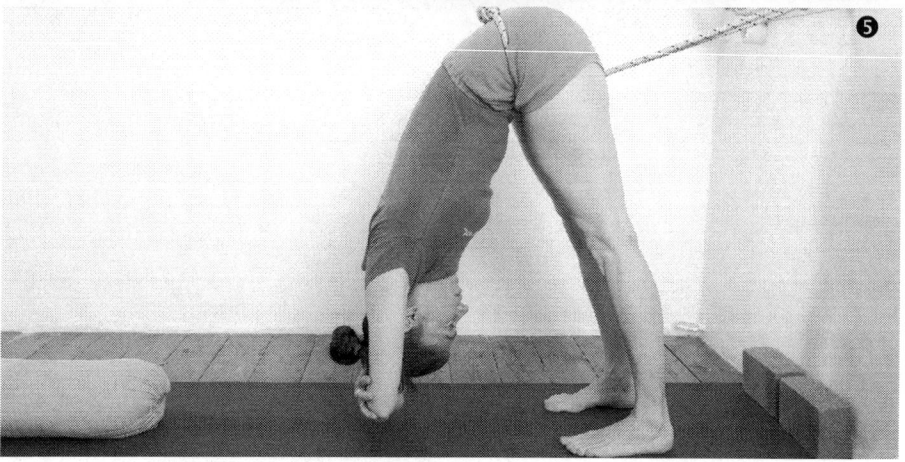

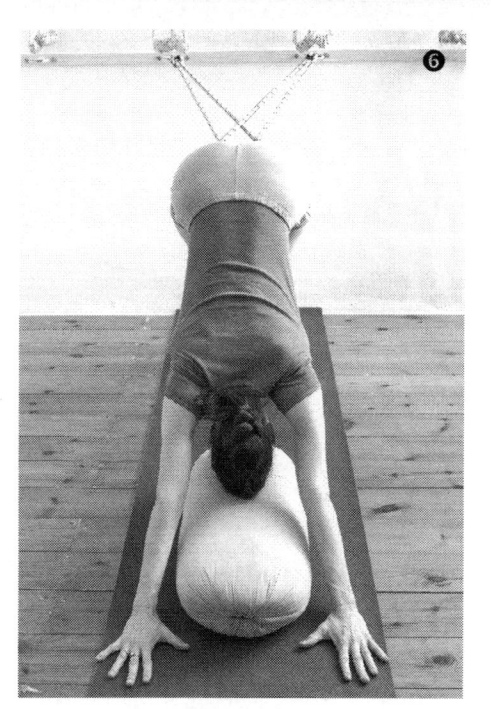

Effects

The rope carries most of the body weight, reducing the load on the legs and the arms. The pose becomes restorative and you can easily stay in it for 5 to 10 minutes. The rope holds the pelvis firmly so the spine gets a good extension; hence this variation is recommended for people suffering from lower back pain.

In the Uttanasana phase, the rope enables you to do the pose with the legs tilted forward; this teaches to roll the buttocks forward and to release the trunk down.

Uttanasana

About Uttanasana

Uttanasana is a 'leg pose' – the legs have to be strong and well lifted while the trunk should be soft and releasing toward the floor. In this pose, there are three imaginary pulleys rolling forward. From the gross to the subtle these pulleys are: the pelvis, the head and the inner ears. The backward movement of the thighs resists the forward rolling and stabilizes the pose. In the following variations we start from the pelvis roll and finish with a restorative variation in which the head is supported. In all of these variations, the legs are spread to pelvic width (unlike the final pose in which the legs are together, see LOY Pl. 48).

Tips

✓ Uttanasana reminds me of a waterfall, the legs being the cliffs from which the trunk is flowing down like water – make the legs strong and tall and the trunk soft and flowing!

⚠ CAUTIONS

If you have spinal disc disorder, practice only the concave back phase of the pose.

Women in advanced pregnancy should also practice only the concave back phase of the pose

Legs and Pelvis

Here are some variations to strengthen the legs, improve the flexibility and to create different effects in the lower part of the body.

Uttanasana
Variation 1

Checking the symmetry: Buttocks against the wall

Props
wall
2 blocks (optional)

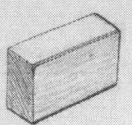

→ Stand with your back to the wall, about 40 cm (15 inches) away from it. To make sure that both feet are at the same distance from the wall, place two blocks between the wall and the feet.

› Lean back until the buttocks touch the wall. Bend foreword and pull the flesh of the buttocks up and sideways until the buttock bones are pressed well against the wall ❶.

› Place your finger tips on the floor and extend forward

› Then, release the back downward and bend into the pose.

› Hold the ankles and use your arms to extend the trunk further down and move it closer to the legs ❷.

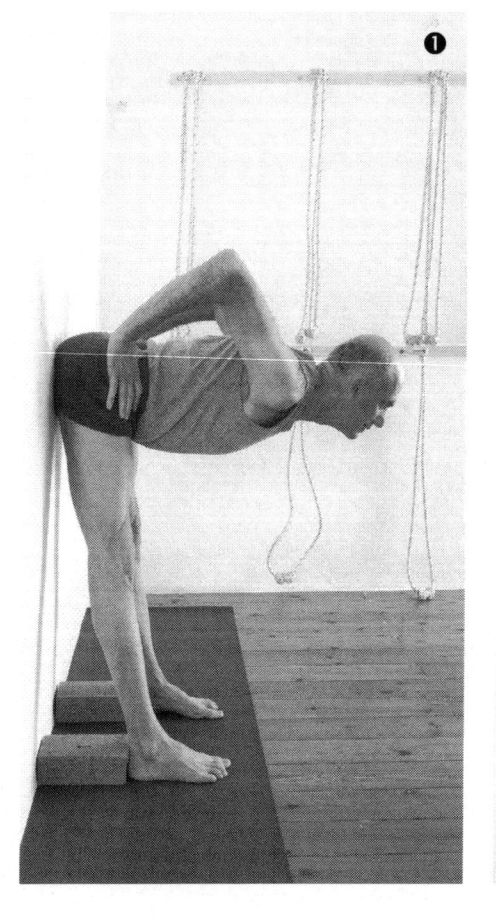

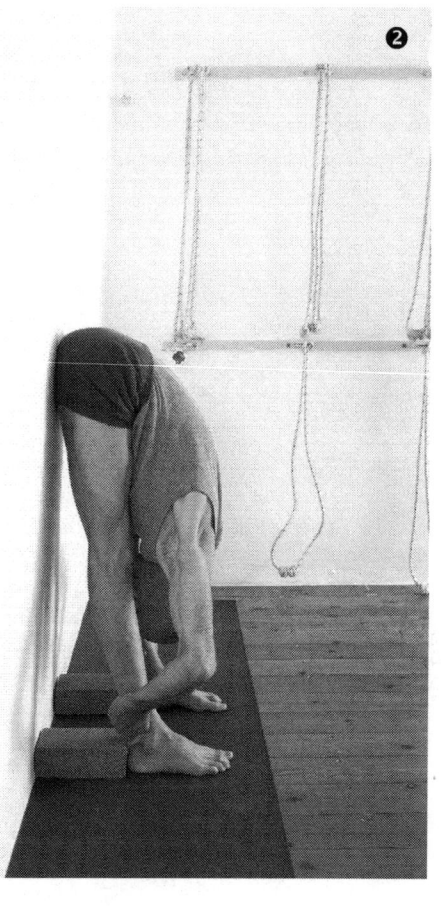

Tips
✓ Check that both buttock bones remain at the same height and are pushing the wall with equal force.

Effects
The wall support makes the pose restful. It also enables you to check the symmetry of the pose. When standing in the middle of the room the pelvis may tilt or turn to one side. It may be difficult to detect such imbalance and it may become habitual. The feedback you get from the wall and the blocks help to correct any mis-alignment and to register the correct alignment in your body.

Uttanasana
Variation 2

Increasing the thighs action: Back of legs against the wall

Props
Wall
2 blocks (optional)

⟶ Stand with your back facing the wall and bend forward into Uttanasana.

› Put your finger tips on the floor and step back until your legs are touching the wall ❶. If your hands do not reach the floor, use two blocks for support.

› Tighten your front thighs and push back so as to leave no gap between the back of the legs and the wall.

› Now raise the fingers from the floor, catch the ankles and bend deeper into the pose ❷.

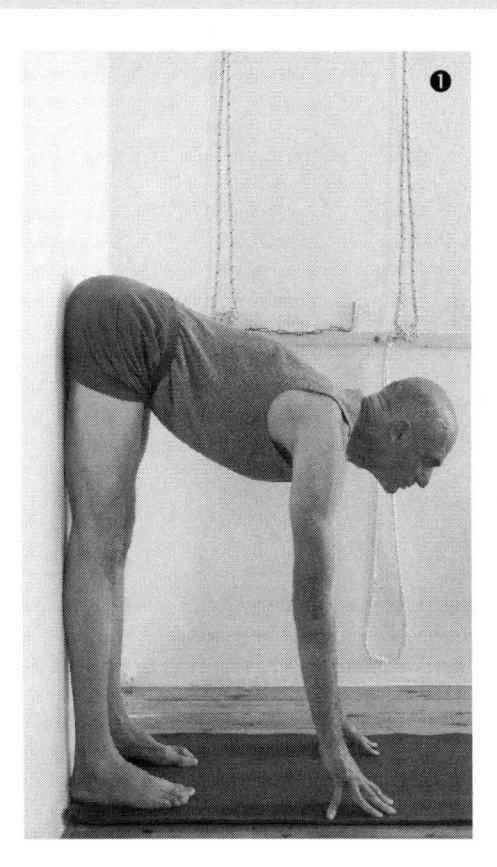

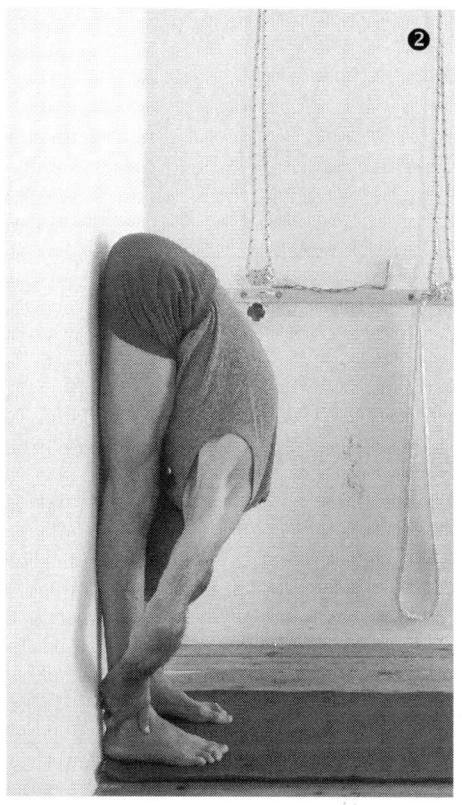

Effects
In Uttanasana the back of the legs should be vertical. When doing the pose in the middle of the room the buttocks tend to lean backward. The wall teaches the verticality of the legs. It also helps to gauge how much the front thighs should go back. Working this way strengthens the thighs.

Tips

✓ Bending into the pose with heels against the wall is challenging – to prevent rolling forward you must tighten and press the front thighs strongly back (into the wall.)

✓ If you still roll forward, support the hands with blocks (not shown).

Props for Yoga / Chapter 1 / Uttanasana 57

Uttanasana Variation 3

Stabilizing the legs: Leaning over the backrest of a chair

Props
chair

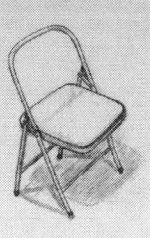

→ Fold the chair and lean its backrest against the front groins. Adjust the height by tilting the chair to the desired angle.

> Bend forward, hold the legs of the chair, concave the back and look forward ❶.

> Now, exhale and bend into the pose; place your forehead on the chair ❷.

> Taller practitioners need to hold the chair at a steeper angle ❸.

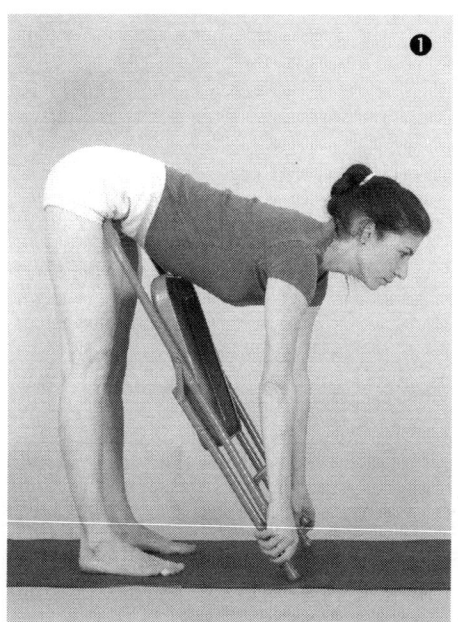

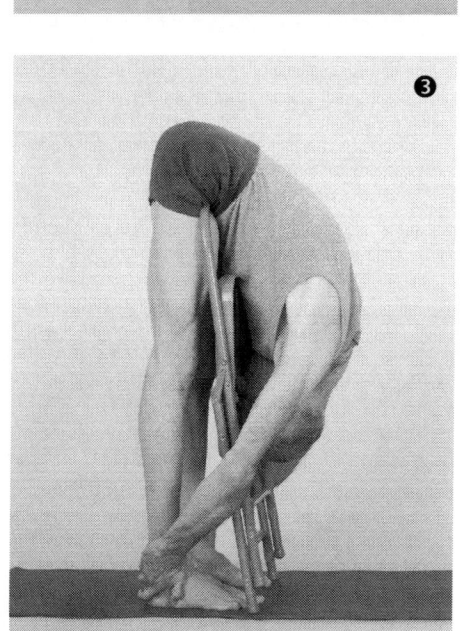

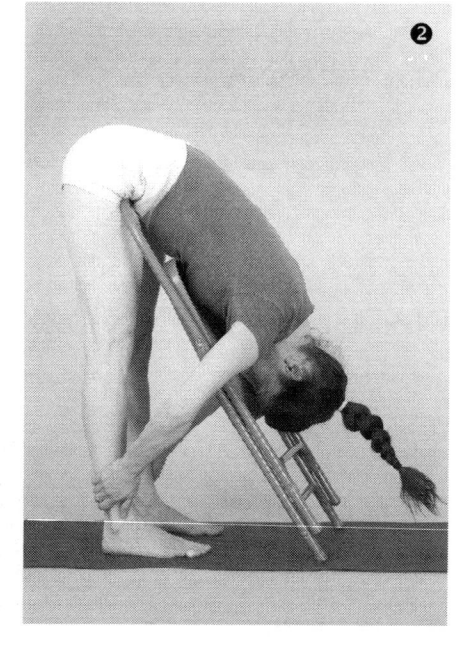

Effects

This variation clarifies the 'waterfall image' of the pose (see tip on page 55): the legs become very tall and stable and the trunk becomes soft and flowing. The support allows the abdomen to become soft; the brain becomes passive.

The touch of the backrest at the front thighs helps to ensure that the pelvis is not tilted and to keep the groins high, thus creating space in the pelvic region.

Tips

✓ Make sure that the two front groins rest evenly on the backrest.

✓ After staying with the support of the chair from 1 to 6 minutes, without getting out of the pose, place the chair on the floor. Try to maintain the same tallness and stability in the legs with the same softness in the trunk.

Uttanasana
Variation 4

Extending the calves: Standing on a slanted surface

Props
chair

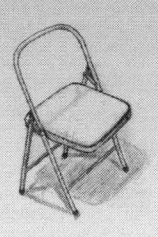

→ Stand on an inverted chair such that the toe mounds are higher than the heels.

▸ Catch the back legs of the chair, concave the back and look forward.

▸ Then grasp the backrest or the sides of the seat and pull the trunk down.

Note: You can create a slanted surface from any board, e.g. a wooden door wing, by placing one end on a higher base. For best results – the board should not be too wide, so that one can grasp its edges in order to pull the trunk down.

Effects
The slope creates a sharp angle between the shins and the feet, hence it increases the stretch in the calf muscles (the Gastrocnemius). This action also develops the feet arches.

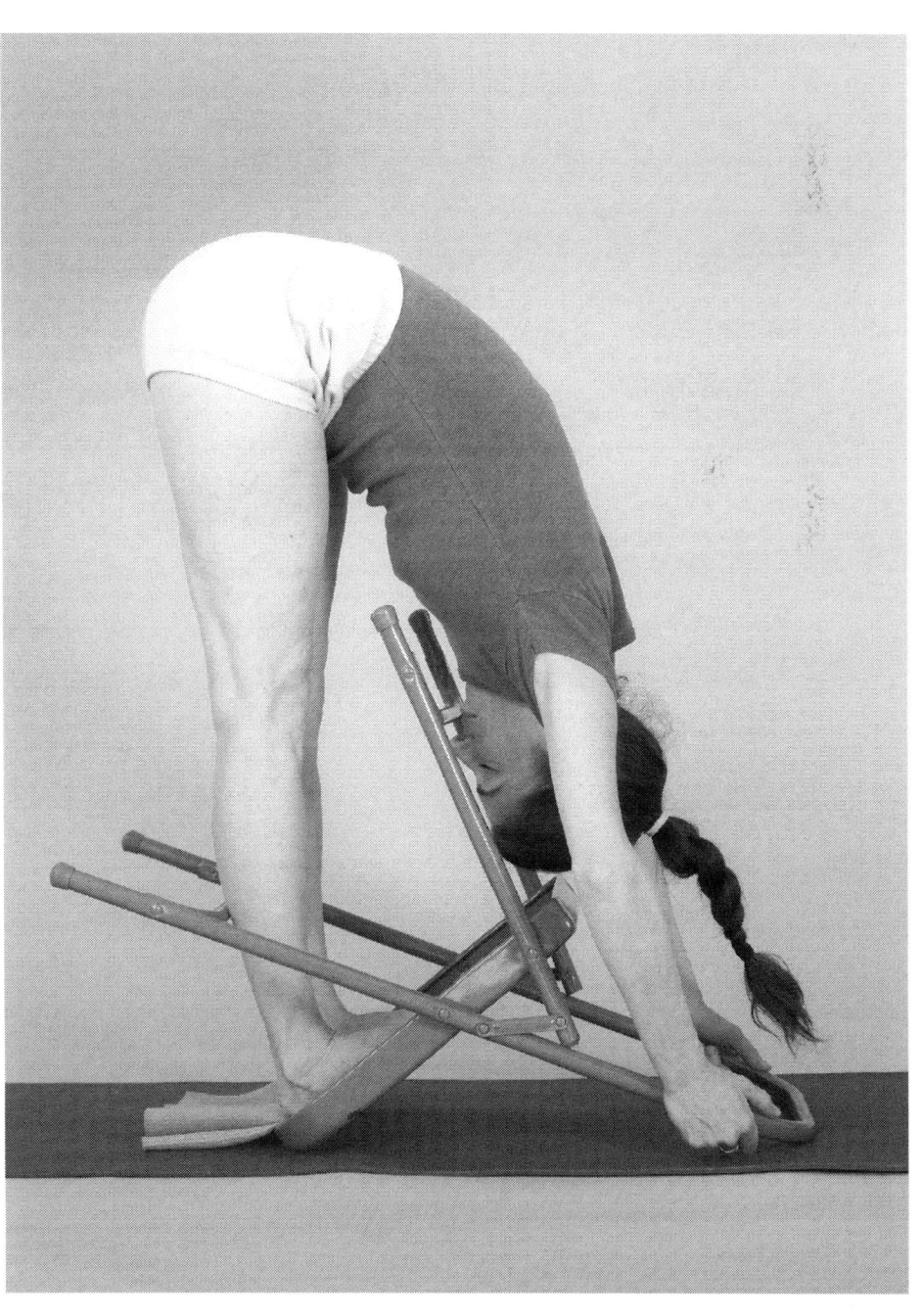

Uttanasana
Variation 5

Stand high; bend low: Standing on a raised platform

Props
chair or 2 blocks

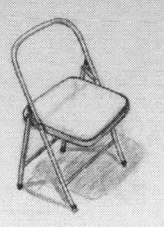

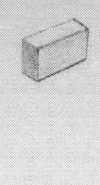

⟶ Do the pose when standing on a chair ❶ or on two blocks ❷.

› Position yourself so that the toes are curling over the rounded edge of the chair or blocks.

› If doing on a chair, grasp the seat of the chair or its legs ❶, and pull the trunk down.

› If doing on blocks, grasp the ankles and pull the trunk down ❷.

Note: It is possible to do this variation on any raised surface that you can stand on its edge. However - a chair is ideal, because the seat and the legs provide many grasping options for the hands. To overcome fear of falling, you can start by facing the backrest and holding its top.

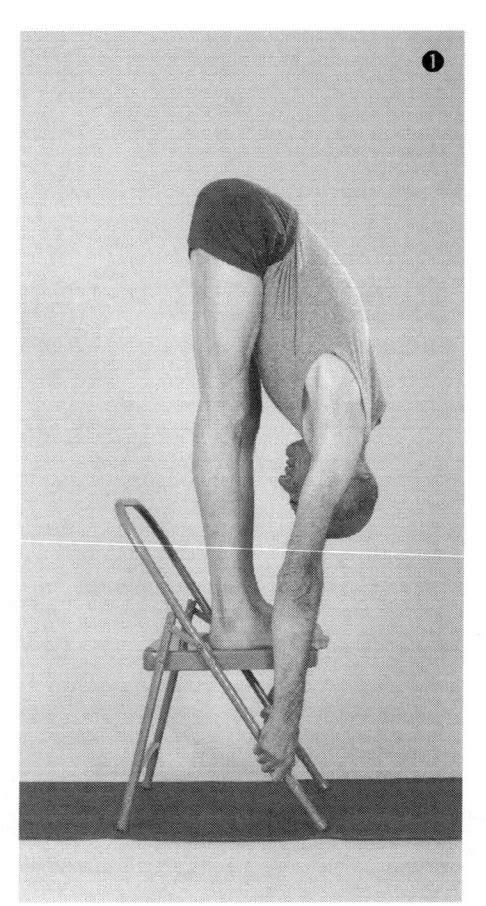

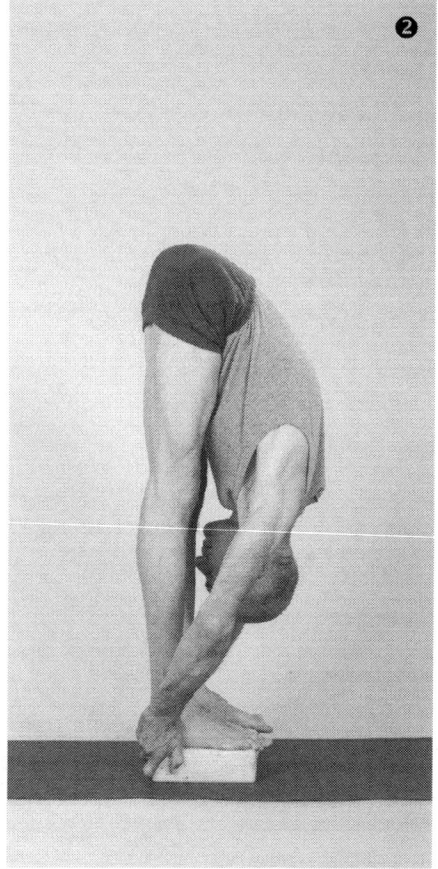

Effects

The resistance of the raised platform activates the legs and makes the bones denser. Releasing the toes down helps to release the muscles of the lower back. A fear of toppling over (especially when the platform is high) may arise and can be overcome with practice.

Tips

✓ Soften the toes and let them bend down, this will induce a downward movement in the trunk.

✓ Roll the buttocks forward until the legs are vertical.

Uttanasana Variation 6

Compact legs: Belt around feet and pelvis

Props
long belt
2 blocks
bandage (optional)

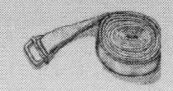

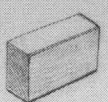

⟶ Enter the pose and loop a belt around the heels and the pelvis.

> Bend your knees slightly and tighten the belt ❶.

> Now, slowly lift the buttocks and straighten the legs against the resistance of the belt ❷.

✓ Adjust the length of the belt until you feel its resistance when straightening the legs.

> Spread the inner legs out to stretch the belt. Lift the inner ankles, the inner knees and hit the inner thighs out.

> Concave the back, place your palms on blocks and look forward ❷.

> Now, maintaining the length in the front body, bend down into the pose ❸.

> To move the sacrum further in, place a rolled bandage between the belt and the sacrum ❹.

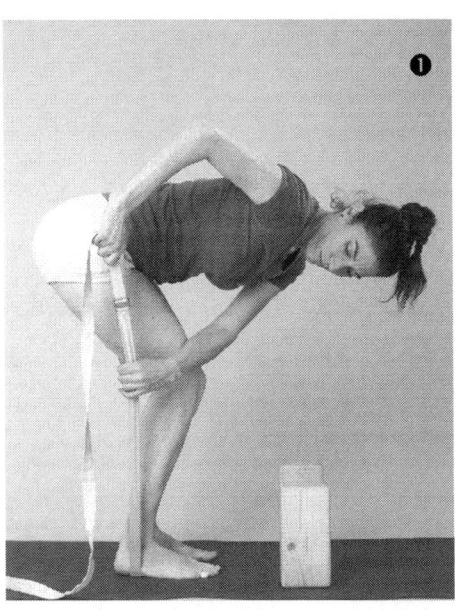

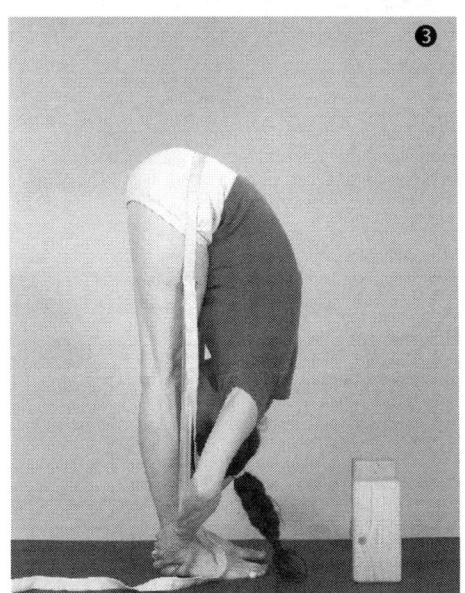

Effects

The belt presses the legs and creates compactness in the legs and the pelvis. The sacrum bone and the femur heads are drawn into the pelvis. This stimulates the organs of the pelvis, including the reproductive organs. The bones of the legs work against resistance which is beneficial for preserving bone density.

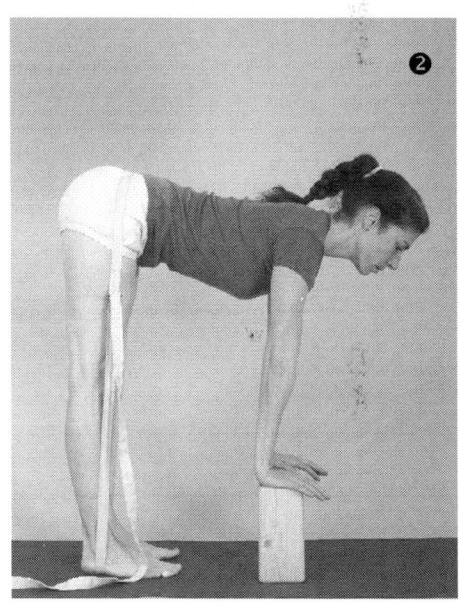

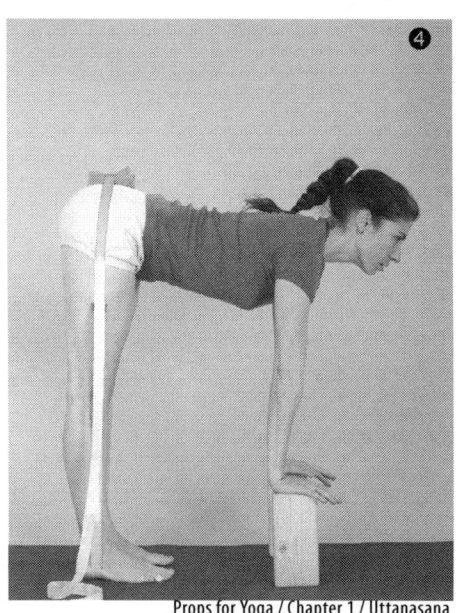

Uttanasana Variation 7

Folding deeply into the pose: Belt around back and legs

Props
belt
wall
chair or stool

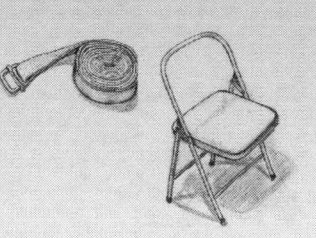

This is an advanced variation for flexible people who wish to bend deeper into the pose.

⟶ Place a chair about one meter (3 feet) away from the wall.

≻ Lean with your buttocks on the wall and bend forward with bent knees.

≻ Bring the trunk as close as possible to the legs and tighten a belt around the central back and the legs ❶.

≻ Now lift the buttocks along the wall to straighten the legs.

≻ Move the trunk away from the wall, concave the back, look forward and place your palms on the chair.

≻ Extend the chest forward and move the thoracic dorsal spine deep in ❷.

≻ After creating length in the front trunk bend down, bring the waist close to the inner thighs, hold the ankles, spread the elbows and fold the body deep into the pose while the buttocks move away from the wall ❸.

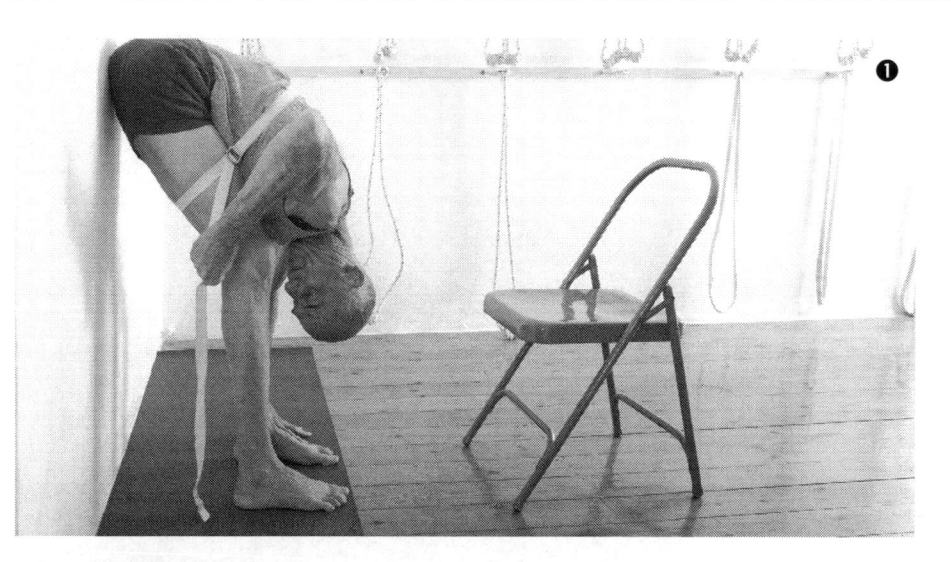

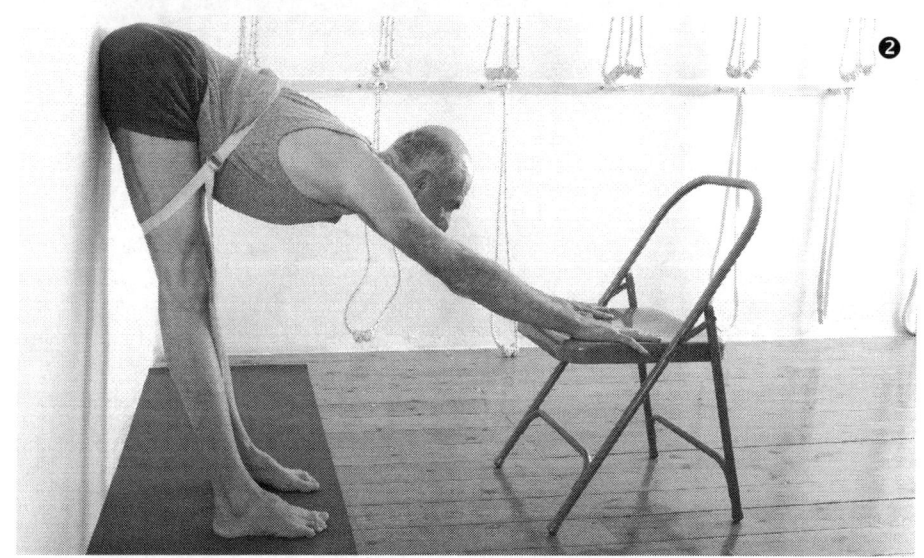

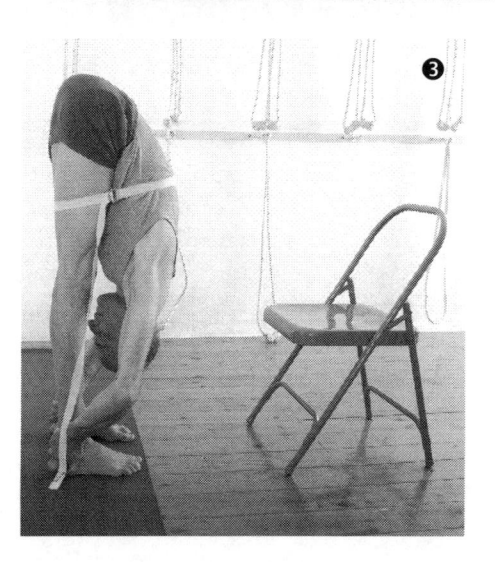

Effects
The first stage (❷) teaches to move the thoracic dorsal spine into the body and to concave the back. When staying in the pose (❸), the belt holds the torso in place; one can thus relax the arms, legs and back muscles while still maintaining the deep forward extension.

Opening the Shoulders

The next variation shows how Uttanasana can be used to create more movement in the shoulders.

Uttanasana Variation 8

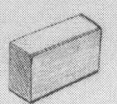

Creating movement in the shoulders: Holding a block behind the back

Props
block or plank

→ Hold a block behind your back and bend into half Uttanasana. Holding the block firmly, stretch the arms and move the shoulders away from the ears ❶.

> Now bend into Uttanasana; keeping the shoulders rolled back, move the arms away from the back ❷.

Effects

Usually this variation is done with the fingers interlocked behind the back. However, people with stiff shoulders may find it difficult to interlock the fingers behind their back. To get some movement in the shoulders they need to keep the hands wider. Holding a block or a plank or using a belt helps to get this movement. It also helps to create firmness in the arms.

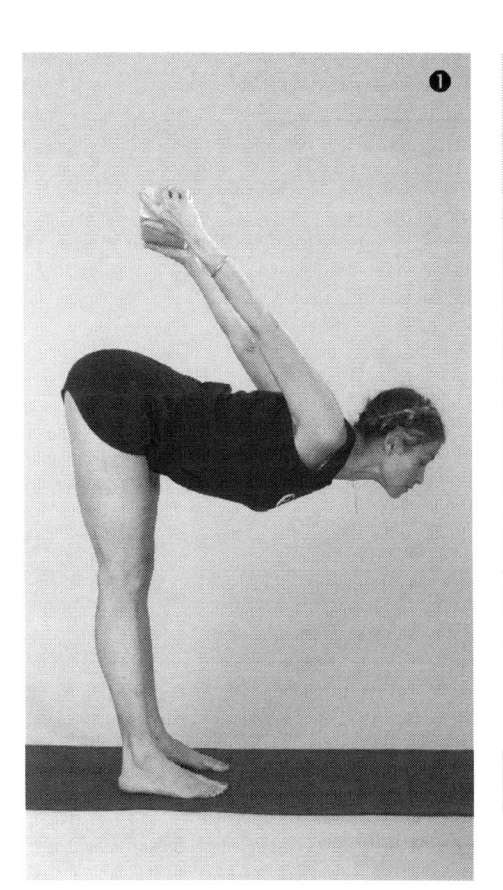

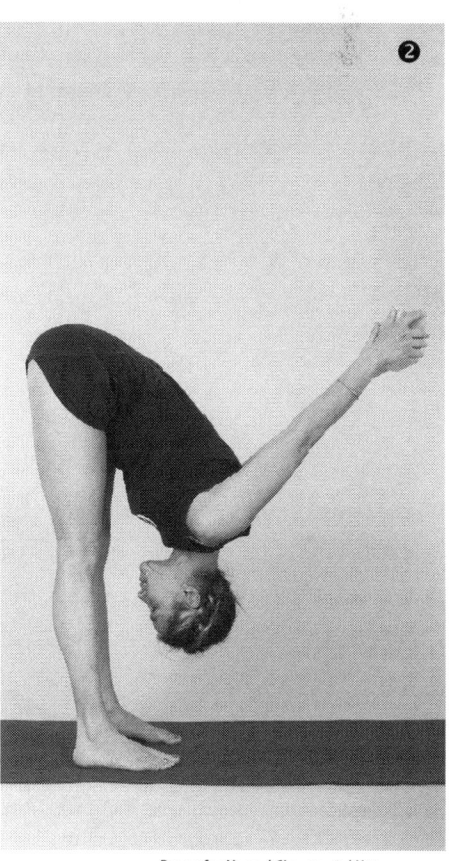

Uttanasana
Variation 8 (cont.)

Creating movement in the shoulders: Holding a block behind

To check the symmetry of the shoulders:

Start the above pose by standing in front of the wall about one meter (3 feet) away from it, holding the block behind your back.

Bend into Uttanasana and move the arms toward the wall.

Keep rolling and stretching the arms until you touch the wall with the block (adjust your distance from the wall if necessary).

Check that the left and right sides of the block reach the wall at the same time ❸.

Ask a partner to check that your arms are parallel to the central line of your body.

If you discover unevenness, correct it, release the pose and then do it again. This will help you correct asymmetries in the shoulder movement.

If your shoulders are stiff, use a wooden plank instead of a block. Hold the plank at shoulder width, palms facing your back ❹. With arms held further apart one gets more movement in the shoulders.

Another option is to place a belt around the elbows to keep them shoulder width apart. Work the arms against the belt.

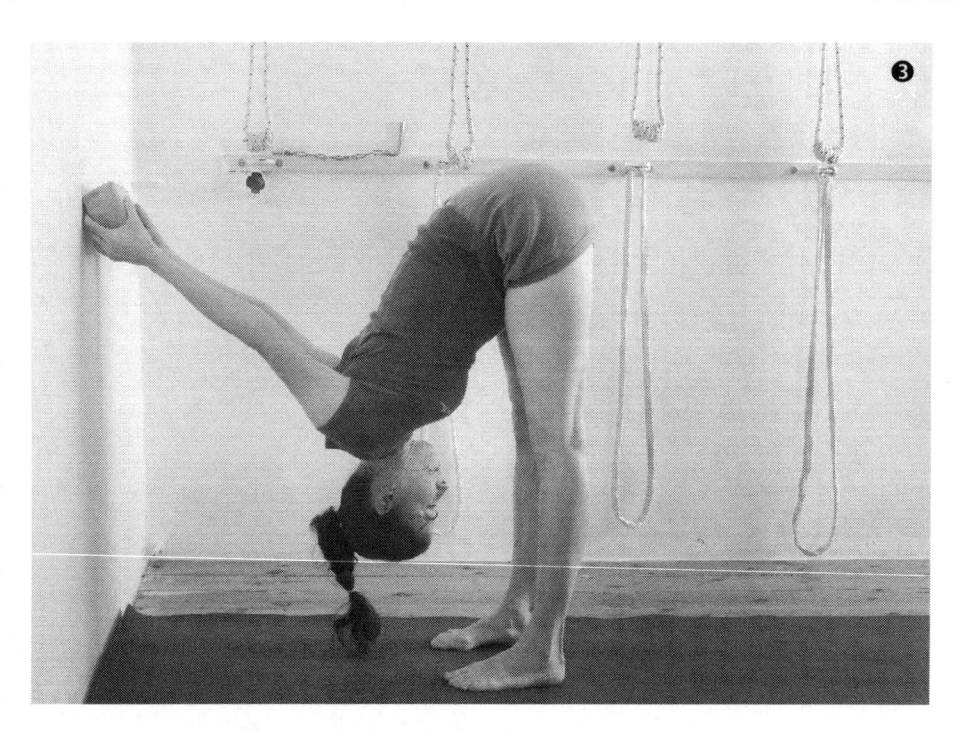

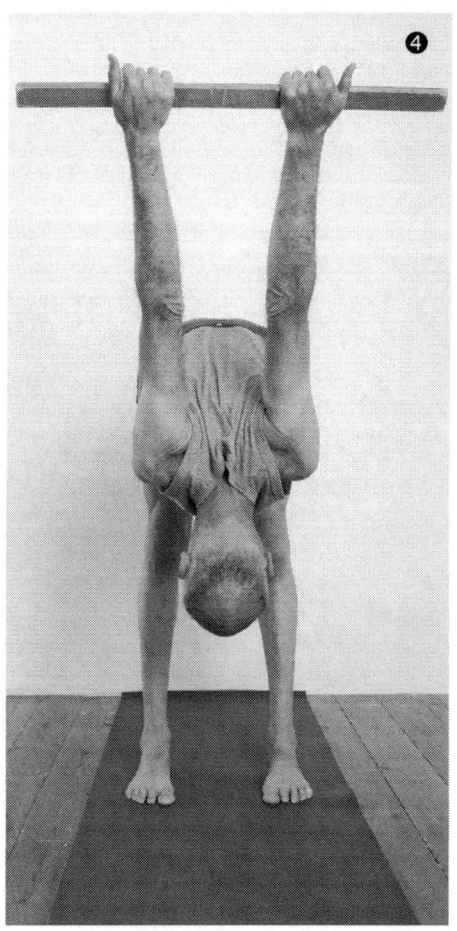

Restorative Uttanasana

These are some of the effects of Uttanasana mentioned by B.K.S. Iyengar:

"The heart beats are slowed down and the spinal nerves rejuvenated. Any depression felt in the mind is removed if one holds the pose two minutes or more. The posture is a boon to people who get excited quickly, as it soothes the brain cells. After finishing the asana, one feels calm and cool, the eyes start to glow and the mind feels at peace." (Light on Yoga, see Pl. 48).

Note, however, that most people require support in order to experience these wonderful effects. Here are a few examples.

Uttanasana Variation 9

Props
wall

Resting in half-inverted pose: Back against the wall

→ Stand in front of the wall, about 40 cm (15 inches) away from it.

› Bend your knees and go into the pose. Tilt forward and position your back against the wall.

› Extend the trunk down with bent knees ❶.

› Now, slowly lift the buttocks and straighten the legs. Keep your back pressed against the wall ❷.

Note: For additional effect, rest the crown of the head on a bolster or folded blankets.

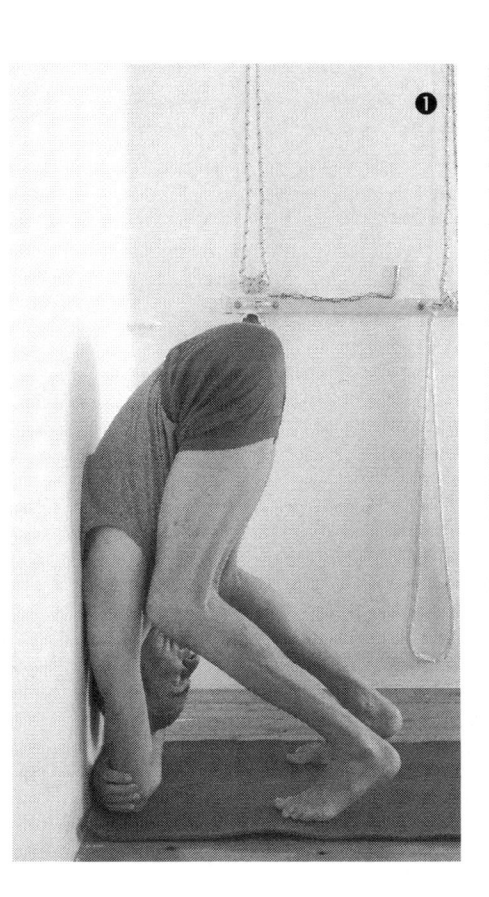

Effects
The wall helps to bend further and draw the trunk closer to the legs. The support of the wall helps to release the back and the back of the head down and makes the pose restful.

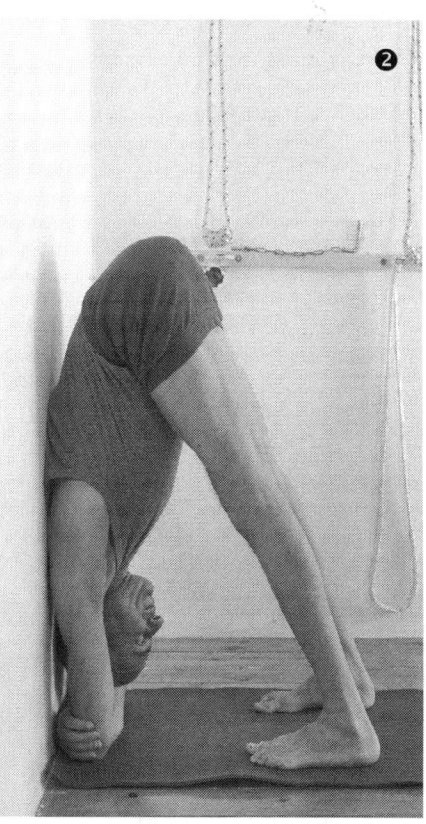

Uttanasana
Variation 10

Relaxing the brain: Top of the Head on block

Props
2 blocks
blanket (optional)

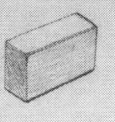

⟶ Bend into the pose and place the crown of the head on top of one or two blocks. Arrange the blocks according to your height and flexibility.

Note: the correct height is reached when you feel the head supported without any compression of the neck. Use a blanket to fine-tune the height if necessary.

❯ Check that your eyes are looking backward, parallel to the floor.

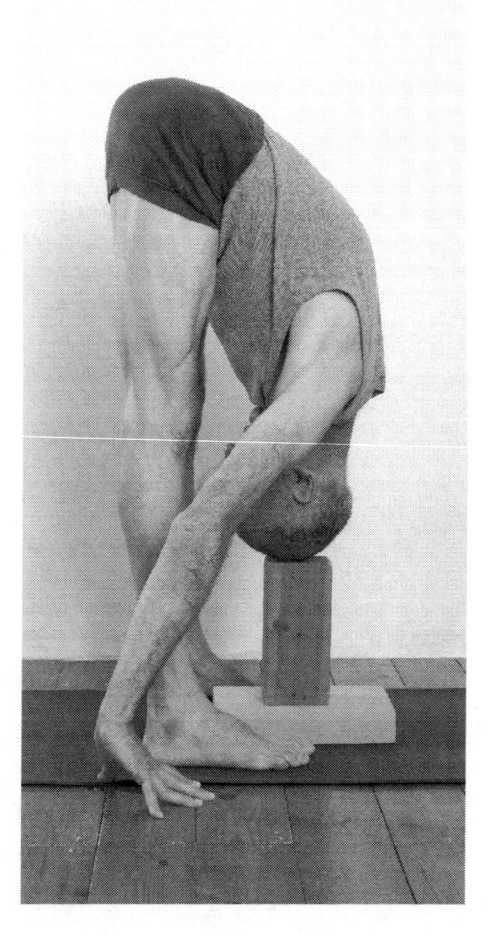

Effects
Supporting the top of the head relaxes the brain. It has a 'Sirsasana effect'. It teaches how to position the head vertically and allows for staying longer in the pose with reduced effort, enhancing the physiological and mental effects of the pose.

Tips

✓ Fine tune the height of the head by changing the distance between your legs: increasing it lowers the head, while decreasing it raises the head.

✓ Check the positioning of the head by the front line of the ears – it should be vertical. Touch the front ears to adjust; if possible, ask a partner to check this.

✓ Learn to position the head on the 'heel of the crown of the head' – i.e., the rear part of the top of the skull. Observe the effect it has on the brain.

Utthita Trikonasana

About Utthita Trikonasana

Utthita Trikonasana is typically introduced as the first standing pose with spread legs. The basic principles of alignment common to all lateral standing poses are introduced here. However, mature performance of the pose requires control and coordination of many subtle actions, which can only be learnt over time.

In the variations we introduce here, the wall and the floor provide reference lines which help to check and correct the alignment; blocks and belts are used in various ways to emphasize the actions of the pose and to create different effects.

Many of the variations described here are applicable to the other lateral standing poses (Virabhadra II, Utthita Parsvakonasana & Ardha Chandrasana) and also to Parivrtta Trikonasana. As always, some of the variations may be combined.

Tips

✓ Imagine doing Utthita Trikonasana in a narrow corridor. The walls in front and behind you do not allow any part of your body to protrude forward or backward. You must maintain the bent body parallel to the walls, aligned with the lateral plane created by your legs.

⚠ **CAUTIONS**

If you are prone to dizzy spells, vertigo, or high blood pressure, look down at the floor in the final pose. Do not turn your head up.

If you have a cardiac condition, practice against a wall (see Variation 12 of this pose). Do not raise the arm, but rest it along your hip.

Aligning the Feet

Utthita Trikonasana is a lateral pose, i.e., the body bends sideways in alignment with the spread legs. Alignment starts from the correct positioning of the feet: the heel of the front foot should be in line with the arch of the back foot. Using a reference line, such as a floor line, a marked centerline on the mat or the edge of a (thin) mat, is an effective way to learn this foot alignment.

Utthita Trikonasana
Variation 1

Correct alignment of the legs: Using a reference line

Props
Floor line
or a sticky mat

→ To do the pose on the right side:

- Stand in Tadasana. Choose a straight line on the floor as mentioned above. Position the middle of the arches of the feet on top of the line. Jump and spread the legs apart to Utthita Hasta Padasana ❶.

- Look at your feet and make sure that the reference line crosses the middle of the arches. Adjust as necessary.

- Turn the right leg out and the left foot in. Position the middle of the right heel and the middle of the left arch on the reference line.

- Bend to the right while keeping the body above the reference line. In particular observe that the left thigh, the right buttock bone, both shoulders and the head are above that line ❷.

- You can also use a belt in the middle of the mat, and if needed a block to support the right palm ❸.

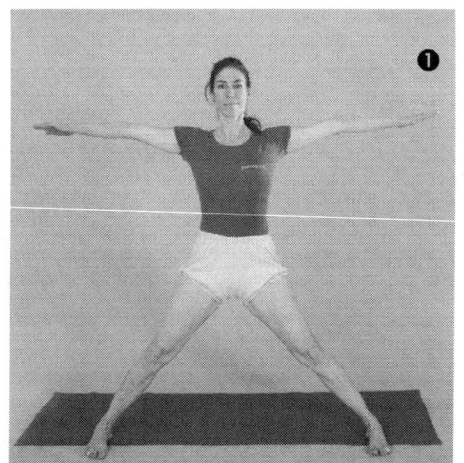

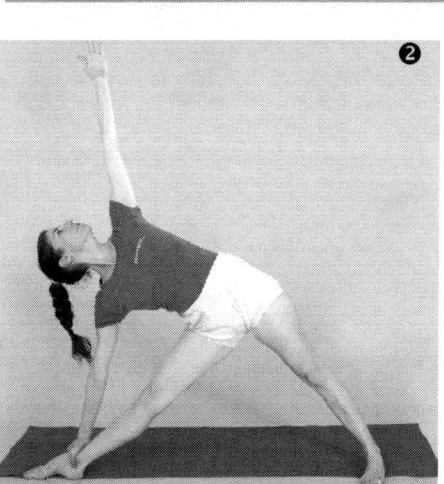

Effects
The reference line allows you to check and correct the alignment of the legs.

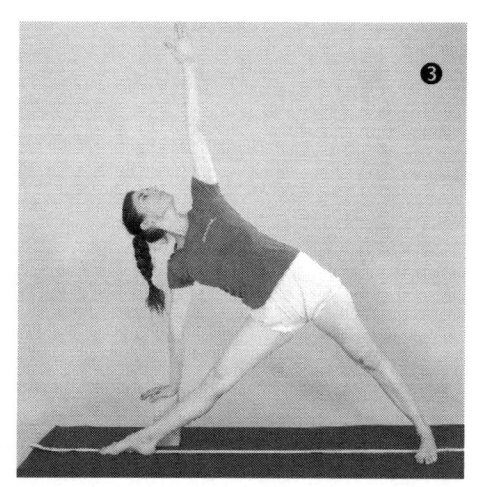

Applicability
All standing poses with spread legs.

Activating the Back Leg

Referring to the standing poses, B.K.S.. Iyengar states that the 'back leg is the brain of the pose'. The following variations help to sharpen the action of the back leg.

Observing the back leg in standing poses teaches us the importance of balance and equanimity in Yoga. When bending into Utthita Trikonasana on the right, our attention is intuitively drawn to the right side because that is the direction of the movement. However, if we neglect the left side, we are missing an important part of the asana. The back leg provides the stabilizing anchor of the pose. Shifting weight from the front leg to the back leg also means spreading our attention more evenly. It makes the pose internalized. As our attention is spread throughout our body, our gaze is softened, our breath cycle stabilizes, and the fluctuations of our mind diminish. The pose can then become more balanced and meditative.

Utthita Trikonasana Variation 2

Anchoring the back foot: Outer foot against the wall

Props
wall
block (optional)

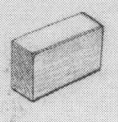

→ To do the pose on the right side:

> Place the left foot against the wall and press its outer side strongly to the floor and against the wall.

> Spread the legs, turn the right leg out.

> Inhale, stretch the arms and as you exhale, enter the pose maintaining the pressure of the left foot against the wall.

> Support the right palm with a block. (The palm can be turned back to induce backward rotation of the shoulder, as shown here).

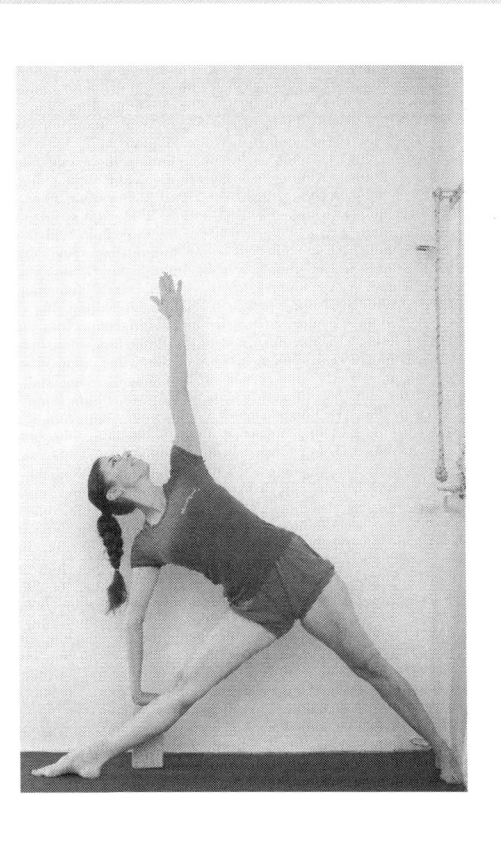

Effects
TThe resistance of the wall activates the back leg and keeps it firm.

Tips

✓ Place the back foot against the wall, before spreading the legs. This will make it easier for you to tuck the outer foot firmly into the corner of the wall and the floor.

✓ After staying in the pose for a while move one inch away from the wall. Check: can you keep the same firmness and stability of the left leg without using the wall?

Props for Yoga / Chapter 1 / Utthita Trikonasana

Utthita Trikonasana Variation 3

Activating the back leg: Foot on belt

Props
belt
partner

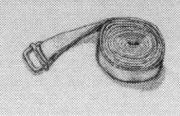

In this variation a thin strip, such as a belt, is placed under the outer foot of the back leg. A helper tries to pull the belt out while the practitioner presses down in order to prevent it from slipping. The more the helper pulls the belt the stronger you need to press on it.

Note: The belt may be replaced by a piece of paper, cardboard or a cloth.

Effects
The challenge of not letting the belt slip away brings awareness to the outer foot of the back leg.

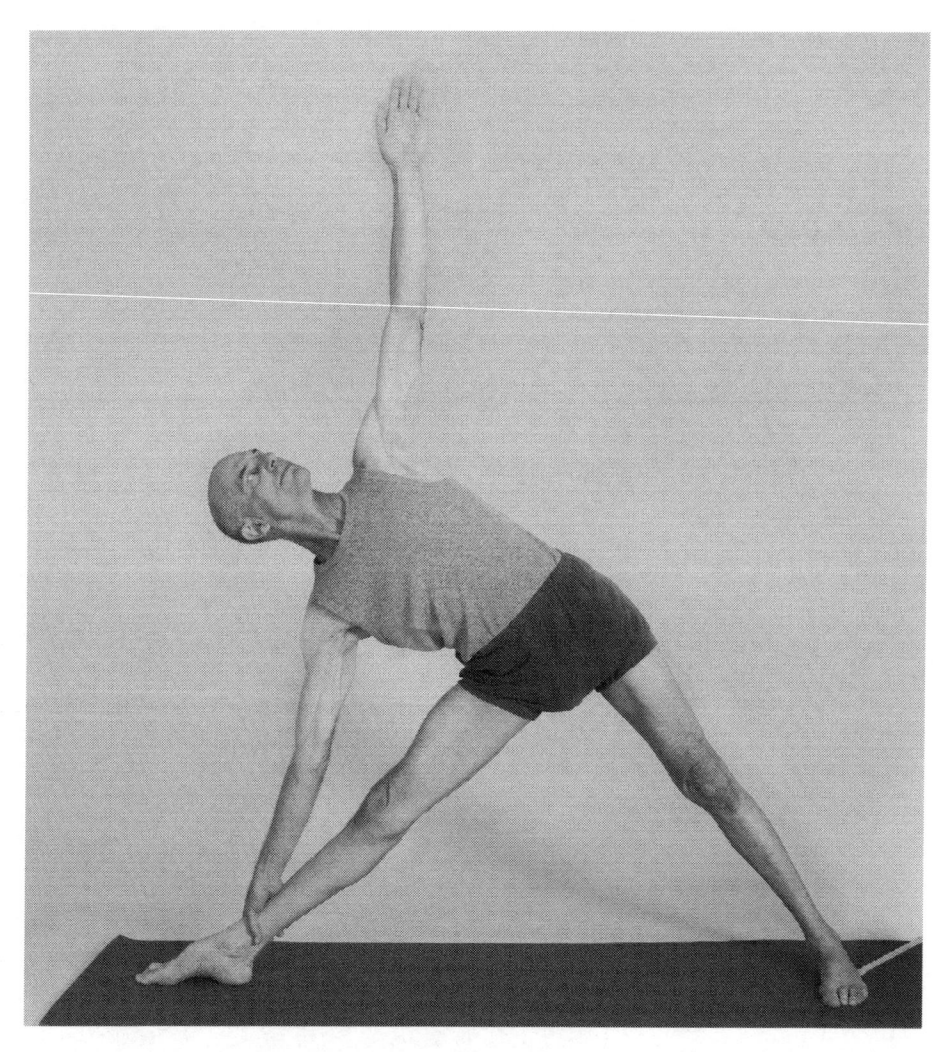

Applicability
Utthita Parsvakonasana, Virabhadrasana II and other standing poses.

Utthita Trikonasana Variation 4

Activating the back leg: Pulling the leg with belt

Props
belt

Another way of activating the back leg is by pulling it with a belt attached to it. Three optional anchoring positions are demonstrated below: the arch of the foot ❶, above the knee ❷ and the groin ❸.

⟶ To do the pose on the right side:

› Tighten the belt around the desired location on the left leg. When anchoring the knee or the thigh, the direction of the buckle should be such that when the belt is pulled it will induce outward rotation of the leg.

› Pull the belt with your left hand and enter the pose.

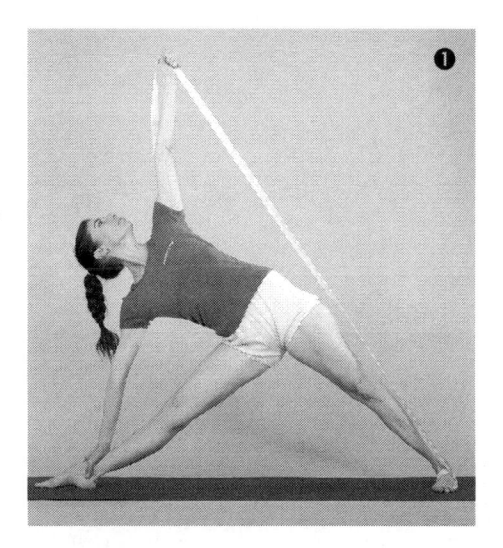

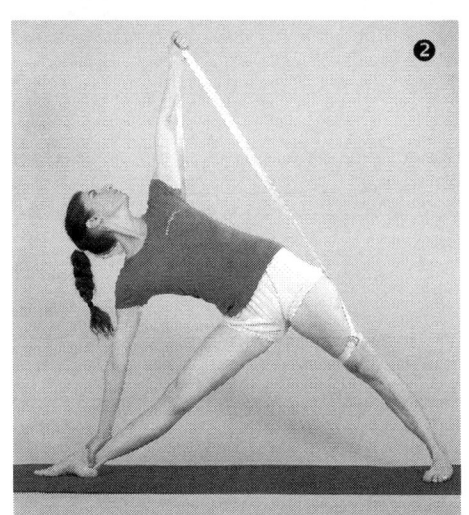

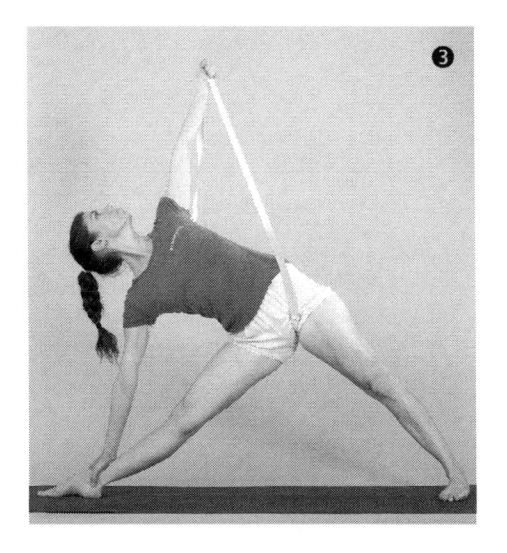

Effects
The above three variations increase the awareness in the back leg and help to keep it stable. Anchoring the knee helps to turn and create space in the knee, while anchoring at the groin lifts and opens the inner groin. This variation is also effective for opening and turning the chest, since the pull of the belt with the left hand helps to turn the chest.

Applicability
The belt here induces outward rotation of the back leg and thus helpful for many lateral standing poses, e.g. *Utthita Parsvakonasana*, *Virabhadrasana II*, and *Ardha Chandrasana*. For poses like *Virabhadrasana I*, the belt should be placed in the other direction, so as to induce inward rotation of the back leg when pulled.

Props for Yoga / Chapter 1 / Utthita Trikonasana 71

Utthita Trikonasana
Variation 5

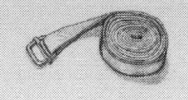

Lifting the inner groin: Partner pulls the back leg

Props
a belt
a partner

To keep the back leg stable you need to press down the outer foot in order to lift the inner thigh and groin. The following variation demonstrates the effect of lifting the groin of the back leg.

⟶ To do the pose to the right (instructions are given for the helping partner):

› Loop a belt around the inner groin of the left leg.

› Place your foot against the outer back heel of the practitioner.

› Gently pull the belt and signal the practitioner to go into the pose ❶.

Notes:
- When placing your foot against the practitioner's outer heel be extremely careful not to "scrape" the skin of the foot, which may be painful.
- Synchronize the pull of the belt with the movement of the practitioner going into the pose.
- When helping a pregnant woman, place the belt on her upper thigh, not on the groin.

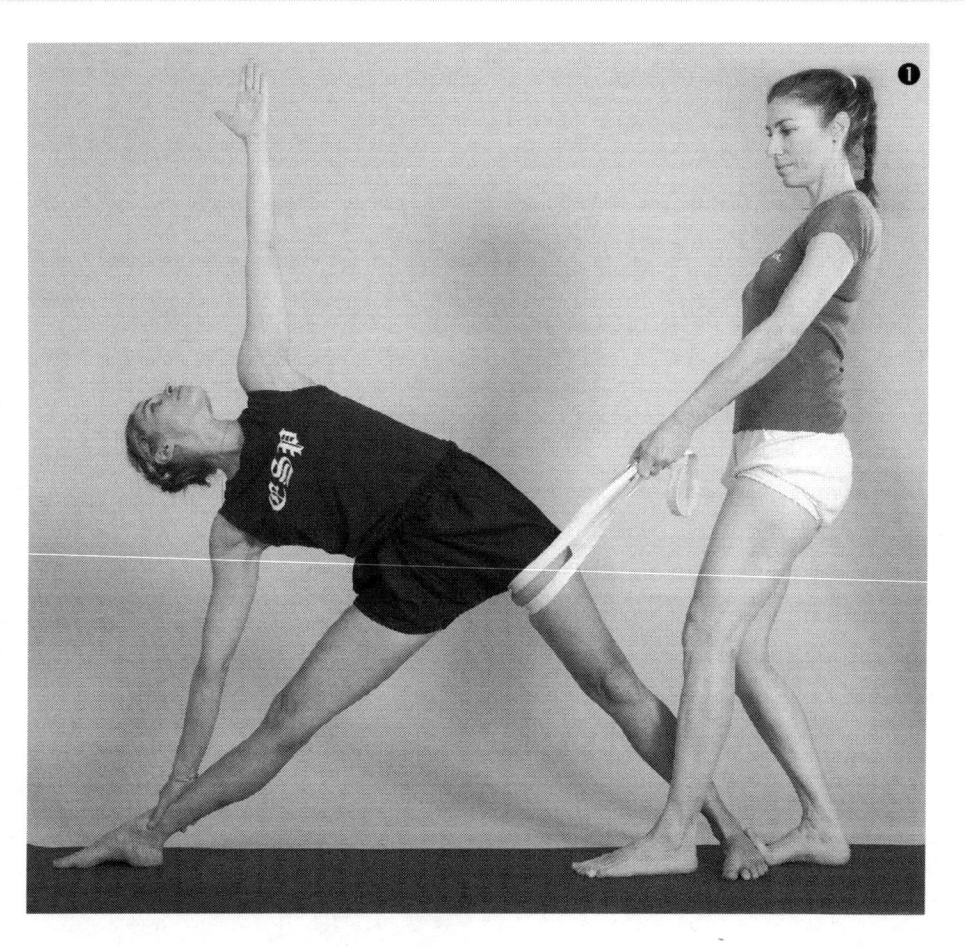

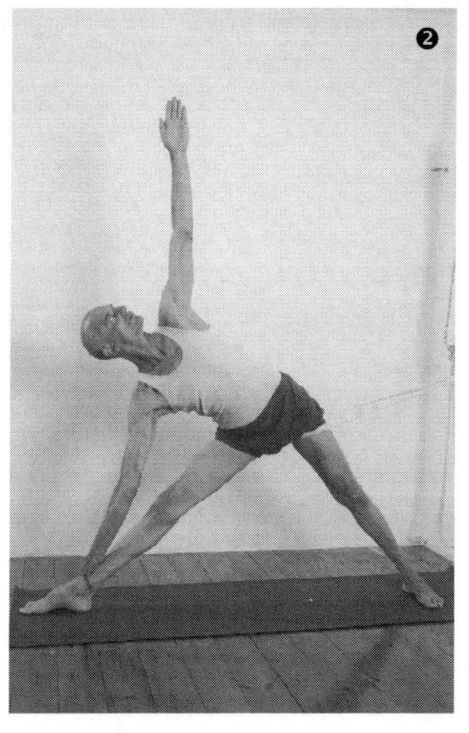

Effects
Pulling the beck leg clarifies the importance of shifting weight to the back leg. It creates space in the pelvis and broadens the organs of the lower abdomen; hence it is especially beneficial for pregnant women. It also makes the pose much easier to sustain.

You can get a similar effect without a partner, by tying a belt or a rope to a wall hook ❷ or to a door handle (see Variation 22, photo 1 of Dog pose.)

Applicability
All lateral standing poses.

Turning the Legs Out

Turning the front leg out from the hip joint is a very crucial action in Utthita Trikonasana. It ensures that the head of the thigh bone will remain in its joint when bending into the pose, and enables moving the tailbone in. Furthermore, if the lower leg, the knee and the upper leg are not aligned, the uneven load on the knee may cause unwanted wear and tear on its ligaments.

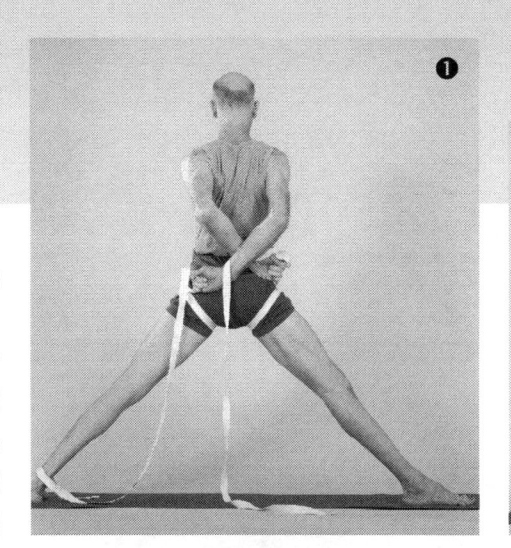

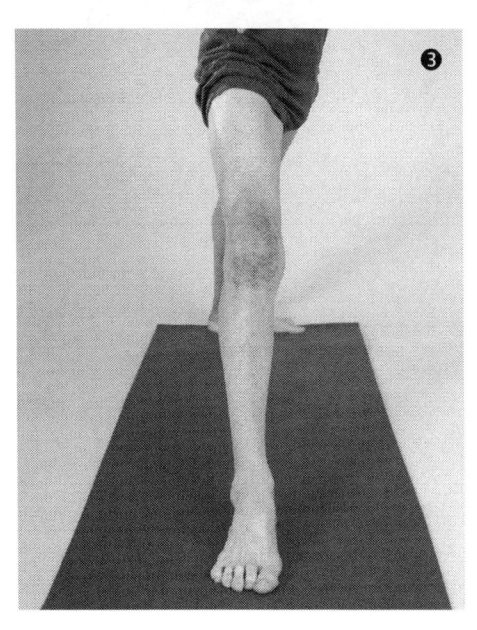

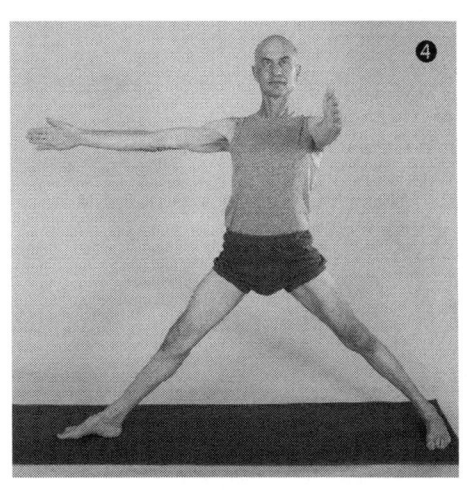

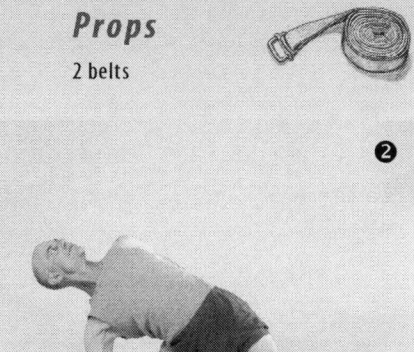

Utthita Trikonasana Variation 6

Turning the legs:
Two belts on the upper thighs

Props
2 belts

➡ To do the pose on the right side:

> Loop one belt around the upper right thigh and another belt around the upper left thigh. Make sure the belts are buckled for outward rotation; i.e., the buckles are placed on the inner thigh and the loose ends of the belts extend to the front.

> Spread the legs and turn the right leg out. Cross the loose ends of the belts behind your back: hold the belt of the right leg with the left hand, and the belt of the left leg with the right hand ❶.

> Pull the belts to turn the roots of the thighs out and bend laterally into the pose.

> *Note:* On page 8 we showed a similar variation for Tadasana. However, for Tadasana the belts are buckled inversely, so as to induce inward rotation of the upper thighs, while here the belts help the outward rotation.

> This variation can also be done with just one belt for the front leg (The turning of this leg is the main action). People with long arms can catch the upper right thigh with the left hand, even without a belt ❷.

Effects
Pulling the belts intensifies the turning action and teaches this crucial action.

Tips

✓ Learn to turn the front leg out from its root (the hip joint) and not from the foot.

✓ The leg should turn out completely – check that the centers of the front ankle, front knee and front thigh are aligned ❸. This prevents undue pressure on the knee.

✓ The front thigh of the back leg should face forward (like in Tadasana); make sure it does not turn in. There should be a 90° angle between the direction of the front-leg knee cap and that of the back-leg knee cap ❹.

Applicability
All lateral standing poses done with spread legs.

Props for Yoga / Chapter 1 / Utthita Trikonasana

Utthita Trikonasana
Variation 7

Turning the front leg out: Foot turned more than 90°

For some people, turning the front leg out does not come easily; if this is your case, turning the foot more than 90° makes it easier to achieve 90° rotation at the root of the front leg.

→ When doing the pose on the right side:

› Turn the right leg 90° out; turn the foot slightly more and roll the muscles of the front thigh out over the femur bone.

› Look at the centerline of the right leg and verify that the front thigh has turned sufficiently; if not, turn the foot slightly more out.

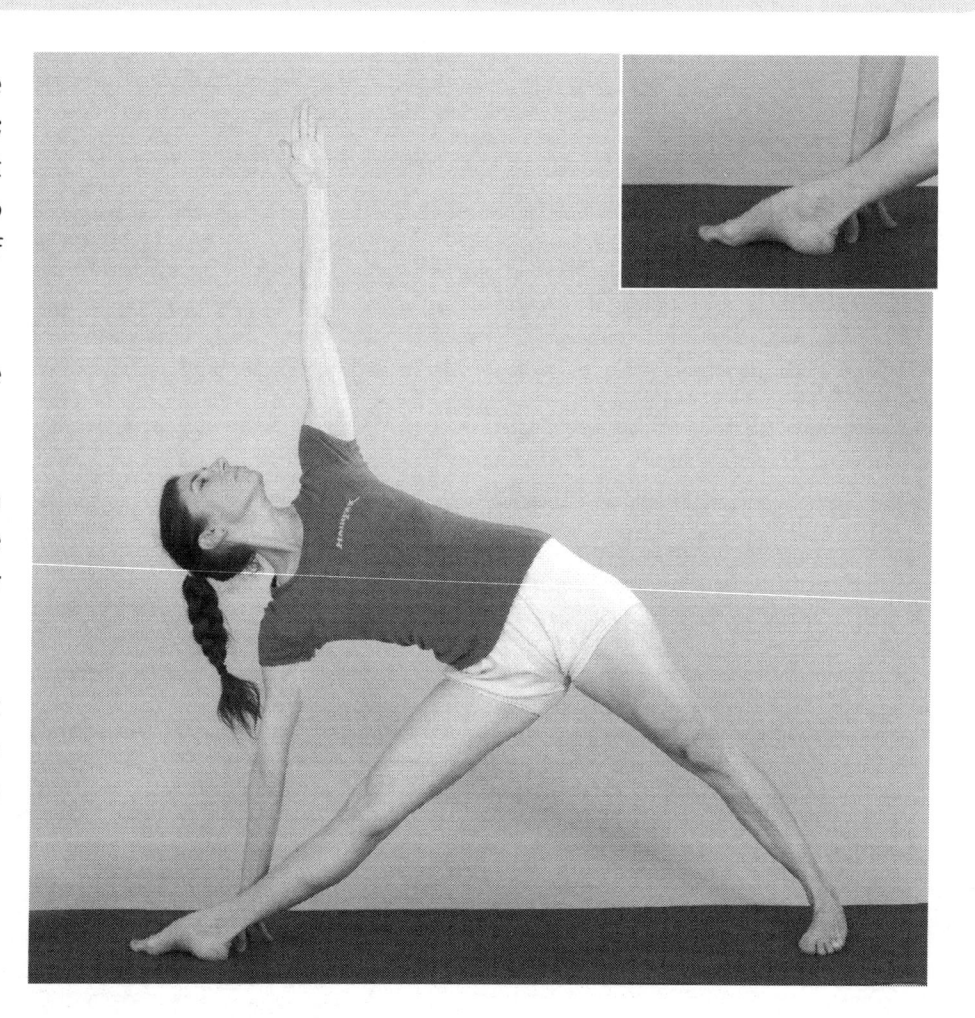

Tips

✓ When turning the front leg out, press the inner foot to the floor and turn the front ankle in.

Utthita Trikonasana
Variation 8

Knee turned out; buttock turned in: Entering from Utthita Parsvakonasana

→ To do the pose on the right side:

› Go to Utthita Parsvakonasana ❶.

› Press the outer right knee against the arm and slowly straighten the right leg ❷.

› Keep turning the knee out and straighten the legs completely to Utthita Trikonasana.

Note: You do not actually need to bend the knee to make a square; even bending half way helps to turn the leg.

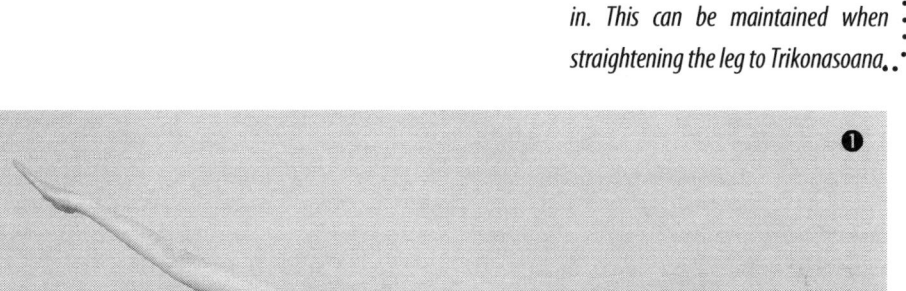

Effects
When the leg is bent it is much easier to turn it out and to roll the buttock in. This can be maintained when straightening the leg to Trikonasoana.

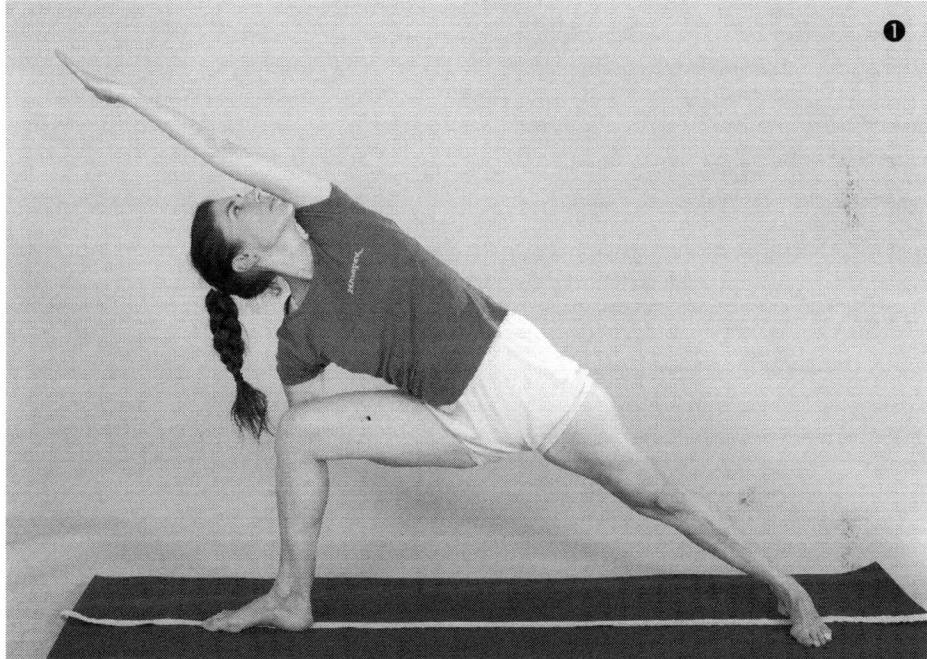

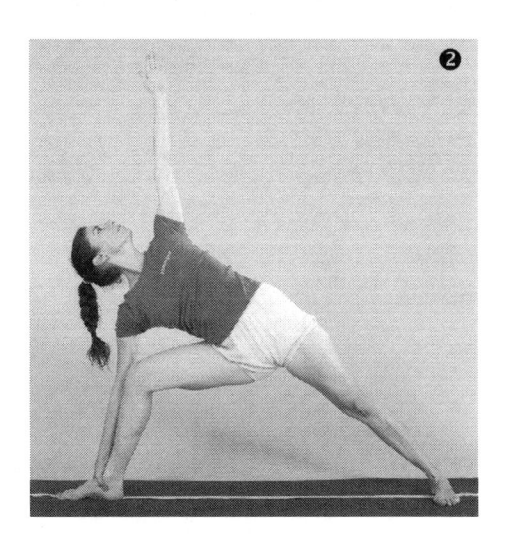

Applicability
All lateral standing poses done with legs wide apart.

Activating the Front Leg

Often, when staying in Utthita Trikonasana, the front leg is not fully straight and its kneecap tends to drop. When awareness fades the leg tends to wobble. The following variations help to activate the front leg and keep it stable.

Utthita Trikonasana
Variation 9

Activating the front leg: Lifting the toe mounds

⟶ To do the pose on the right side:

› Raise the toes and the sole of the right foot from the floor while pressing the heel against the floor.

› Enter the pose maintaining the lift of the toes and sole up ❶.

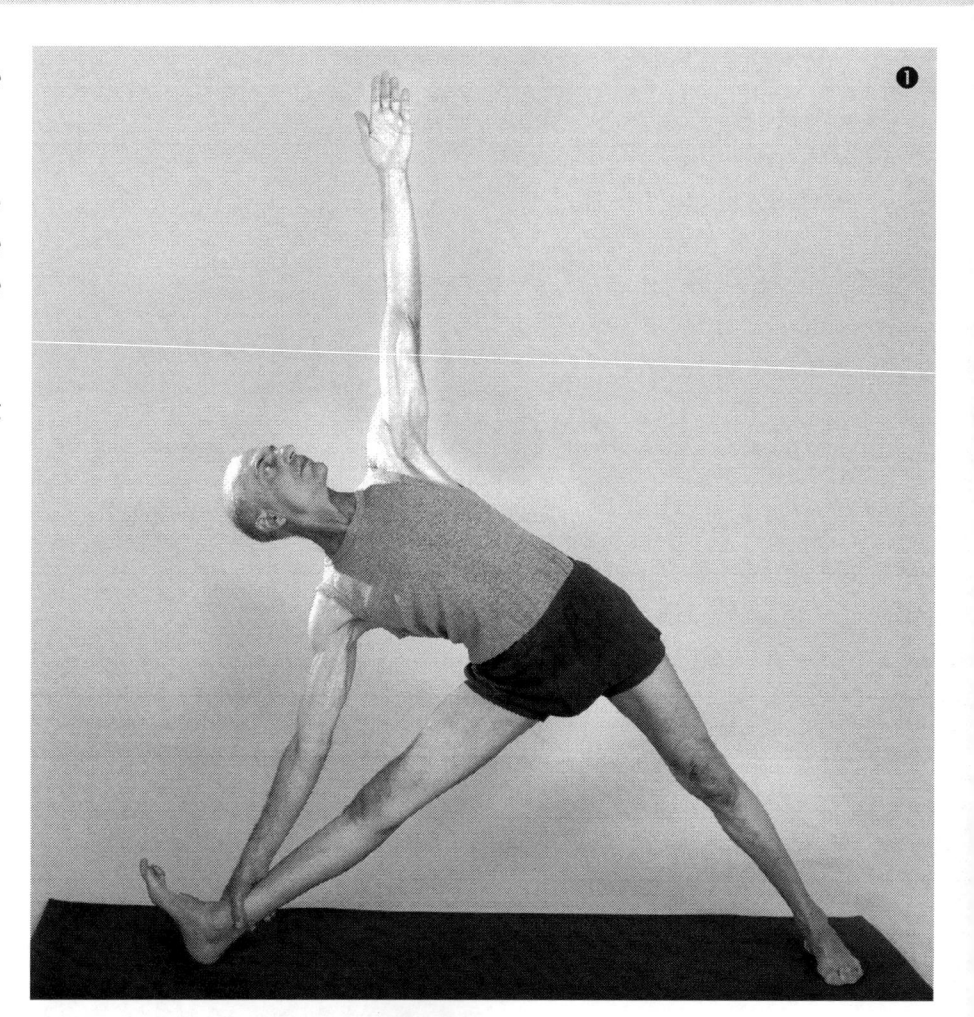

› Some people find the above variation difficult due to pain in the heel. This pain can be avoided by supporting the raised sole on a rounded block (if available) ❷.

› You may also place the heel on a rectangular block and the toe mounds against a wall, as explained in the following variation.

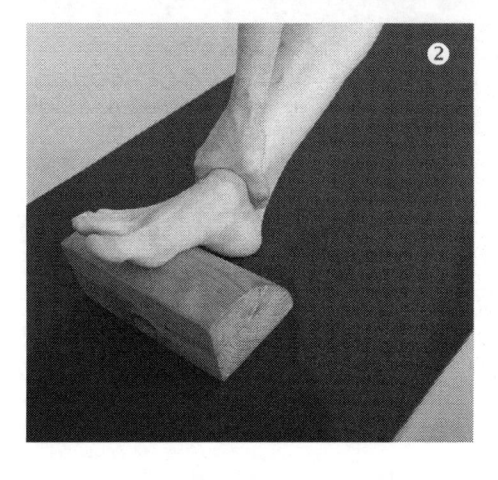

Effects
Raising the sole of the foot activates the entire leg.

Utthita Trikonasana
Variation 10a

Activating the front leg: Heel on block

Props
2 blocks
wall

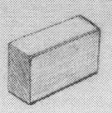

⟶ To do the pose on the right side:

> Put a block flat next to the wall and position another block about 25 cm (10 inches) away from the wall.

> *Note:* You can replace the block by a higher box, a low stool, or even a seat of a chair, this will intensify the effect.

> Place the right heel on the flat block and lean the toe mounds against the wall.

> Activate the right leg by pushing against the block and the wall.

> Bend into the pose and place the right palm on the second block ❶.

> Extend the left arm over the head and place the finger tips on the wall. Use the wall to turn the chest from right to left ❷.

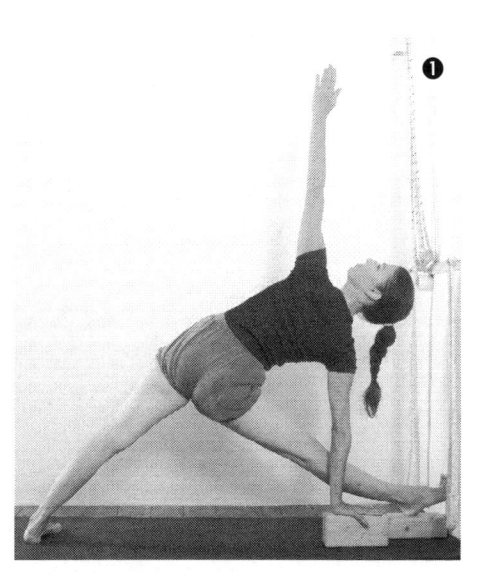

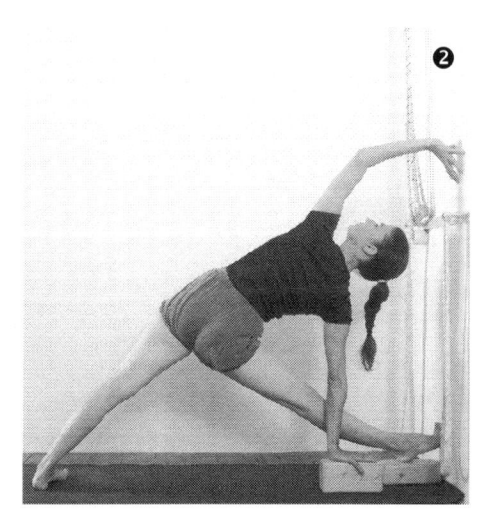

Effects

This variation is useful for people that have the following conditions in the leg joints:

- *Flat feet:* Pressing the heel and the mounds help to increase the arch of the foot.
- *Ankle pain:* The positioning of the foot reduces the pressure on the ankle. In particular, people suffering from pain in the Achilles tendon will find relief in this variation.
- *Knee pain:* The load on the front leg is reduced and the knee is activated. This can be intensified by raising the foot on a higher support.
- *Hip joint:* The femur head is drawn into its place in the hip socket.

Tips

✓ Learn how to activate the front leg by stretching the foot.

✓ Activate the foot against the wall to activate the entire leg.

✓ Observe how the front-leg's knee cap is drawn into place, the back of the knee is opened and the head of the femur (thigh bone) is moved deep into the hip socket.

Applicability

All standing poses with spread legs except for the balancing poses (Ardha Chandrasana, Parivrtta Ardha Chandrasana & Virabhadrasana III).

Utthita Trikonasana
Variation 10b

Props
wall

Stretching the front leg; Sole against the wall

A further stretch and activation of the front leg can be achieved by placing the entire sole against a wall.

⟶ To do the pose on the right side:

> Kneel as if doing Parigasana at an appropriate distance from the wall. Place the entire sole of the right foot on the wall, such that the heel is pushed into the corner of the wall and the floor.

> Press the sole of the foot firmly against the wall ❶.

> Now, slightly bend forward over the right leg ❷ and use the hands on the floor to lift and straighten the left leg into Utthita Trikonasana ❸.

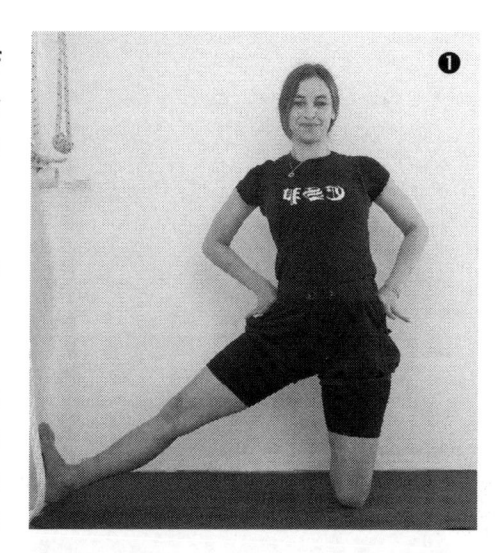

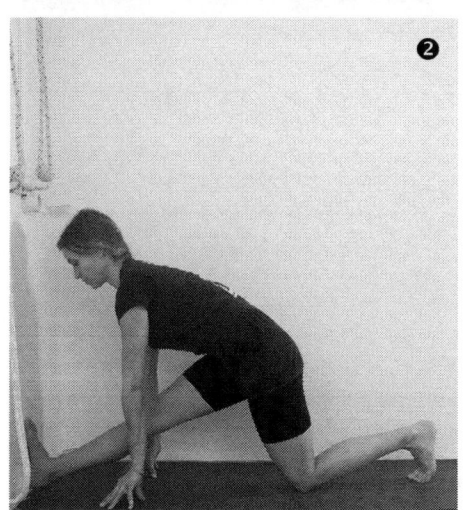

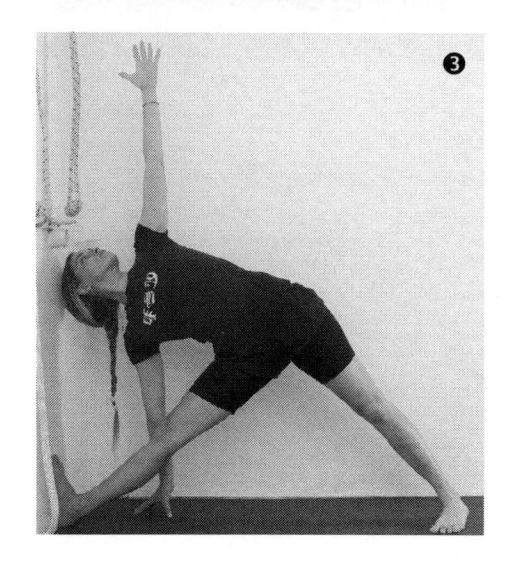

Effects
This stronger variation further opens the back of the knee, stretches the calf muscle and activates the entire leg.

Applicability
Parsvottanasana, Parivrtta Trikonasana.

Opening the Pelvis

In order to widen the pelvis in the lateral standing poses, you need to move the buttock of the front leg strongly in, while moving the thigh of the back leg backward. The main action should be around the hip joints and the pelvic girdle – If this area works correctly and the tailbone is moved deep into the pelvis, then there will be no pressure on the lower back.

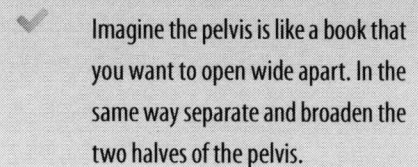

✓ Imagine the pelvis is like a book that you want to open wide apart. In the same way separate and broaden the two halves of the pelvis.

✓ Learn to extend the lower spine toward the upper spine.

Here are three ways to develop these actions.

Utthita Trikonasana Variation 11

Opening the groins: Diagonal alignment

Props
block

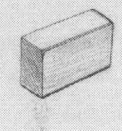

→ To do the pose on the right side:

› Do the pose as usual, in the center of the mat. Place the right palm on a block ❶ (the belt in the photo mark the centerline of the mat).

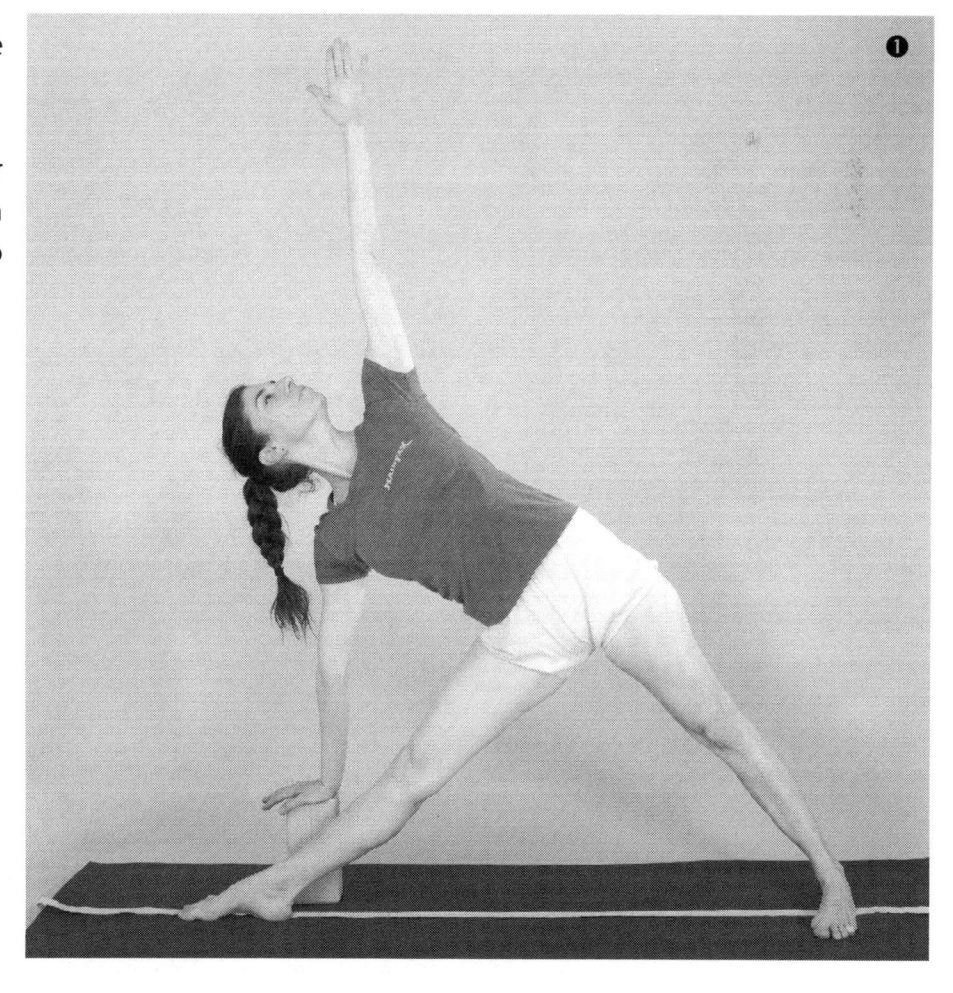

Props for Yoga / Chapter 1 / Utthita Trikonasana 79

Utthita Trikonasana Variation 11 (cont.)

Opening the groins: Diagonal alignment

Props
block

> Now move the right leg so that its inner foot aligns with the front edge of the mat. Move the right buttock in, along with the foot. Move the block closer to the foot ❷.

> Next move the left leg back so that its heel is aligned with the back edge of the mat. Move the left front thigh back along with the leg.

> The legs are now positioned diagonally ❸.

> Press down the inner side of the right foot and move the right buttock in; at the same time press the outer side of the left foot down and move the left thigh back, while keeping the tailbone tucked in.

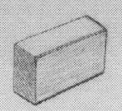

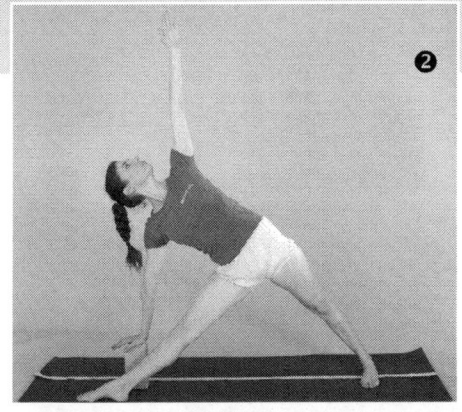

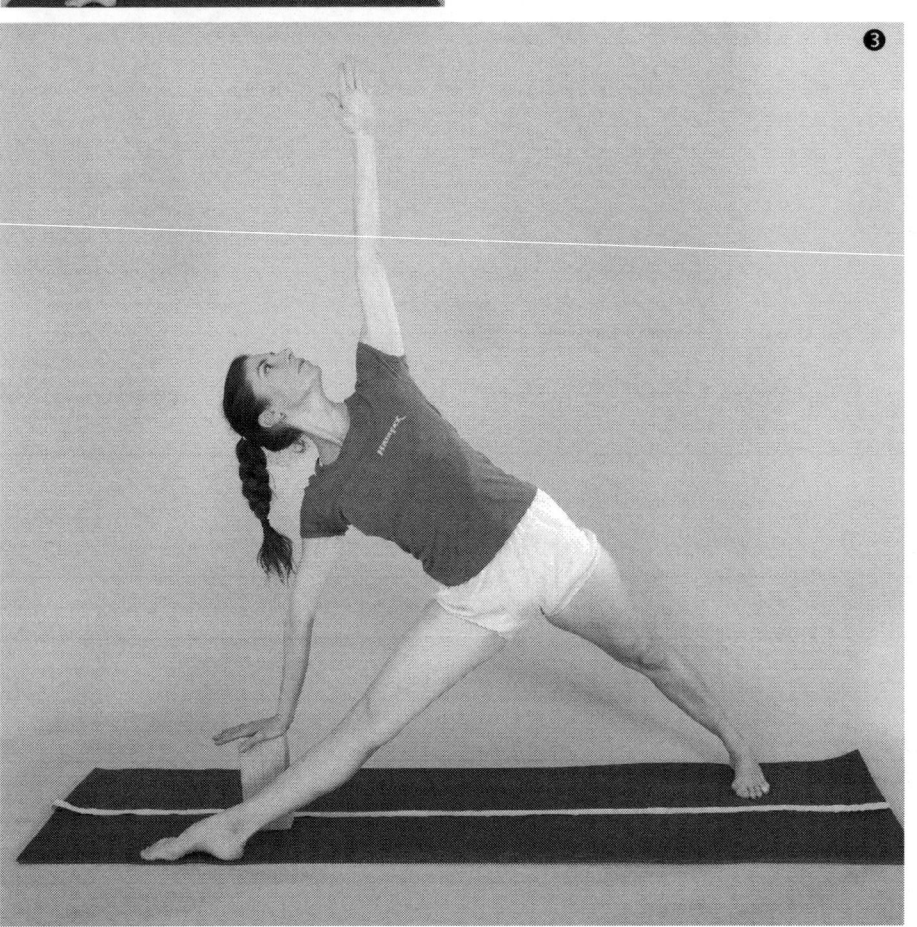

Effects
The diagonal alignment opens the groins and broadens the pelvis. One learns to move the buttock of the front leg in, while moving the thigh of the back leg backward.

Tips
✓ To verify that the tailbone and right buttock are actually pushed in, place the left palm on the pelvis; move the left elbow back and use the left thumb and fingers to feel the shape of the pelvis. Then straighten the left arm right up.

Applicability
All lateral standing poses with spread legs.

80 Props for Yoga / Chapter 1 / Utthita Trikonasana

Utthita Trikonasana
Variation 12

Ensuring lateral alignment:
Back against the wall

Props
wall
rope or belt
(for the helping partner)

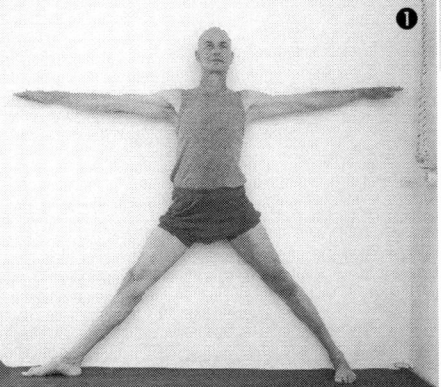

The wall provides feedback on the lateral alignment of the pelvic and shoulder girdles.

→ To do the pose on the right side:

> Stand with your back to the wall, spread your legs and turn the right leg out to Parsva Hasta Padasana ❶.

> Move left heel to touch the wall and position the right foot parallel to the wall, aligned with the arch of the back leg - about 5 cm (2 inches) away from the wall.

> Push the right buttock away from the wall and move the left thigh toward the wall.

> Touch the wall with the back of the shoulders and the back of the head.

> Now slide your back against the wall as you bend to Utthita Trikonasana. Keep both sides of your back in contact with the wall ❷.

A partner can help you do these actions:

Position yourself with your back to the wall as before.

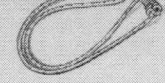

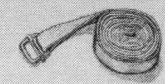

Effects

When doing the pose in the middle of the room, it is difficult to know if the body is aligned correctly. The wall gives immediate feedback and is very useful in the learning stages.

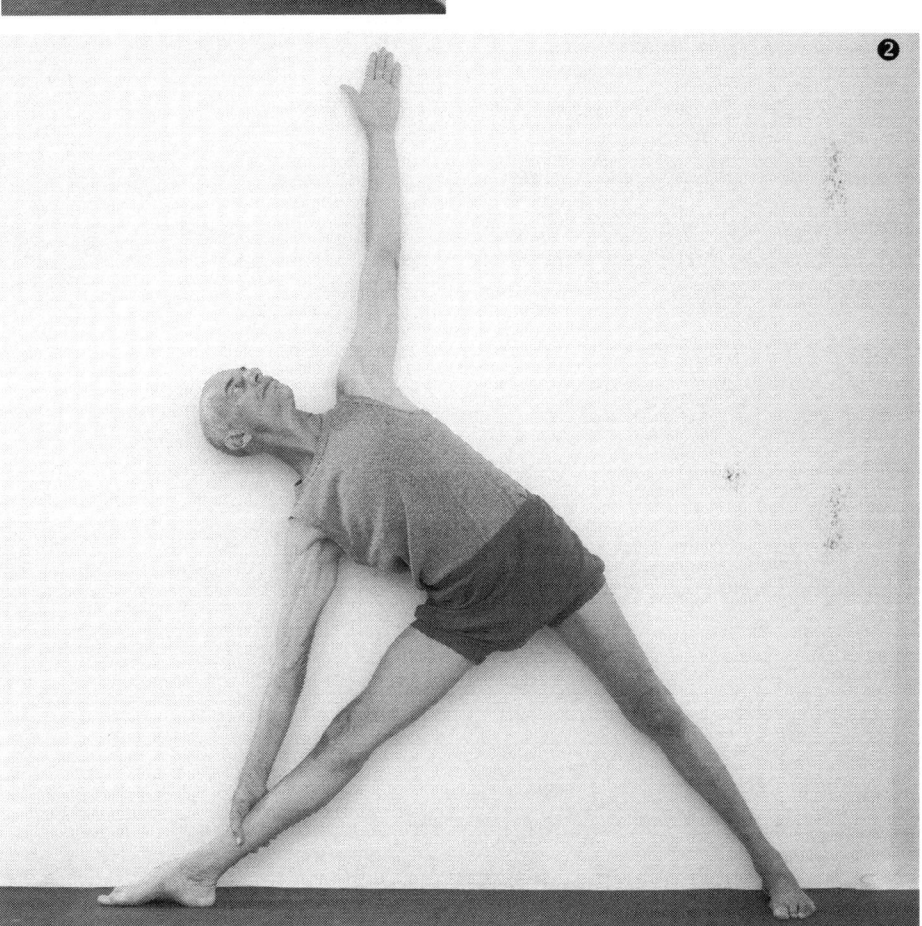

Tips

✓ As you tighten your right buttock away from the wall, can you still touch the wall with your left buttock? What about the back of the left leg?

Applicability
All lateral standing poses.

Utthita Trikonasana Variation 12 (cont.)

Ensuring lateral alignment: Back against the wall

Props
wall
rope or belt
(for the helping partner)

Instructions for the helper:

> After practitioner enters the pose with the back against the wall: Sit in front of the practitioner and place the rope around his/her right buttock (See ❷ for the correct position of the rope on the buttock.)

> Place your left foot just above the practitioner's right knee and your right foot on his/her left thigh, near the front groin.

> Pull the right buttock of the practitioner while using your feet to prevent him/her from falling towards you. To help the practitioner turn the buttock in, pull the lower part of the rope a bit stronger than the upper part. ❷

> Maintain these actions as the practitioner bends into the pose.

> After a while you can slowly release and allow the practitioner do the pose on his/her own.

Notes:
- Do not pull the rope before you place your feet on the practitioner's thighs.
- As always be cautious and sensitive when working with other people. Do not pull and push too strongly; look at your partner to see how much he/she can take.

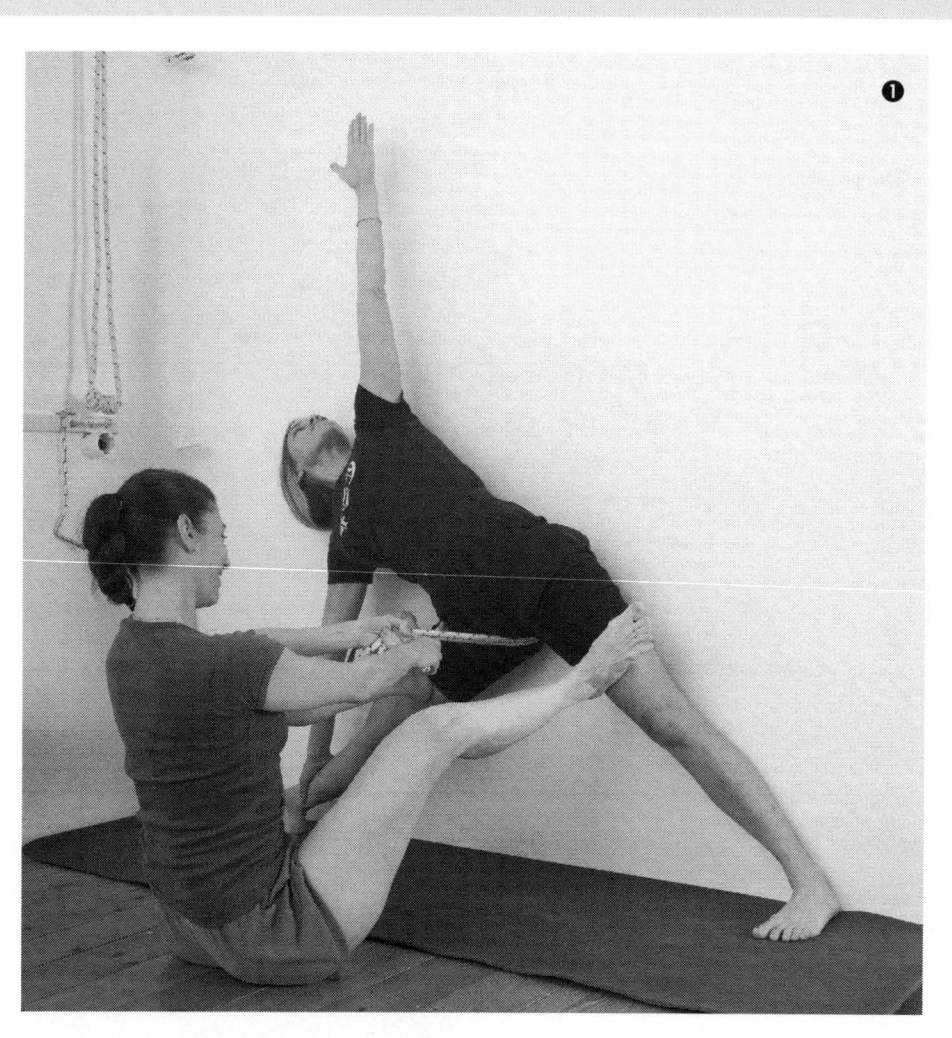

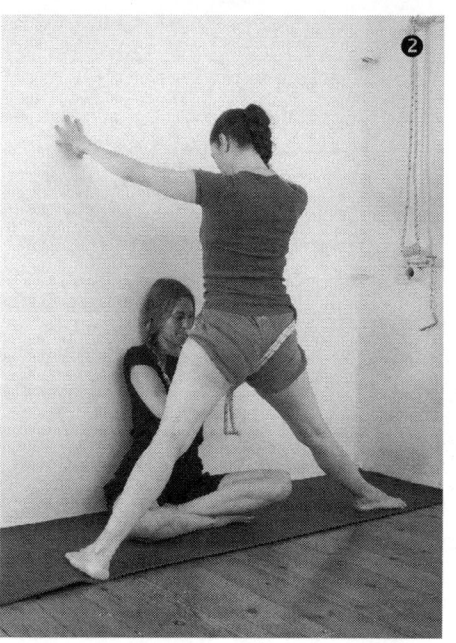

Effects
The external pull clarifies the extent to which the buttock should go in. This cellular memory can guide you when doing the pose on your own.

Applicability
All lateral standing poses.

Utthita Trikonasana
Variation 13

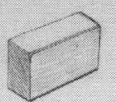

Broadening the trunk and relaxing the eyes: Facing the wall

Props
block

⟶ Another way of using the wall as a reference is to do the pose facing the wall. To do the pose on the right side:

> Stand facing the wall, spread your legs and turn the right leg out.

> Place a block between the right foot and the wall.

> Move the left leg toward the wall, until the tips of the toes touch the wall.

> Press the right foot against the block and move the right buttock toward the wall.

> Bend into the pose. Push the wall with the left hand to help turn the chest from right to left.

Effects
The wall gives a reference plane for the correct alignment of the body. Indeed, B.K.S. Iyengar often says that the best 'guru' is the wall. The proximity of the wall and the limited field of vision create a special effect: nowhere to look externally so vision is drawn inwards. The support for the top hand helps to turn the trunk, broadening the pelvis and the abdomen.

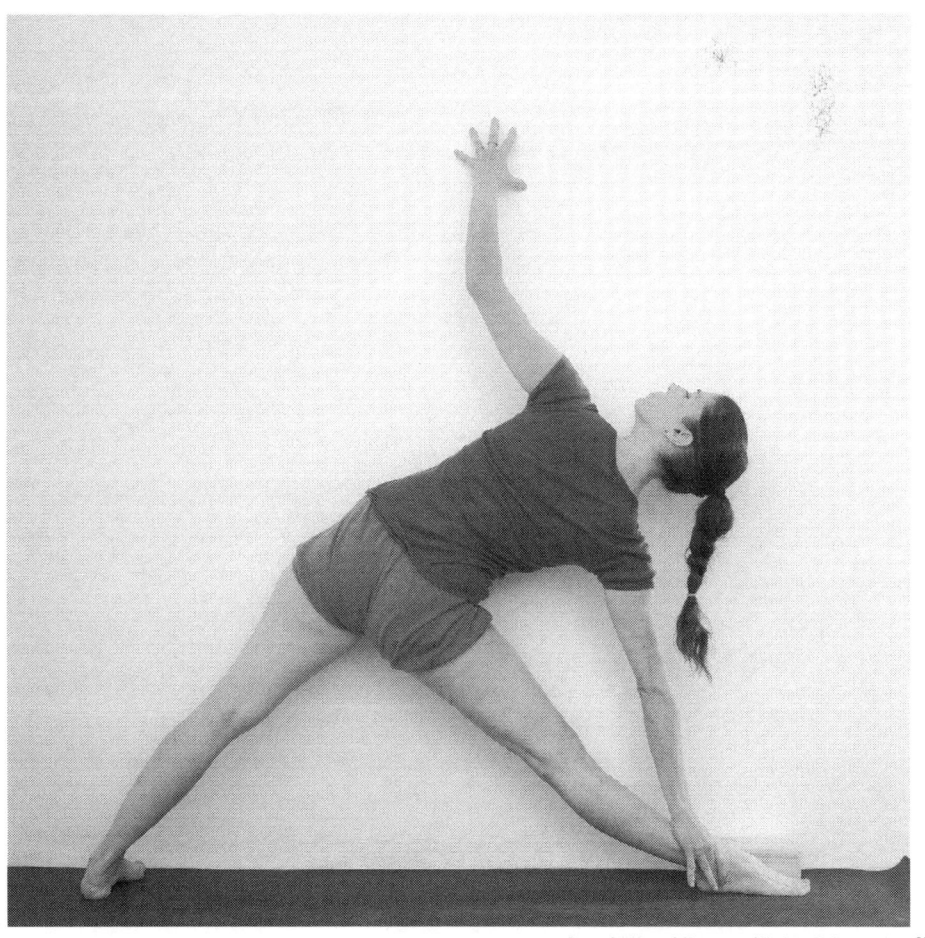

Applicability
All lateral standing poses.

Maintaining Length Along the Sides of the Trunk

In Utthita Trikonasana both sides of the trunk should maintain their full length. When bending into the pose on the right side, the right side of the trunk tends to shorten, as shown here:

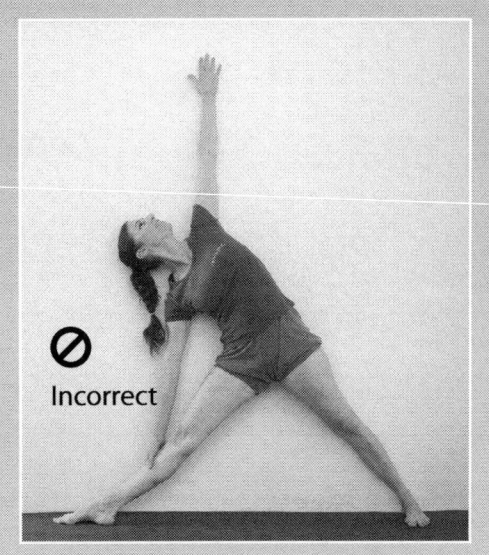

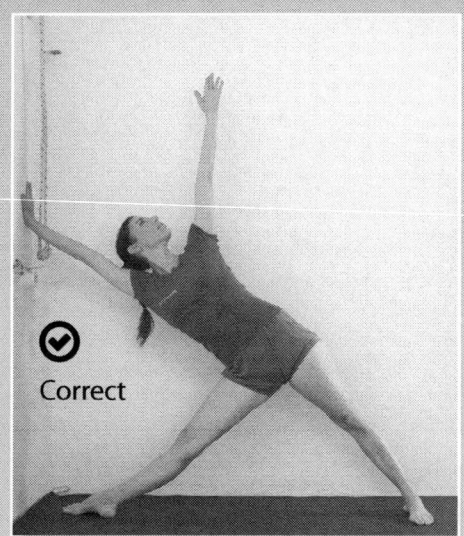

Incorrect

Correct

To keep that side long, the bending must start from the hip joints, not from the waist. Here are several ways to learn this action.

Utthita Trikonasana
Variation 14

Props
wall

Extending the sides of the trunk: Front hand on wall

→ To do the pose on the right side:

> Stand with legs apart, with the right foot about 20 cm (8 inches) away from the wall.

> Turn the right leg out, lift the right arm to extend the right side of the trunk and bend into the pose.

> Place the right palm on the wall so that the right side of the trunk and the right arm form a straight line.

> Pushing the wall bend further by moving the right buttock away from the wall and in, tilting the pelvis directly above the right leg without shortening the right side of the trunk ❶.

> After practicing with the wall, try to do it without placing the palm on the wall.

> To do the pose on the right side, start by placing the right palm on the right front groin and push the groin in while maintaining the length from the front groin to the armpit ❷.

> If while bending you feel the right side of the trunk shortening and the ribs protruding to the left, lift the right arm and stretch it to create length in the right side, at the same time move the left arm close to the body and stretch it to prevent the left side from over-extending ❸.

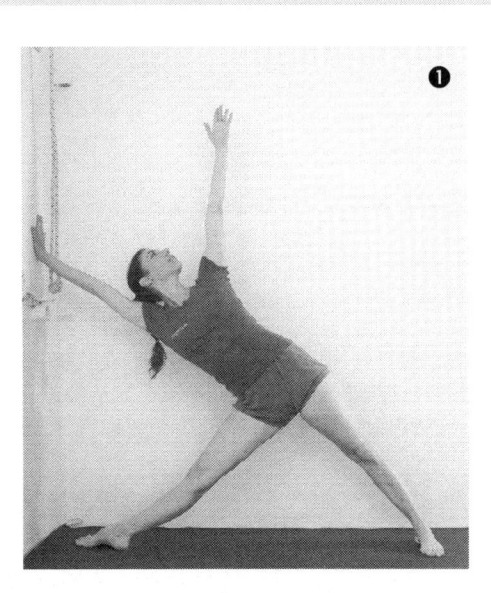

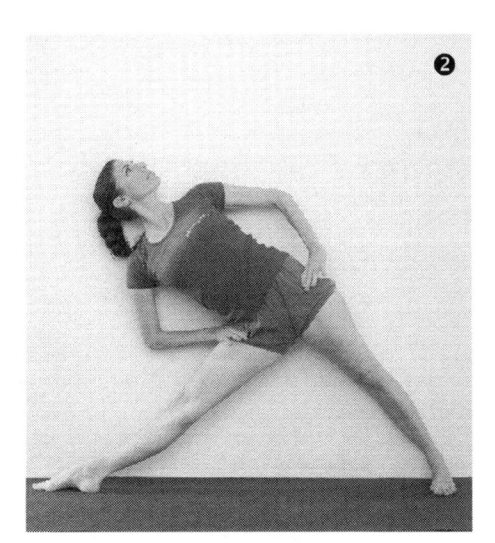

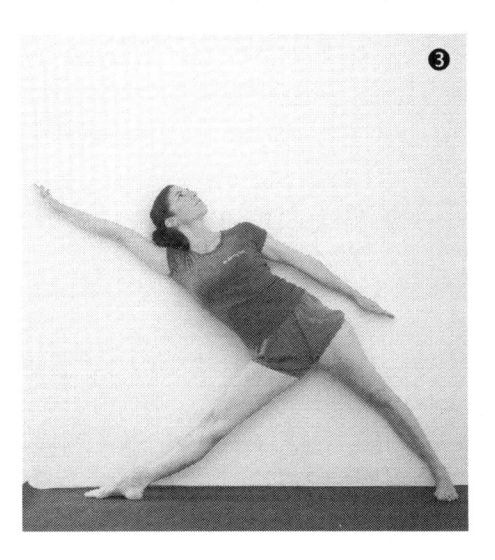

Tips

✓ Use your breathing to gauge the evenness of the trunk extension: before bending into the pose take a few slower and deeper breaths, sensitizing your lungs. Slowly move into the pose and keep monitoring the sensations of the breath in the lungs. Check the volume and intensity of the breathing in both lungs. If you feel that the breath in the right lung is less pronounced, expand it: extend the right trunk from the hip to the armpit and broaden the space between the ribs on the right side.

Applicability
Utthita Parsvakonasana.

A partner can help to induce the correct movement. Here are two ways to do that:

Utthita Trikonasana
Variation 15a

Bending from the hips: Partner pulls the front hip

Props
belt
partner

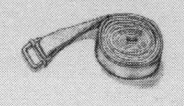

Bending to Utthita Trikonasana should commence from the hip joints, not from the waist. When bending to the right side, the front groin of the right leg should move deeply in.

→ To do the pose to the right (instructions are given for the helper):

> Stand on the left side of the practitioner and place an open belt around his/her pelvis.

> Hold the two ends of the belt and gently pull it while the practitioner goes into the pose.

> Pull the right side of the belt slightly stronger in order to help the practitioner turn the right thigh out and take the right hip joint in.

Effects
The belt anchors the right hip in place, helping with the extension of the lower side of the trunk as well as its rotation.

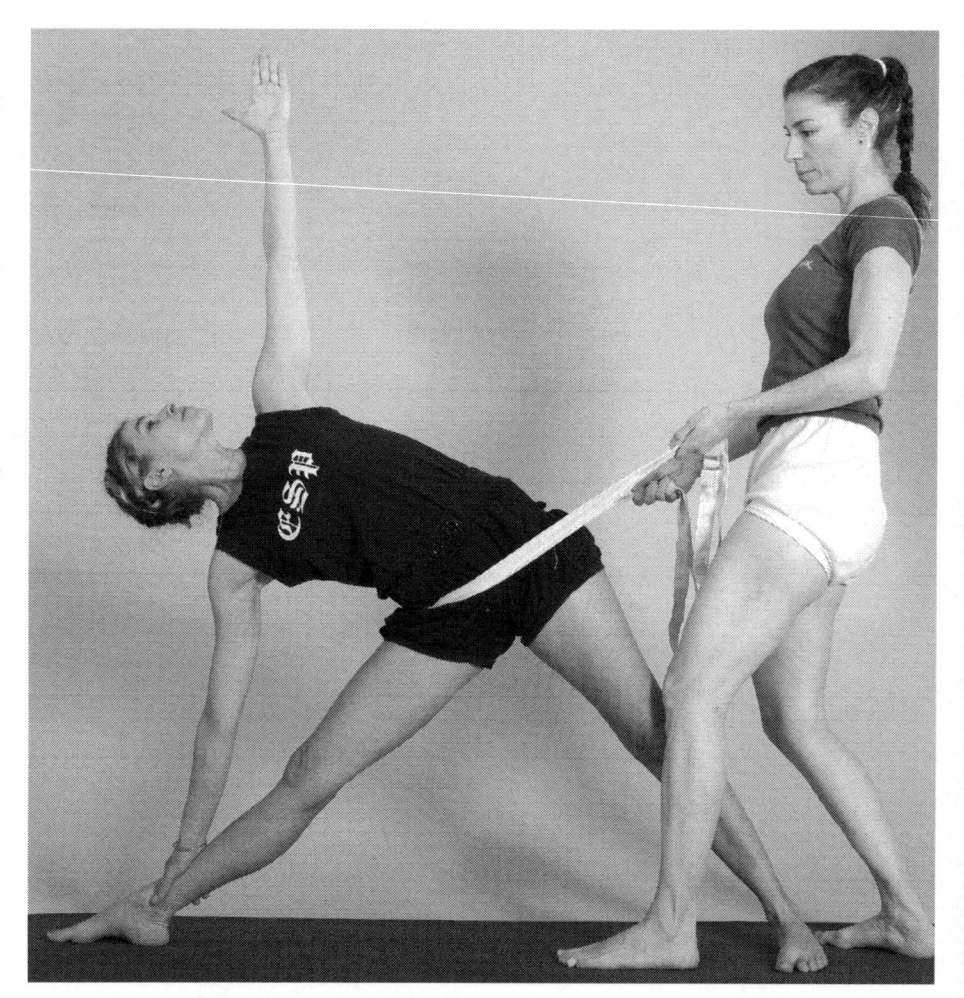

Utthita Trikonasana
Variation 15b

Pulling the front groin while stabilizing the back leg

Props
belt
partner

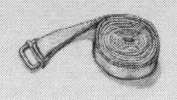

This is a slight improvement of the previous variation which helps to move the right buttock in and the left thigh back at the same time.

→ To do the pose on the right side:

> Stand on the left side of the practitioner and place the belt as in the previous variation.

> Pass the right end of the belt in between the practitioner's legs from back to front and hold it with the left end.

> The belt should now be looped behind the right buttock and in front of the practitioner's left thigh.

> Gently pull the belt as the practitioner moves into the pose.

Note: Pull the belt with care. Always be sure to keep the practitioner's center of gravity in between the two feet to prevent him/her from falling backwards.

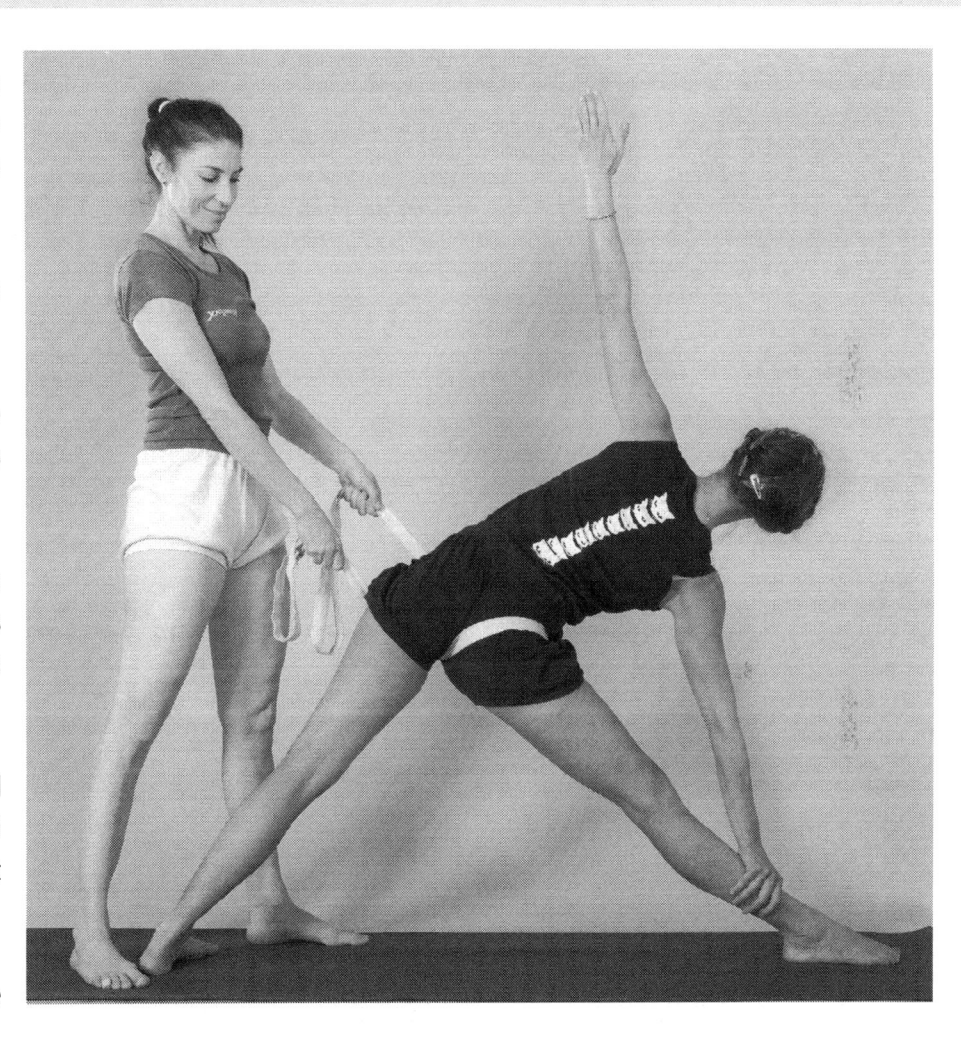

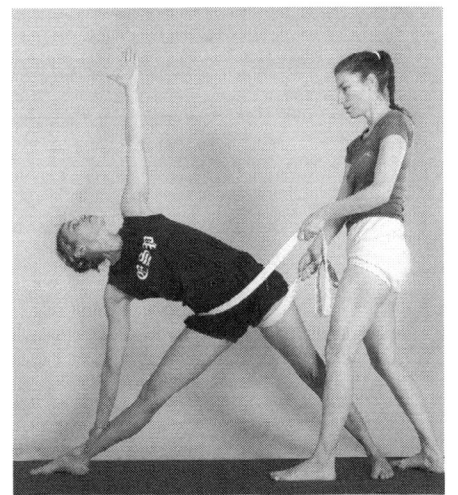

Effects
The belt anchors the right hip in place while preventing the left thigh from moving forward. This helps to extend the trunk while keeping it on the same lateral plane with the legs.

Applicability
Utthita Parsvakonasana.

Correcting Hyper-extended Knees

Some people suffer from excessive flexibility in the legs. When doing Trikonasana, such hyper-extension is typically manifested by the calf of the front leg which sinks excessively toward the floor and 'locks' the knee. Over time, this unhealthy pressure on the knee may lead to injury. People who have this structure must learn to straighten the leg by activating the thigh muscles while reducing pressure on the shin bones. We'll show first how to learn this in an active way, and then how to support the calf.

Utthita Trikonasana Variation 16

Active work for hyper-extended knee: Pressing the foot against the wall

Props
wall
block (optional)

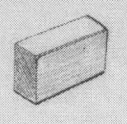

⟶ When doing the pose on the right side:

› Before bending into the pose, slightly bend the right leg and shift weight to the toe mounds.

› Press the mounds strongly to the floor and the calf muscle toward the shin bone.

› To straighten the leg, lift the thigh bone into the pelvis while resisting the tendency of the calf to move back.

› Lift the knee cap without pushing the knee back.

Using a block and a wall can help to learn this:

› Place the toe mounds on a wall and bend the knee.

› Press the mounds against the wall to straighten the leg. Activate the calf muscle to resist the backward movement of the shin.

Effects
Pressing the toe mounds against the wall stabilizes the leg and makes it easy to control the movement of the knee.

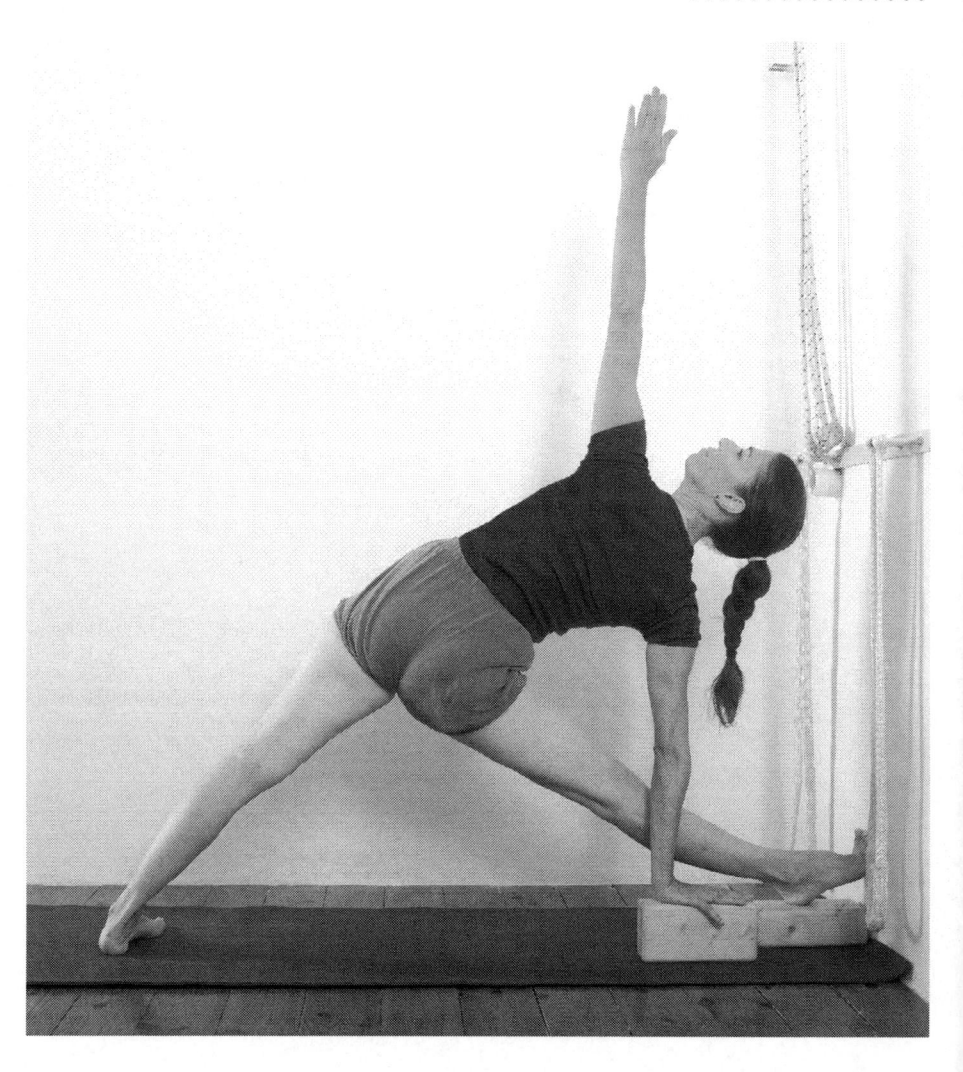

Utthita Trikonasana
Variation 17

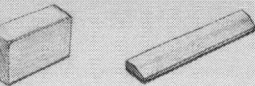

Stabilizing hyper-extended knee: Supporting the calf with block

Props
block
slanting plank (optional)

→ When doing the pose on the right side:

> Enter the pose and bend the right leg slightly. Place a block diagonally under the shin so that the top of the block supports the calf muscle.

> Straighten the leg and move the front thigh muscles back (into the thigh bone and up toward the pelvis).

> Position the block so that it stops the downward movement of the shin and keeps the leg straight ❶.

> A slanting plank can be added to stabilize the block ❷.

Note: Another option is to do the pose with the back against the wall and to place a rolled bandage between the calf of the back leg and the

Effects
The block prevents the excessive movement of the knee and helps to activate the quadriceps (front thigh muscles)

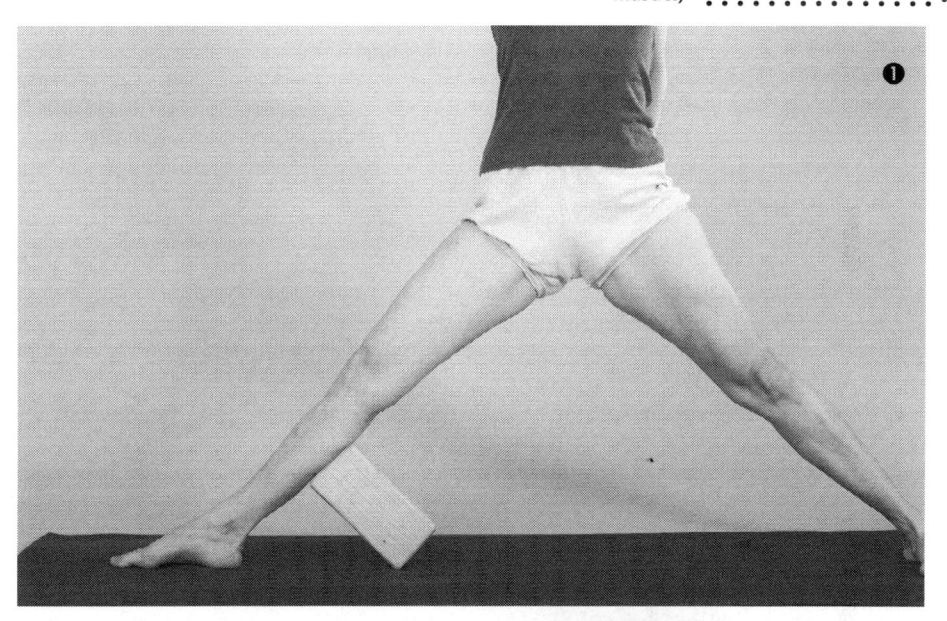

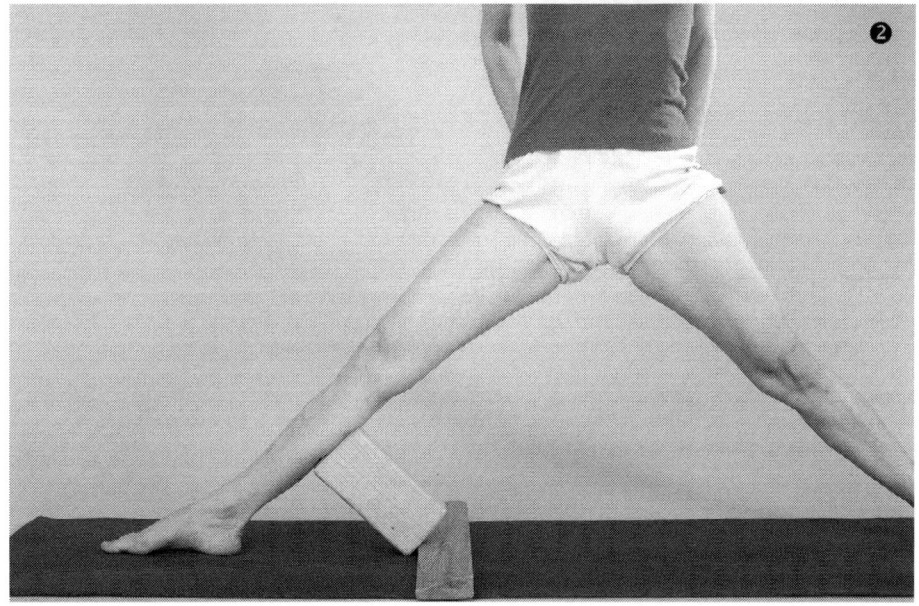

Tips
✓ Move the quadriceps toward the thigh bone and pull them up toward the pelvis.

Applicability
Parsvottanasana.

Props for Yoga / Chapter 1 / Utthita Trikonasana 89

Working the Upper Body

Here are a few variations that intensify the actions of the upper body in Utthita Trikonasana.

Utthita Trikonasana
Variation 18

Turning the chest: Upper hand holds weight

Props
wooden block

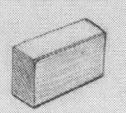

→ To do the pose on the right side:

> Hold a wooden (heavy) block in the left hand.

> *Note:* Use a heavy block but be careful not to drop it! The block can be substituted by another object weighing 1-2 Kgs (2 to 4.5 pounds), such as a small hand weight which is easy to grasp.

> After entering the pose, stretch the left arm up and move it backward.

> Use the movement of the left arm to turn the chest from right to left. ❶

> Once the chest has turned, turn the head up and look towards the ceiling.

> After a while move the left arm back to its vertical position and stretch it up, looking towards the left hand. ❷

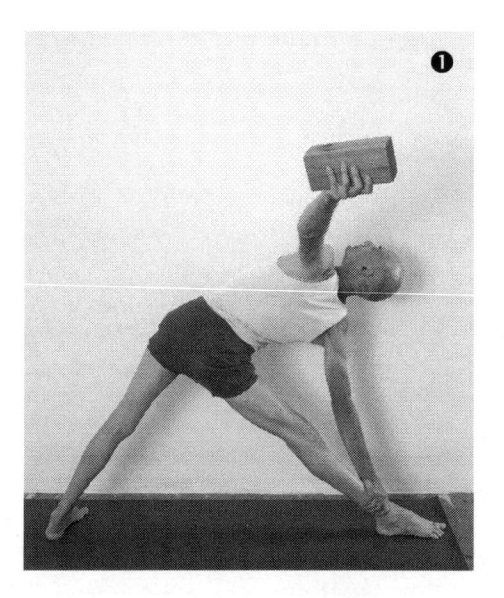

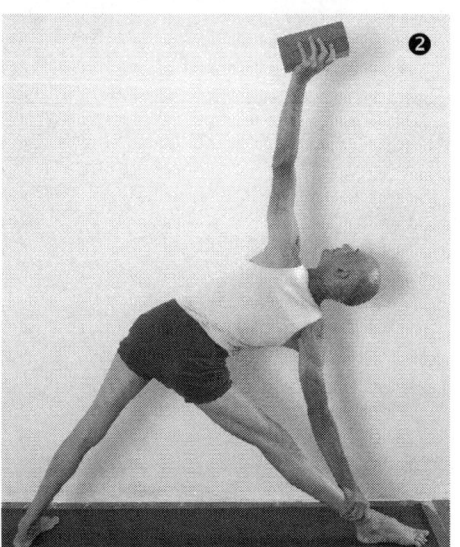

Effects
The weight on the upper arm helps to create movement in the top shoulder and turn the chest. People with stiff shoulders can use it to develop movement in the shoulder girdle.

Tips

✓ Turn the chest until both sides of the trunk are facing the wall in front of you.

✓ Relax and soften the eyes, jaws and face. The pupils of the eyes should remain in the center; the gaze upward should be relaxed. The eyes should remain soft and receding toward the back of the skull, which should be pointed to the floor.

Applicability
Utthita Parsvakonasana.

Utthita Trikonasana
Variation 19

Turning the chest: Hands holding a chair from behind

Props
chair

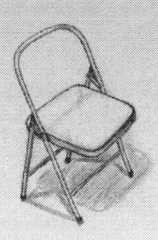

→ A chair can be used to support and align the pose as shown in the photo (see *A Chair for Yoga* for more details):

Effects
The chair supports the pose enabling longer stay. Catching the backrest helps to roll the top shoulder back. The chair also provides a reference line for checking the alignment of the body.

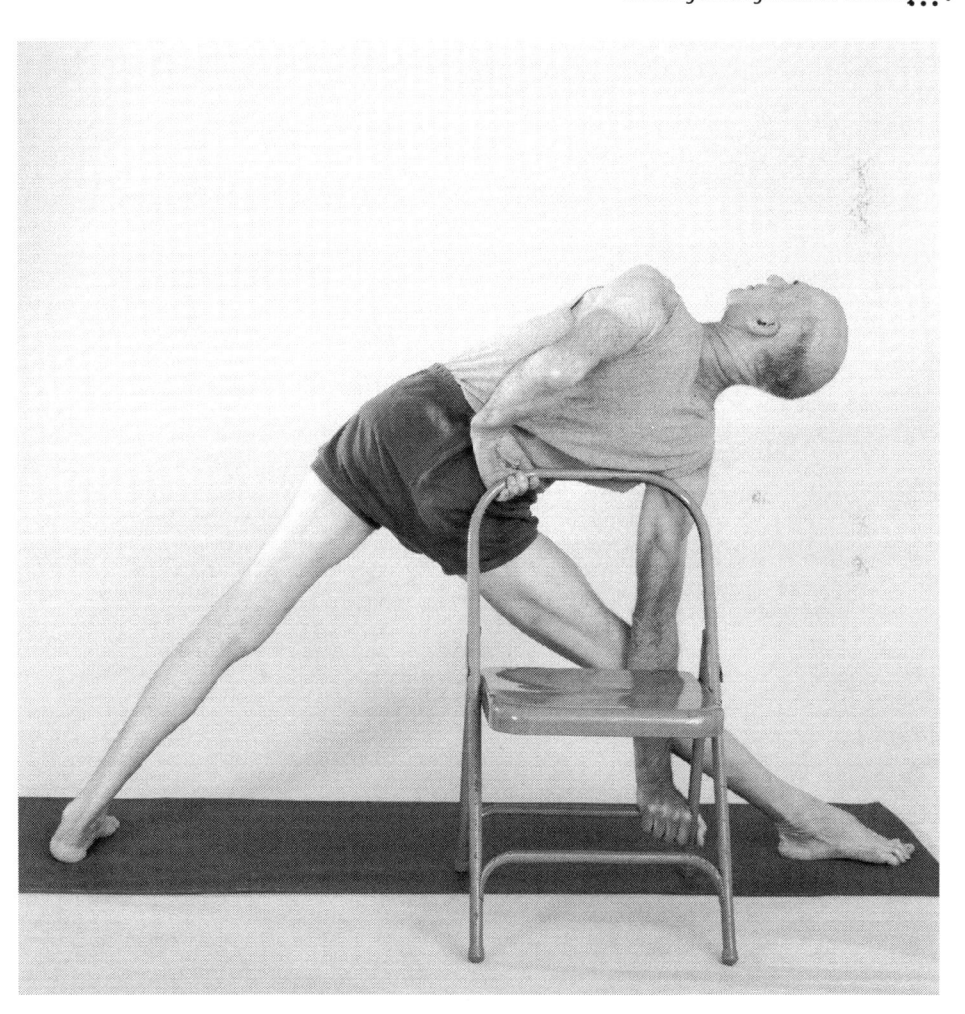

Applicability
All lateral and twisting standing poses.

Utthita Trikonasana Variation 20

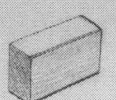

Rolling the shoulders back: Bottom palm on block

Props
block

⟶ To do the pose on the right side:

> Place a block next to the right shin.

> Go into the pose; turn the right arm from inside out and place the palm on the block such that the fingers are pointing backward.

> Using this turning of the arm, roll the shoulder back and draw the shoulder blade in.

> Turn the chest from right to left and look up.

Effects
Turning the arm so that the biceps is rolling out and the triceps is rolling in is a key action that enables rolling the shoulder back and moving the shoulder blade in. Turning the palm intensifies and clarifies this action.

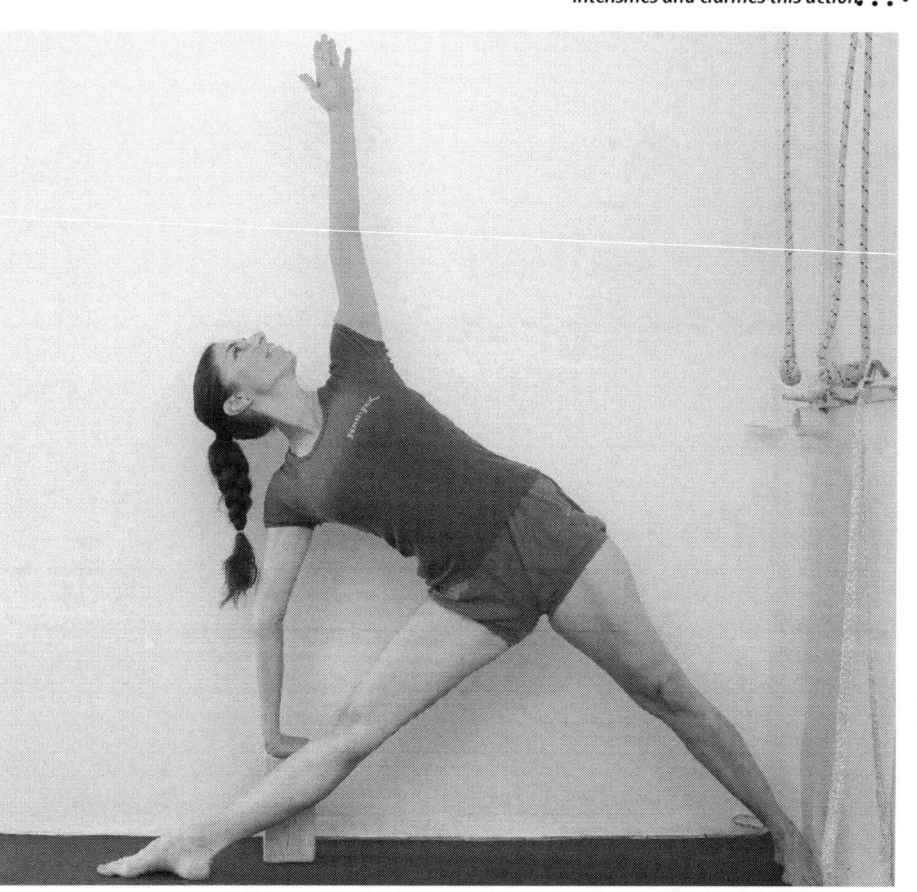

Tips

✓ Learn to turn the biceps muscle from inside out and the triceps muscle from outside in.

✓ Both the right knee cap and the right biceps should face your right side.

Applicability
Utthita Parsvakonasana, Ardha Chandrasana.

Utthita Trikonasana
Variation 21

Moving the shoulders back: Arms behind the back

In classic Utthita Trikonasana the arms are stretched along the same plane as the body. Interlocking the arms or the fingers behind the back moves the shoulders back. Photos ❶ - ❺ show different ways of interlocking the arms.

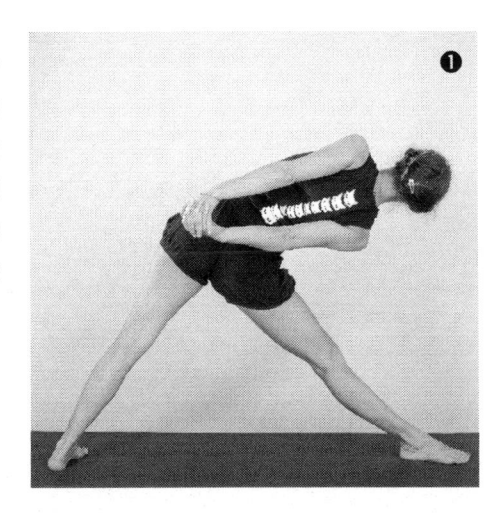

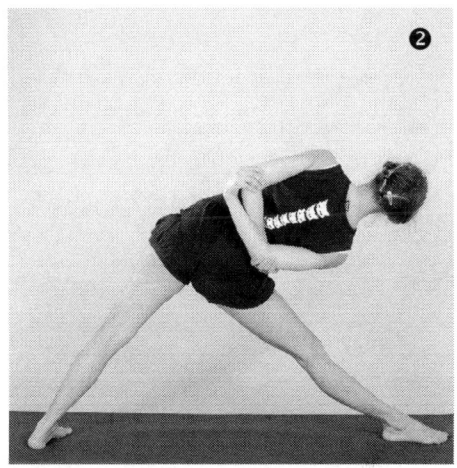

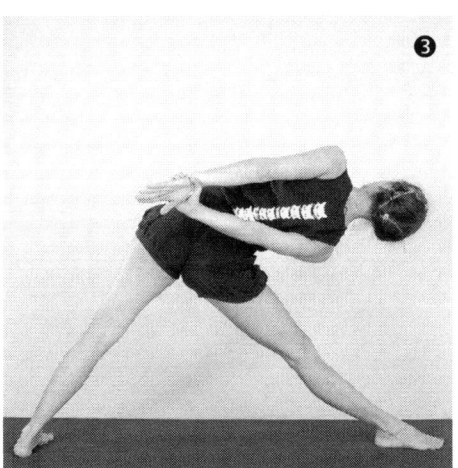

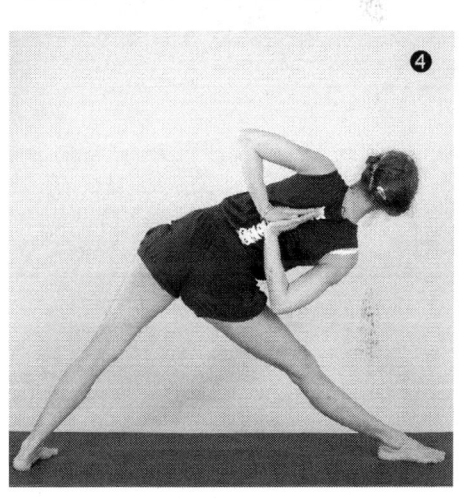

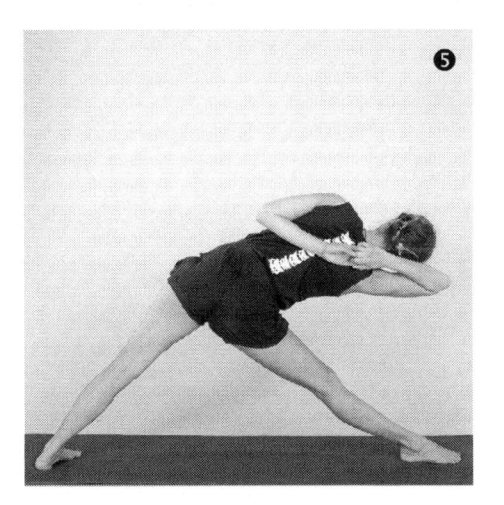

Effects
stretching the arms behind the back moves the shoulders back and thus helps to open the chest.

Tips
✓ After staying in the pose for a few moments with arms behind the back, change to the regular arm position while retaining the openness in the shoulders and in the chest.

Applicability
All standing poses.

Stretching the Top Arm

Stretching the top arm helps to open the chest in Utthita Trikonasana; holding a rope clarifies this action.

Utthita Trikonasana Variation 22

Stretching the top arm: Holding a rope

Props
a rope attached to a ceiling or wall hook

⟶ To do the pose on the right side:

> Stand under a rope attached to the ceiling and hold it with your left hand.

> Stretch the left arm and hold the rope tightly.

> When going into the pose, let the palm slide down the rope without releasing the grip. The palm should move with resistance in order to keep the left arm stretched.

> Use the stretch of the arm to turn the chest from right to left ❶.

> After a while release the rope and stretch the left arm vertically up.

> A wall rope can also be used as in ❷.

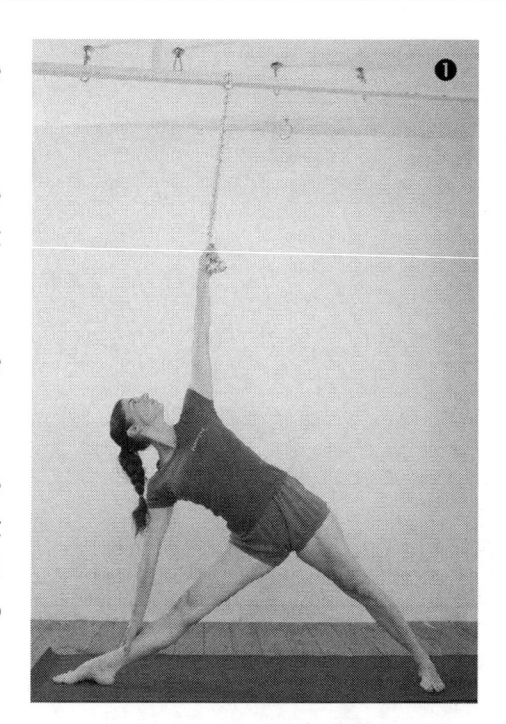

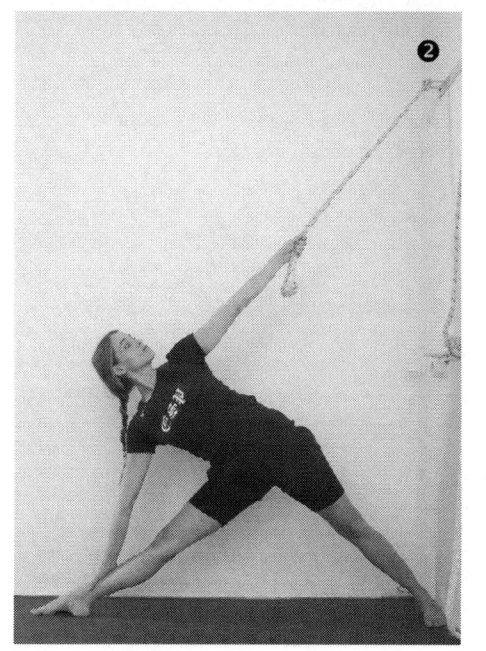

Effects

Pulling the rope helps to experience and understand the role of the top arm in opening and turning the chest. When doing the pose on the right side, the stretch of the left arm also helps to extend the right side of the trunk.

Tips

✓ Learn to use the top arm in order to turn and broaden the chest.

Applicability

All standing poses done with raised arm; in *Virabhadrasana I & II*, lift the arms and catch the rope with both hands.

Virabhadrasana II

The Virabhadra poses (I, II & III) are more strenuous compared with other standing poses. In these poses, the body weight must be carried by the feet alone without hand support.

The first three variations focus on bending the front leg to 90º. The other variations help to maintain the chest open when going into the pose.

> **⚠ CAUTIONS**
>
> Do not practice this asana if you have a cardiac condition, palpitations, heartburn, diarrhea, or dysentery. Women with menorrhagia and metrorrhagia should avoid this asana.

Bending the Knee to Form a Square

Many beginners find it difficult to release the buttock of the front leg down, in order to form a 'square' (i.e., 90º between the shin and the thigh).

Virabhadrasana II
Variation 1

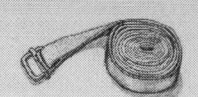

Squaring the front leg: Belt from knee to back leg

Props
long belt

→ To do the pose on the right side:

> Loop a belt from the left foot to the right knee.

> Bend the right leg half way and place the belt just under the knee cap. Tighten the belt.

> Now bend the leg to 90°. The belt should be well stretched. Keep the buckle accessible so that you can adjust the length of the belt as required.

> Look at the upper thigh of the right leg and make sure it is horizontal.

> Stretch the left leg to resist the pull of the belt.

> Stretch your arms sideways and stay in the pose for a minute or so.

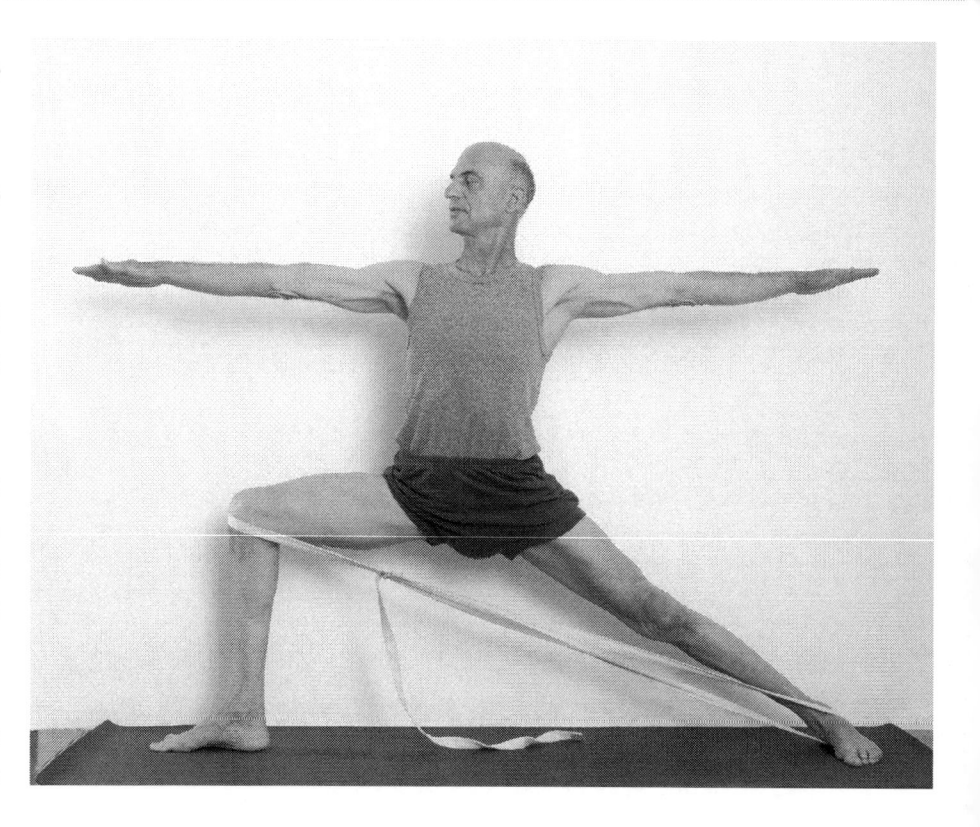

Tips

✓ Move the tailbone in, extend the spine upward and open the chest to allow for smooth breathing.

✓ Learn to extend your stay in this pose. Make sure your breath is flowing without interruption.

✓ When turning the head to the right side, mentally connect the right side of the brain with the left palm and the left side of the brain with the right palm.

✓ Look with soft eyes over the nails of the right palm towards infinity.

Effects

The belt stabilizes the front knee and helps to release the front buttock down while transferring body weight to the back leg, thus making the pose less strenuous. It helps to move the head of the femur (thigh) bone into its socket. The belt also activates the back leg which should provide resistance.

Applicability

Virabhadrasana I,
Utthita Parsvakonasana.

Virabhadrasana II
Variation 2

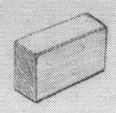

Squaring the front leg: Supporting the knee with a block

Props
wall
foam or cork block

→ To do the pose on the right side:

> Do the pose with your right side to the wall so that after bending the leg, the right knee is about 25 cm (10 inches) from the wall.

> Place the block between the front of the knee and the wall. If necessary, adjust your distance from the wall to ensure that when your knee is square, the block is pressed well against the knee.

Note: Use a lightweight foam block or a cork block. If only a wooden block is available, cover the foot with a folded mat or blanket to protect it in case the block slips down.

> Align the front thigh with the block and make sure both are horizontal.

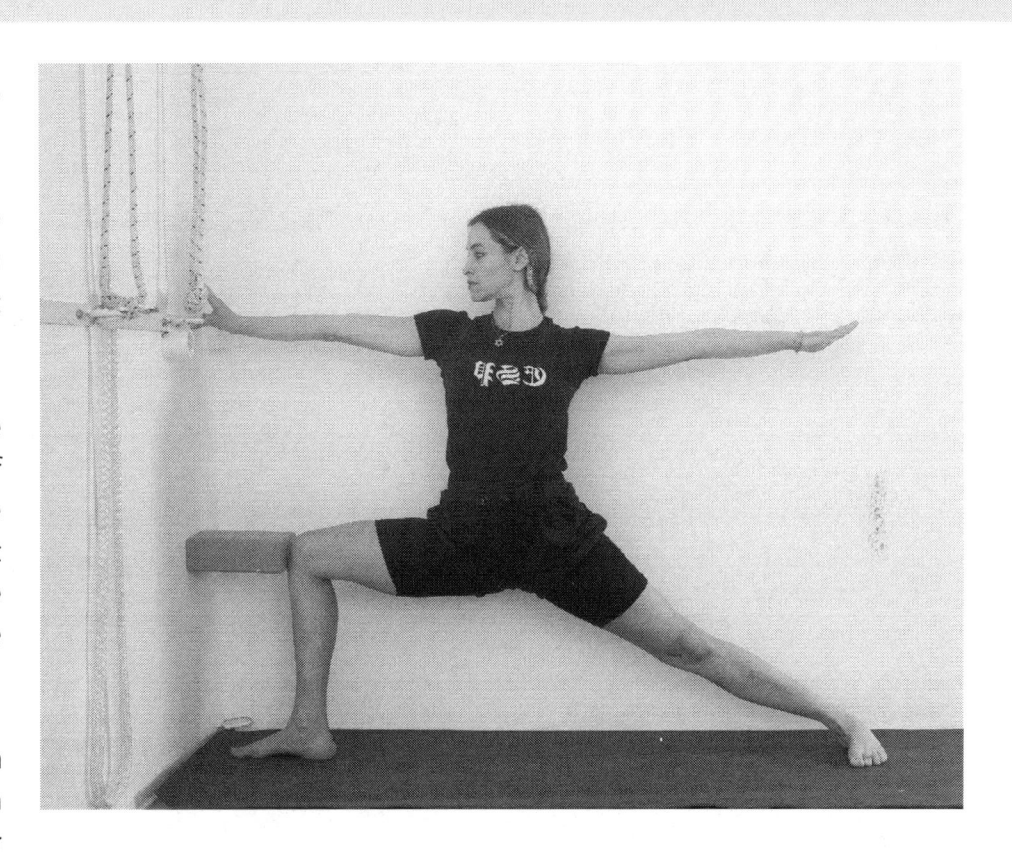

Tips

✓ When bending the front leg to Virabhadrasana II, concentrate on releasing the buttock down rather than on the forward motion. Resist the tendency of the knee to move forward. In fact the head of the shin bone should be drawn backward; otherwise the forward movement will shift excessive weight to the front leg.

✓ Observe the front thigh and make sure it is parallel to the floor and aligned with the block.

Effects

The block stabilizes the front leg and helps shift weight to the back leg. This helps to lower the buttock and reach 90° while keeping the back leg firm on the floor. This variation also helps to check the alignment of the bent leg: the buttock bone, knee and heel should all be on the same vertical plane of the block.

Applicability

Virabhadrasana I,
Utthita Parsvakonasana.

Virabhadrasana II
Variation 3

Reducing muscular effort: Resting the buttock on a chair

Props
chair

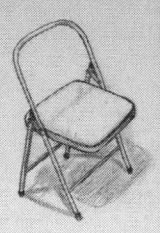

A chair can be used to support the buttock of the front leg. This reduces the muscular effort required to hold the pose but allows experiencing the intense stretch that the pose brings about.

⟶ To use the chair on the right side:

> After spreading the legs, place a chair in front of you and align the front edge of the seat with your right thigh.

> Turn the right leg out and pull the chair closer to it.

> Bend the right leg; move the chair with you as needed to support the right buttock and thigh.

> Keep the left leg well stretched.

> Hold the backrest and use the arms to turn the chest from right to left and lift it upward ❶.

Pulling the chair closer to you between your legs helps to spread the thighs and open the inner groins.

> If the seat of the chair is lower than the bottom of your knee, place on it a folded blanket or a foam block ❷.

> Adding height to the chair can also help people with tight groins. The extra height helps to open the groins and straighten the back leg.

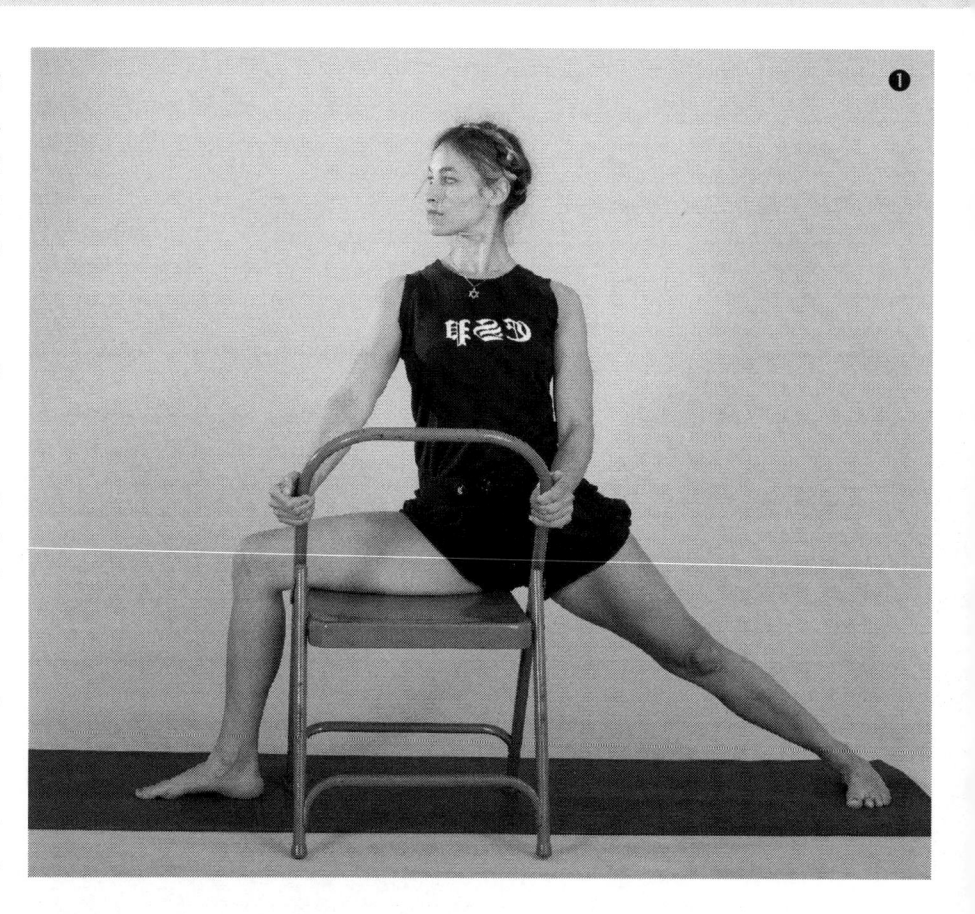

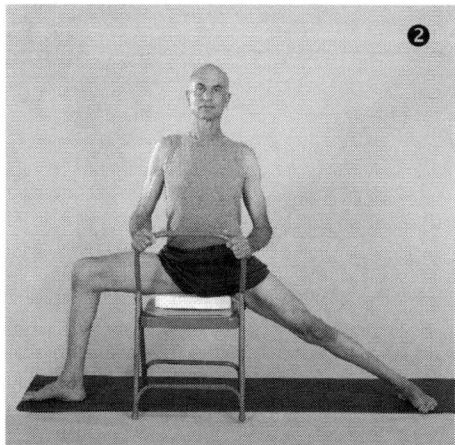

Effects

In the above three variations, much of the body weight is taken by the prop. With reduced effort on both legs, one is able to stay longer and work on the details of the pose. When doing on the right you can work on: stretching the left leg and moving it backwards, rolling the right knee from inside out and making sure it is bent to 90°; creating width in the pelvis, lifting the lower abdomen and turning the chest from right to left.

Applicability

Utthita Parsvakonasana,
Virabhadrasana I.

98   Props for Yoga / Chapter 1 / Virabhadrasana II

Stretching the Back Arm

In Virabhadrasana II the chest should be aligned vertically above the pelvis. The following two variations help to prevent the tilting of the trunk toward the front leg.

Virabhadrasana II
Variation 4a

Props
wall

Activating the back arm: Back palm against the wall

⟶ To do the pose on the right side:

› Stand with your left outer foot against the wall, stretch your arms sideways and place the left palm against the wall. At this stage the left arm will be lifted ❶.

› As you bend into the pose, slide the left palm down while you keep pushing it against the wall ❷.

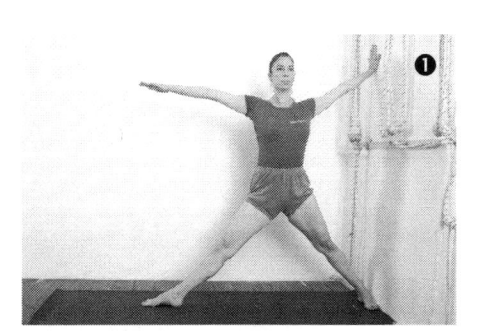

Effects
Stretching the back arm to the wall activates it and ensures that the trunk will not tilt sideways toward the front leg.

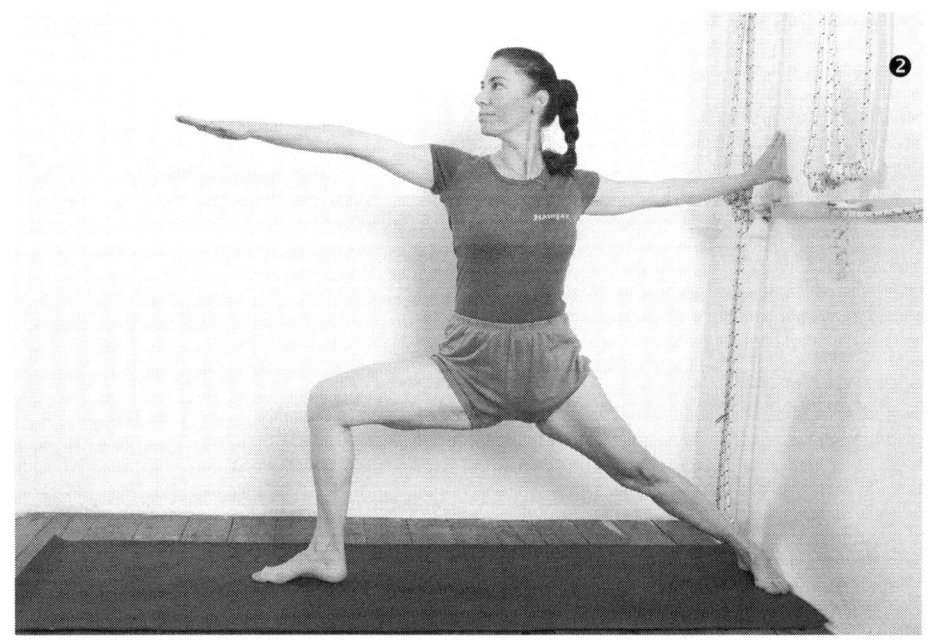

Tips

✔ Learn to stretch the back arm; do not allow the palm to move away from the wall.

✔ As you bend to the pose, move the femur head of the back (straight) leg into its socket, lift the side trunk from there to the armpit and stretch from the armpit to the palm.

Virabhadrasana II
Variation 4b

Aligning the chest above the pelvis: Back hand holds a wall rope

Props
wall hook & rope

One of the challenges of standing poses is to balance the body weight on the two legs. In the beginning, the body weight tends to shift to the front leg. This is true especially for poses like Virabhadrasana II, in which the front leg is bent. Pulling the rope helps to shift weight to the back leg. Splitting the bearing of the body weight between the two legs lightens up the pose and enables a longer, more relaxed stay. This variation teaches the important role of the back arm in the pose.

→ To do the pose on the right side:

> Stand with your left side to the wall and hold a rope attached to the wall.

> As you bend into the pose let the left hand slide along the rope.

> In order to maintain the stretch of the left arm, keep grasping the rope strongly as the palm slides down with resistance.

> Stay in the pose for a while, then let go of the rope and remain in the pose for another 40-60 seconds.

Note: Any firm object to which you can tie the rope can substitute for the wall hook.

Effects
Holding the rope helps to keep the trunk vertical when bending the front leg. This develops flexibility in the hips and groins and opens the chest.

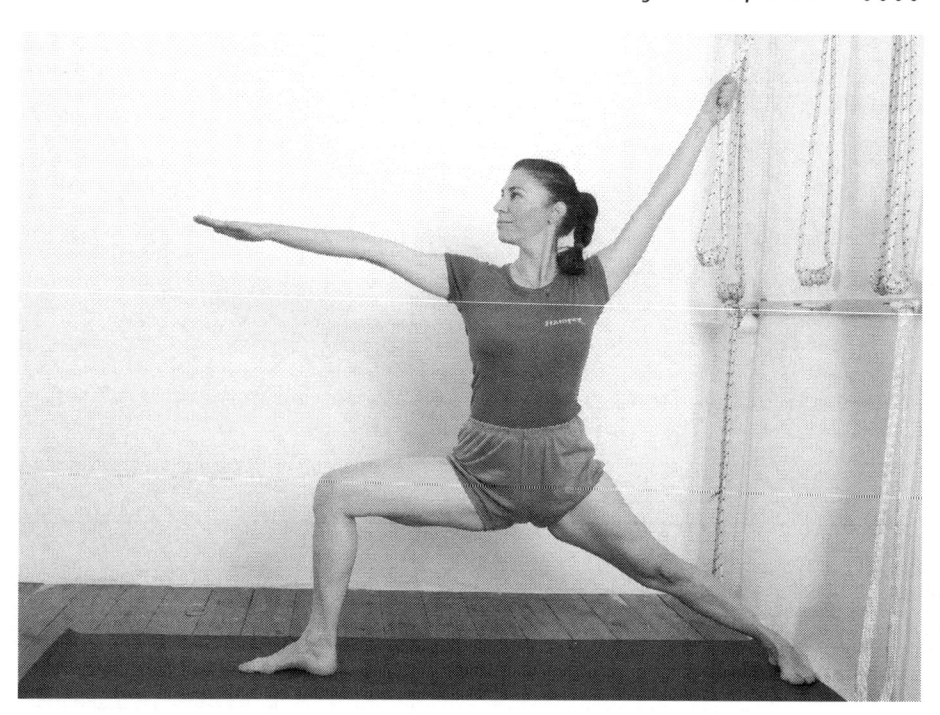

Tips
✓ When bending the right leg, do not allow the chest to tilt to the right; observe and check that the left armpit is just above the left hip.

100 Props for Yoga / Chapter 1 / Virabhadrasana II

Virabhadrasana II
Variation 5

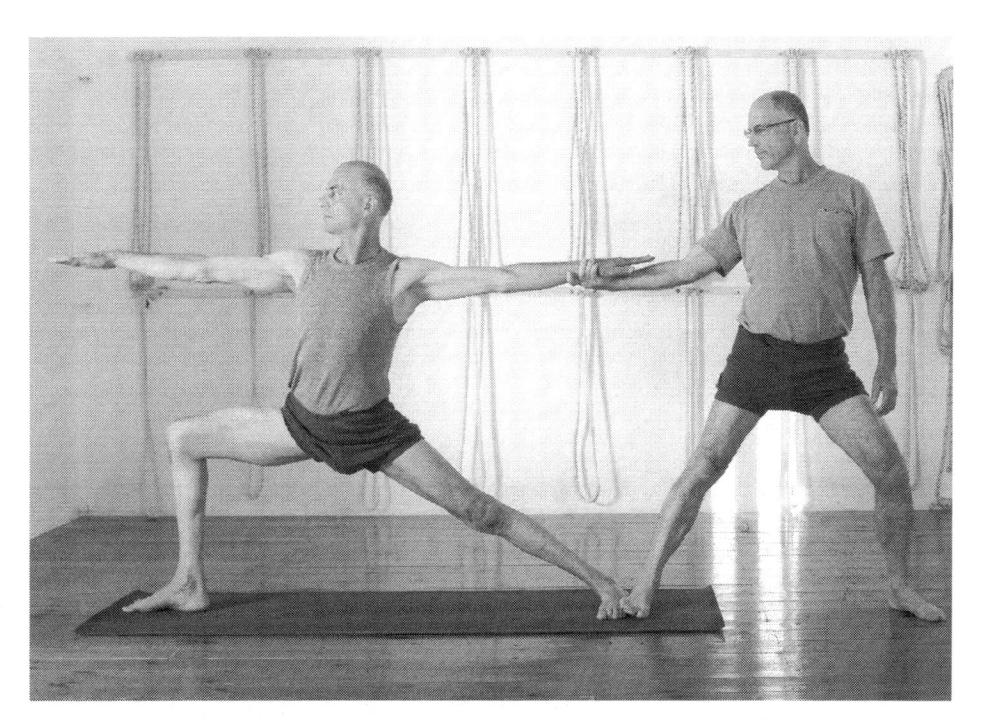

Aligning the chest above the pelvis: Partner holds the back arm

This variation is similar to the previous one; but instead of a rope, a partner holds the back arm and pulls it. The partner also uses his foot to support the practitioner's back foot.

Effects

Similar to the previous variation. The partner can adjust the pull to provide adequate resistance. He/she also provides anchoring for the back foot.

Lifting & Opening the Chest

Virabhadrasana II is useful for learning the work of the arms, shoulder blades and shoulders. Stretching the arms sideways broadens the chest, while stretching them up lifts the chest.

Virabhadrasana II
Variation 6

Lifting the chest: Holding a block

Props
block

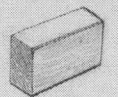

⟶ To do the pose on the right side:

> Stand in Utthita Hasta Padasana, interlock the fingers or hold a block. Stretch the arms upward.

> Turn the right leg out and go into the pose. ❶

> Make sure that when releasing the right buttock down you are not shortening the trunk. Keep extending the arms upward to keep the length of the spine and the lift of the chest.

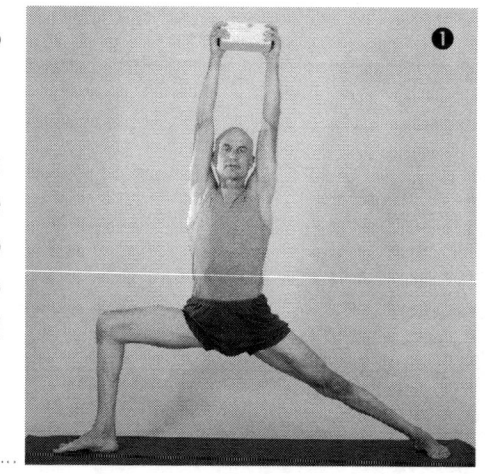

Photos ❷-❺ illustrate how to apply four variations that were shown for Utthita Trikonasana for this pose.

In ❸ the pose is done with back against the wall.

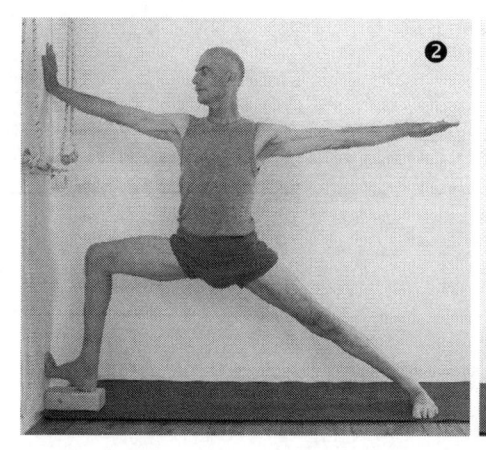

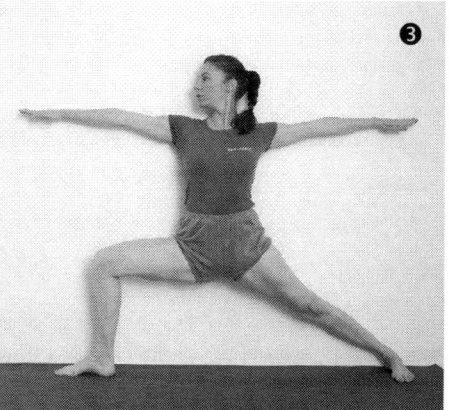

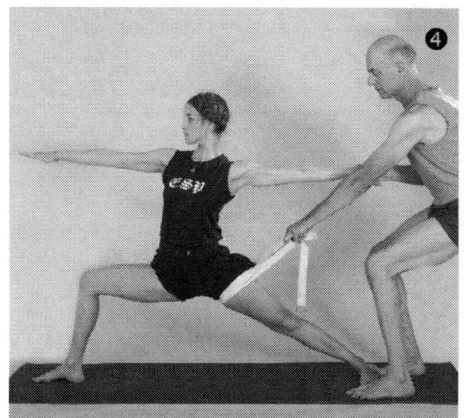

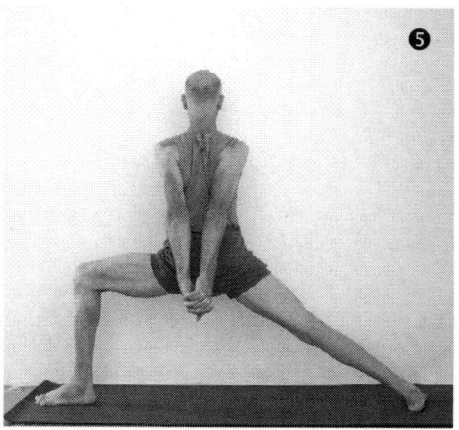

102 Props for Yoga / Chapter 1 / Virabhadrasana II

Virabhadrasana I
About Virabhdrasana I

In Virabhadrasana I, the body turns 90º sideways. The back leg is the anchor of the pose; it should be strong and stable. At the same time, the trunk should be lifted upward and moved forward from its base. The pose stretches the muscles connecting the trunk with the back leg. Often these muscles are tight. As a result the spine is pulled by the back leg and the lower back is compressed. Virabhadrasana I prepares for back bends because it extends the muscles of the back leg; once you get sufficient length in those critical muscles, your back will be less vulnerable. B.K.S. Iyengar used to say mastering Virabhadra I is a key to understanding back bends. Remember that back bends are very healthy for the back, provided you bend from the right place.

Tips

✓ Virabhadrasana I is a challenging pose. Often students ask: "What is more important: to keep the heel of the back leg on the floor or to turn the pelvis 90º sideways?" My response is that every stretch involves pulling between two ends. Ultimately, the stretch is achieved by insisting on pressing the heel down while turning the pelvis – when you give up one, the stretch is lost and the pose will never improve. There are no shortcuts! Progress is achieved with persistence, judicious effort and….a lot of patience! However, in the learning stages, you can choose to concentrate on one of these two actions.

⚠ CAUTIONS

Do not practice this asana if you have high blood pressure or a cardiac condition.

Turning Sideways

In Virabhadrasana I one should turn the body so that the two sides of the pelvis are aligned; this means that both are equidistant from the wall you are facing. Often this turning is taught first in Parsvottanasana. In Virabhadrasana I however, the challenge is greater since the legs are spread wider apart and the front knee is bent. The following variations help to turn the back leg and the trunk in Virabhadrasana I.

Virabhadrasana I
Variation 1a

Learning the sideways orientation: Entering by stepping back

Props
slanting plank

In this variation enter the pose by taking one leg backward.

⟶ To do the pose on the right side:

› Stand in Tadasana near the front edge of the mat, place the hands on the hips, move the elbows back and place the thumbs close to the tailbone and the fingers on the buttocks.

› Keeping the body facing the front, take the left leg far back. Do not allow the left side of the pelvis to move back. Use your hands to check this and keep both sides of the pelvis facing forward ❶.

› Use your thumbs to stick the tailbone in, and your fingers to extend the gluteus (buttocks) muscles downward and broaden the left buttock outward (away from the tailbone).

› Keep the fingers on the hips when bending the right leg to form a square. Sense with the fingers the position of the tailbone, the buttocks and the lumbar.

› Then lift the arms up, roll the head back, look up and stay in the pose for a while.

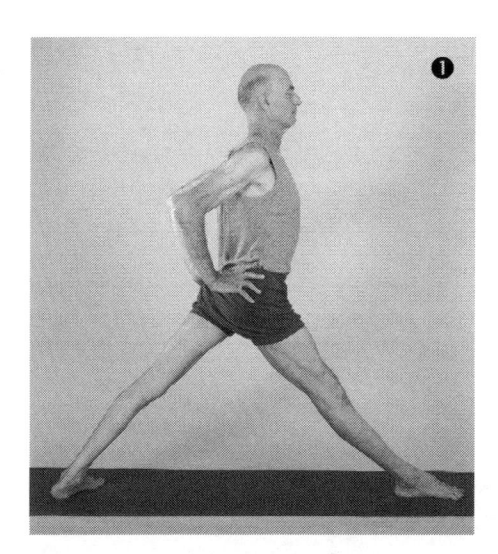

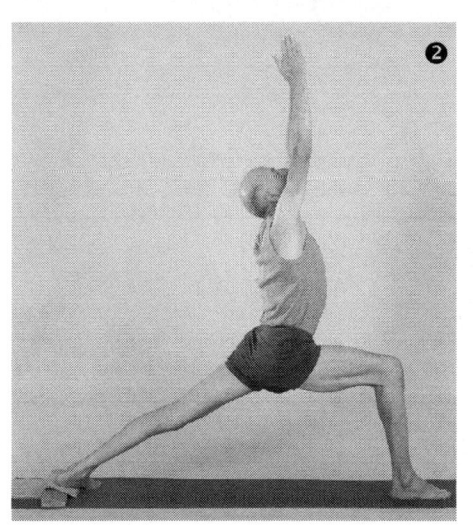

Effects
In entering the pose this way you do not need to turn the body sideways – your initial position is already facing the side; all you have to do is to retain this orientation when stepping back. This is easier than turning sideways with spread legs, as required in the classic pose. You can experience the full turning that is required in the final pose.

Note: In order to activate the heel of the back leg, you can use a plank placed under the heel and press against it ❷.

Tips
✓ Imagine that your two ilium crests (on two front sides of the pelvic bone) are the front lights of a car. Work your body such that the light beams will continue to project directly forward on the road ahead of you, even after you have taken your leg back. Resist the tendency of the ilium bones to tilt down and to the back leg side.

Applicability
Parsvottanasana.

104 Props for Yoga / Chapter 1 / Virabhadrasana I

Virabhadrasana I
Variation 1b

Turning sideways: Entering from Vimanasana

→ Go to Vimanasana and check that the line of the chest and arms is parallel to the wall in front of you.

› Check also that the pelvis has turned completely and is facing the same wall.

› Then roll the shoulders and arms back, lift the arms and look up.

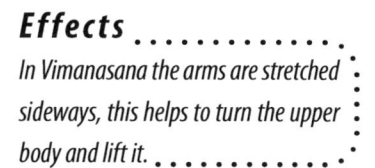

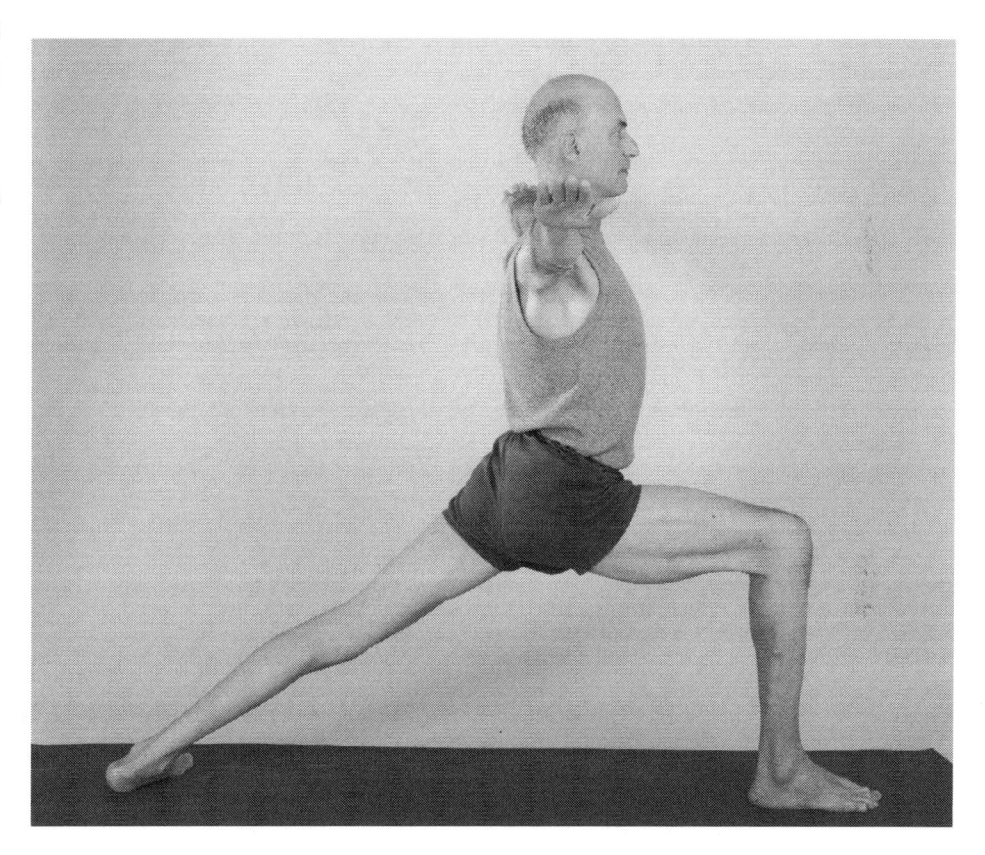

Effects
In Vimanasana the arms are stretched sideways, this helps to turn the upper body and lift it.

Tips
✓ Look at the palms to ensure that they are in line

Virabhadrasana I
Variation 2

Opening the chest:
Belt attached to the back leg

→ To do the pose on the right side:

- Tie a belt around the left groin or just above the left knee; the belt should be adjusted for inward rotation of the leg.

- Spread the legs apart; turn the left leg in and the right leg out (you can also enter the pose by stepping back as described above).

- Catch the loose end of the belt from the inner side of the leg. Pull it to turn the left thigh from outside in (outer thigh should be moving forward). ❶

- Keep stretching the belt as you bend the right leg into the pose. ❷

    Note: If the back heel cannot be held on the floor firmly, support it with a block, plank or wall, as shown in Variation 4.

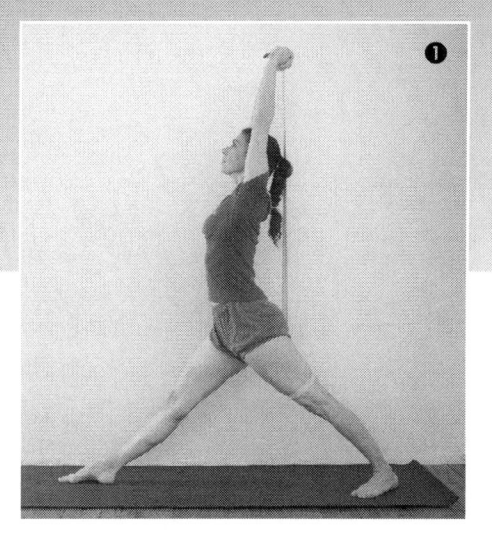

Props
belt

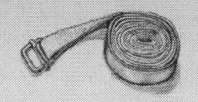

Effects
The pull of the belt helps to straighten the back leg and to turn the thigh inward. It also helps to arch the back, open the chest and stretch the arms.

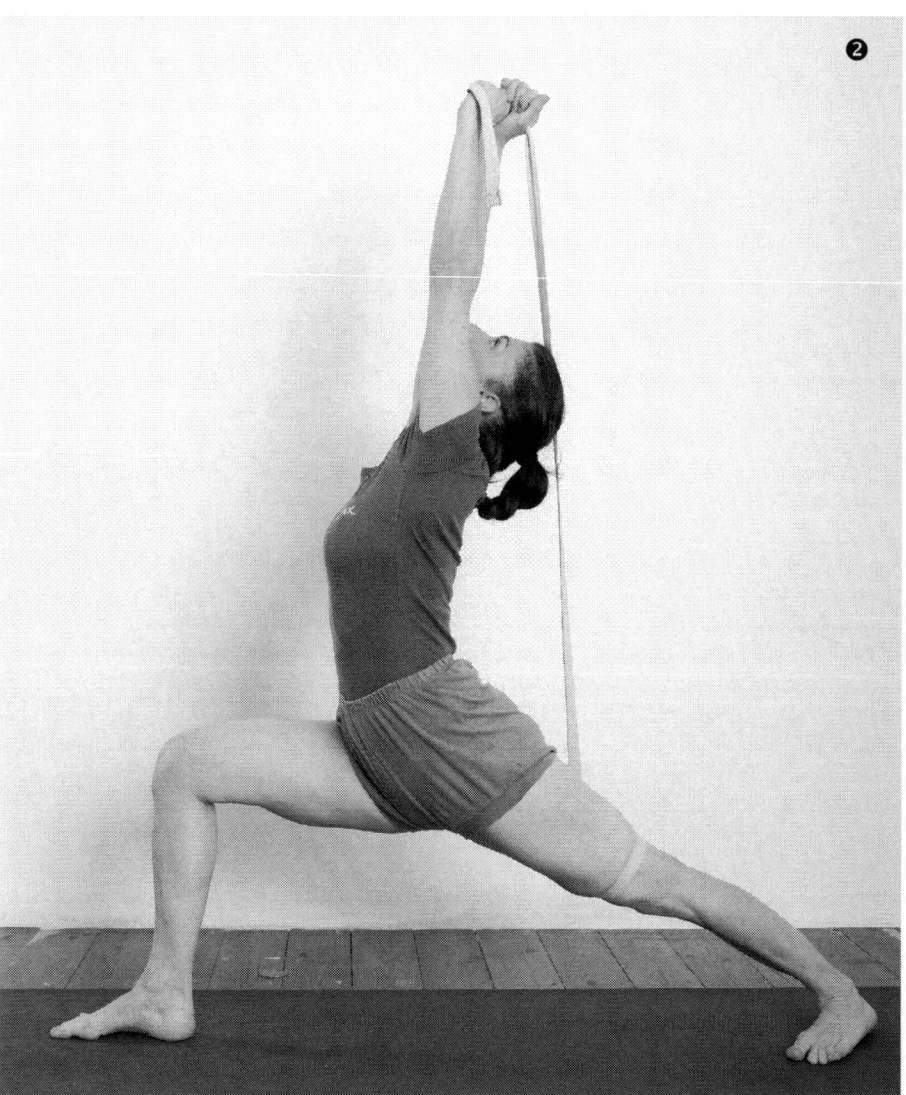

Tips
✓ Use your legs to align the pelvis: push the left hip forward and move the right outer thigh backward until the two Ilium bones are on one plane, parallel to the wall in front of you.

Applicability
Virabhadrasana III,
Parsvottanasana.

Virabhadrasana I
Variation 3

Arching back: Hands against the wall

Props
wall
foam block (optional)

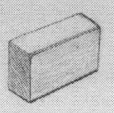

⟶ To do the pose on the right side:

> Face the wall and place the toes of the right foot against the wall.

> Move the left leg backward, keeping the pelvis and the chest aligned in parallel to the wall.

> Start bending the right leg and place the finger tips on the wall in front of you. Make sure the two hands are equidistant from your centerline.

> Press your fingertips against the wall to lift and turn the chest; roll the shoulders back, arch your neck and look upward.

> You can use a foam block to support the front knee by the wall.

Effects
The wall stabilizes the pose and gives a reference plane. It helps to move the shoulders back and to lift and turn the chest. The resistance of the wall helps to move the tailbone in.

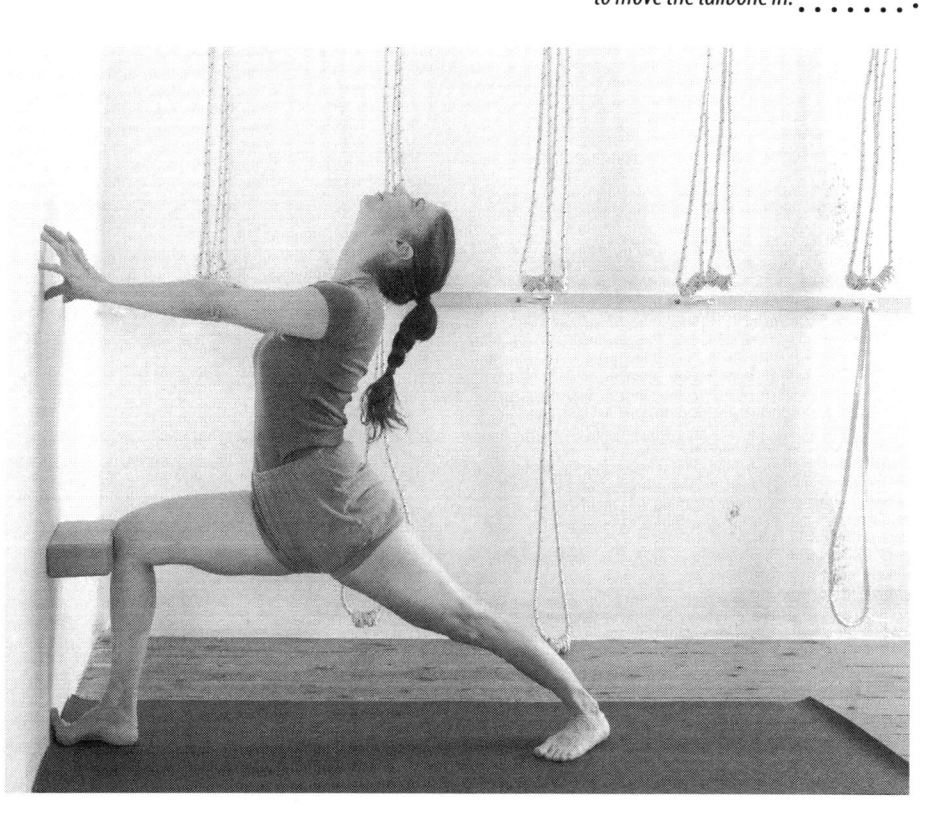

Tips

✓ Learn to move the tailbone into the pelvis, lift the lower abdomen and move the lumbar spine back (away from the wall).

✓ Before rolling the head back, lift your cheek bones and by this action, lift the sternum further and extend the neck. Then roll the head and mentally observe the middle of your back. Soften the eyes and relax the forehead.

Props for Yoga / Chapter 1 / Virabhadrasana I

Virabhadrasana I
Variation 4

Activating the back leg: Supporting the heel

Props
block
or slanting plank
or wall

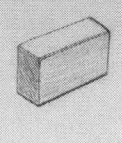

Most people find it difficult to turn the pelvis 90° and at the same time keep the back heel heavy on the floor. At the learning stage, pressing the heel against a raised surface enables one to turn the pelvis without compromising the stability of the pose (which occurs when the heel is up in the air). The choice between block or slant or wall depends on how far down one can extend the heel while keeping the frontal alignment of the pelvis.

⟹ To do the pose on the right side:

> Place the left heel on the block / wall ❶ / slant ❷.

> Step the right leg forward and bend into the pose.

> Keep stretching the back leg by press the heel down and moving the hip joint forward.

> Gradually learn to lower the heel down until you can press it into the bottom of the wall ❸.

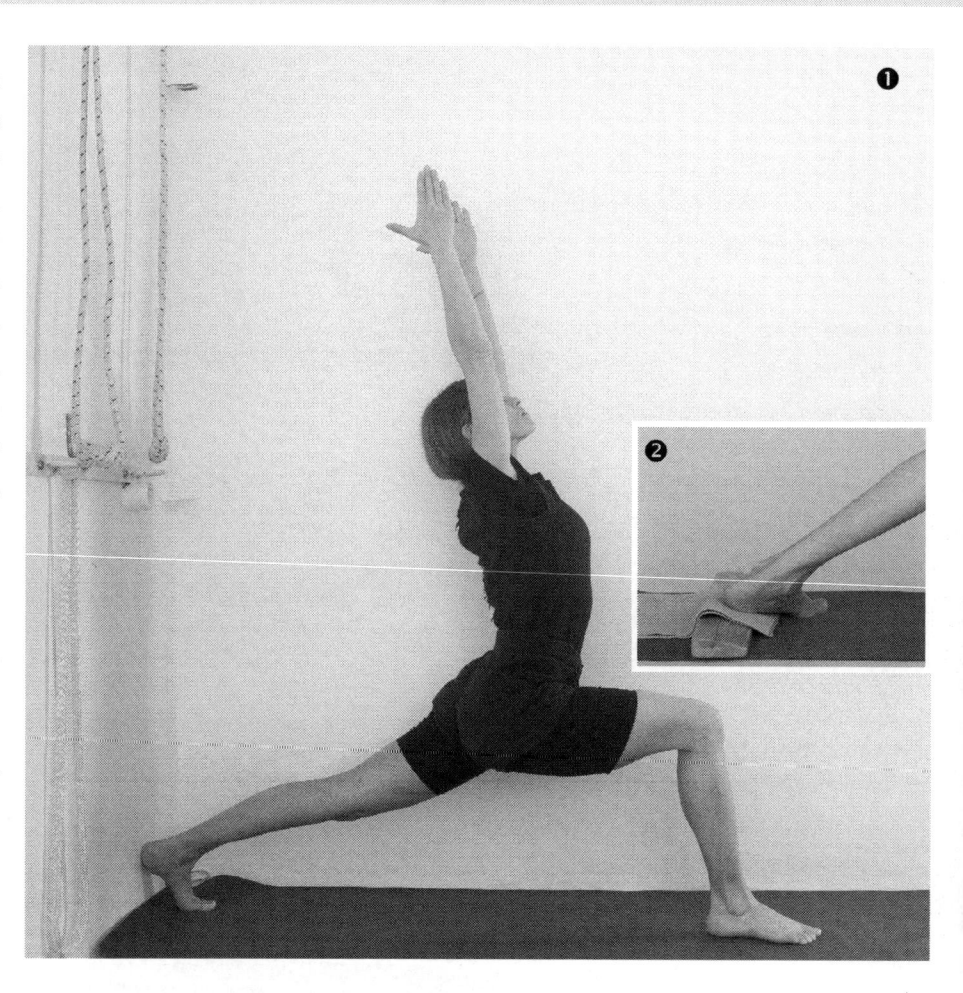

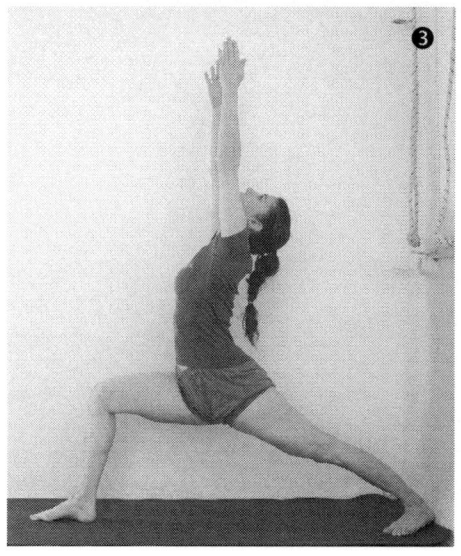

Effects

This variation is particularly helpful in intermediate stages; it allows you to rotate the pelvis while keeping the back leg stretched. The wall gives stability and helps to draw the awareness to the back leg. People suffering from lower back pain can do the pose with the heel raised against the wall as in ❶.

Virabhadrasana I
Variation 5

Reducing muscular effort: Front thigh rests on chair

Props
chair

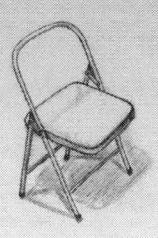

→ To use a chair on the right side:

> Stand facing the chair and insert the right leg under the backrest.

> Bend the right leg to 90º and place the buttock on the chair. If needed, place a folded blanket or foam block on the seat to adjust the height (see Virabhadrasana II on page 98).

> Lift the left heel and turn the leg and the pelvis from left to right. Move the tailbone into the pelvis.

> Move the left buttock away from the tailbone and the left front groin forward to touch the seat.

> Hold the backrest to lift the chest and bring it to the correct vertical alignment, which is directly above the pelvis and facing forward.

> Keeping the shoulder blades in, push the backrest to roll the shoulders back; then roll the head back and look up.

Note: You can also place the heel of the back leg against a wall; this helps to turn the pelvis to the front while maintaining the stretch of the back leg.

Effects

The chair bears the weight of the body and allows you to stay in the pose with reduced load. This allows working on the challenging actions of this pose, like: keeping the back leg stretched, turning the pelvis, extending the spine up and lifting the chest. Gradually, with practice, the front groins will lengthen and these rather difficult actions will become possible.

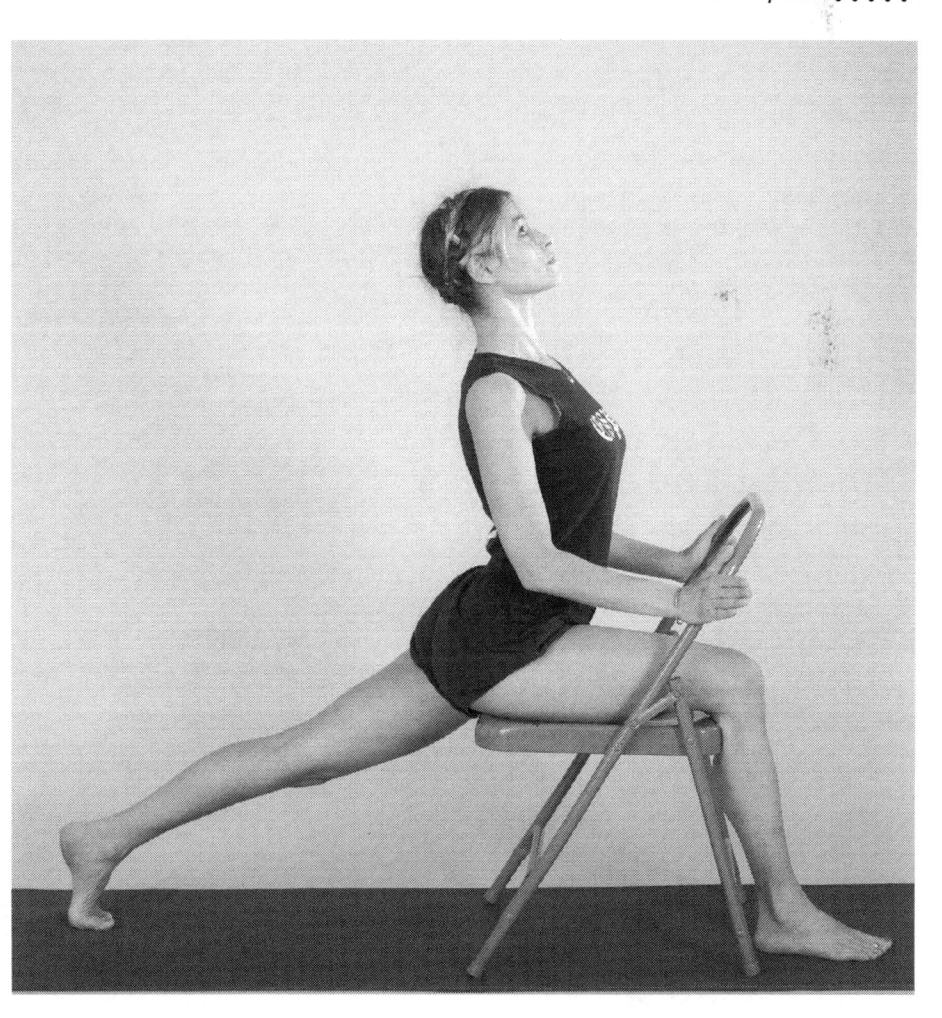

Applicability
Virabhadrasana II, Utthita and Parivrtta Parsvakonasana.

Props for Yoga / Chapter 1 / Virabhadrasana I

Virabhadrasana I
Variation 6

Moving the tailbone in: Pubic bone against a wall corner

Props
wall
or a rectangular column,
block

When bending into the pose, the pelvis should move forward from its base; this means that the forward movement should start from the tailbone; the spine and the pubic bone should move forward and up. To better feel the position of the pubic bone you can use a wall edge or a rectangular column.

⟶ To do the pose on the right side:

> Stand facing the wall edge (or column); Align the inner right groin with the right side of the wall.

> Place a block to support the heel of the left (back) leg.

> Move the right leg forward and touch the wall with the inner right leg. Move the left leg backward, stretch it and press the heel down onto the block.

> Bend into the pose, pressing your inner right thigh against the outer plane of the wall, as you slide along it. Keep moving the tailbone forward so as to touch the wall with the left side of the pubic bone.

Effects
this is a challenging variation; it really makes you move the pelvis from the tailbone and teaches how much the pubic bone should move forward and up. It also enables you to check if the pelvis and the abdomen have been sufficiently rotated.

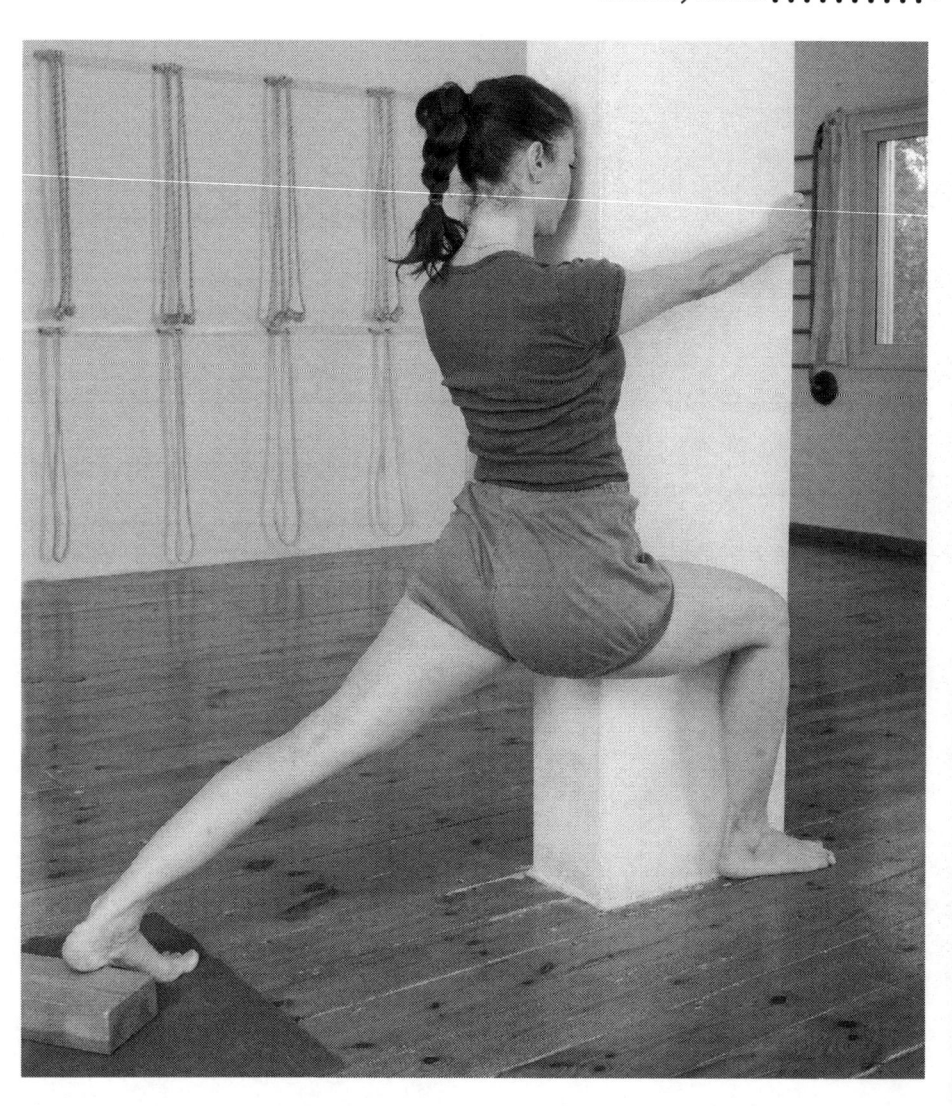

Tips
✓ Once the action is learnt, try to do it without the support for the back heel.

Virabhadrasana I
Variation 7

Experiencing lightness: Helpers lift the groins

Props
2 helpers
2 belts (or ropes)

While bending into Virabhadrasana I, it is important to maintain the height of the inner groins. This will enable the upper body to extend up more freely. This lifting action can be learnt while working with two helpers (instruction for the helpers):

→ Place a belt (or rope) on each inner groin of the practitioner and pull up and sideways.

› When the practitioner bends the front leg, allow him to descend, but keep pulling to resist gravity and to help lift the groins.

Note: The helpers should balance their pull to the sides.

› After a while, release the belt and let the practitioner stay in the pose on his own for a while.

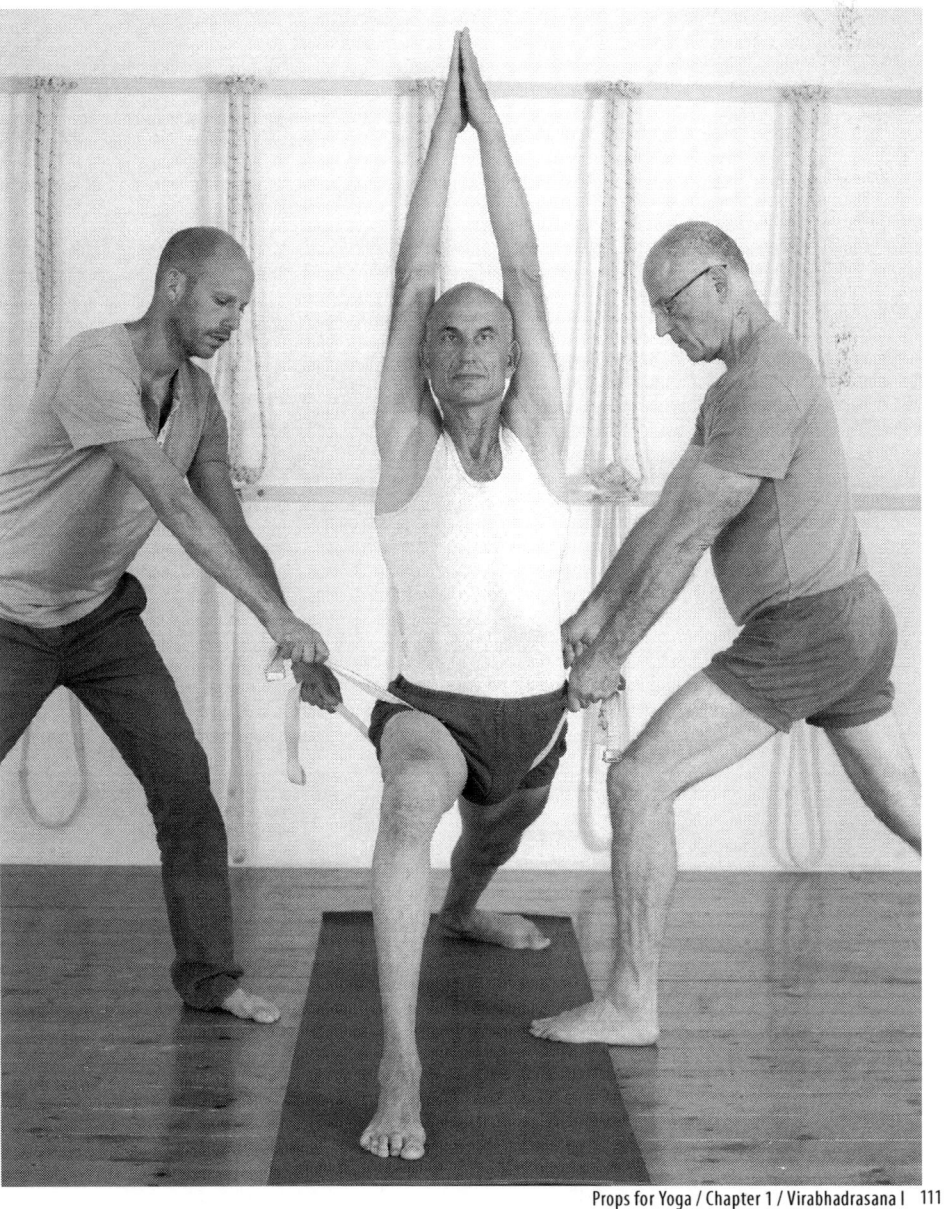

Effects

In Virabhadrasana I, the abdominal organs tend to drop, especially in the back leg side. Pulling the ropes helps to lift the trunk from the groins so that the organs are kept in place and remain soft. The pose becomes almost effortless. This feeling of lifting from the base of the trunk will guide you when doing the pose on your own.

Upper Body

In Virabhadrasana I one must use the arms for lifting the trunk and open the chest. This prevents pressure on the lower back and helps the breathing while maintaining the pose. Here are some variations to strengthen the arms and help in arching the upper body.

Virabhadrasana I
Variation 8

Activating the arms:
Belt around the elbows

Props
belt

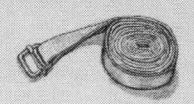

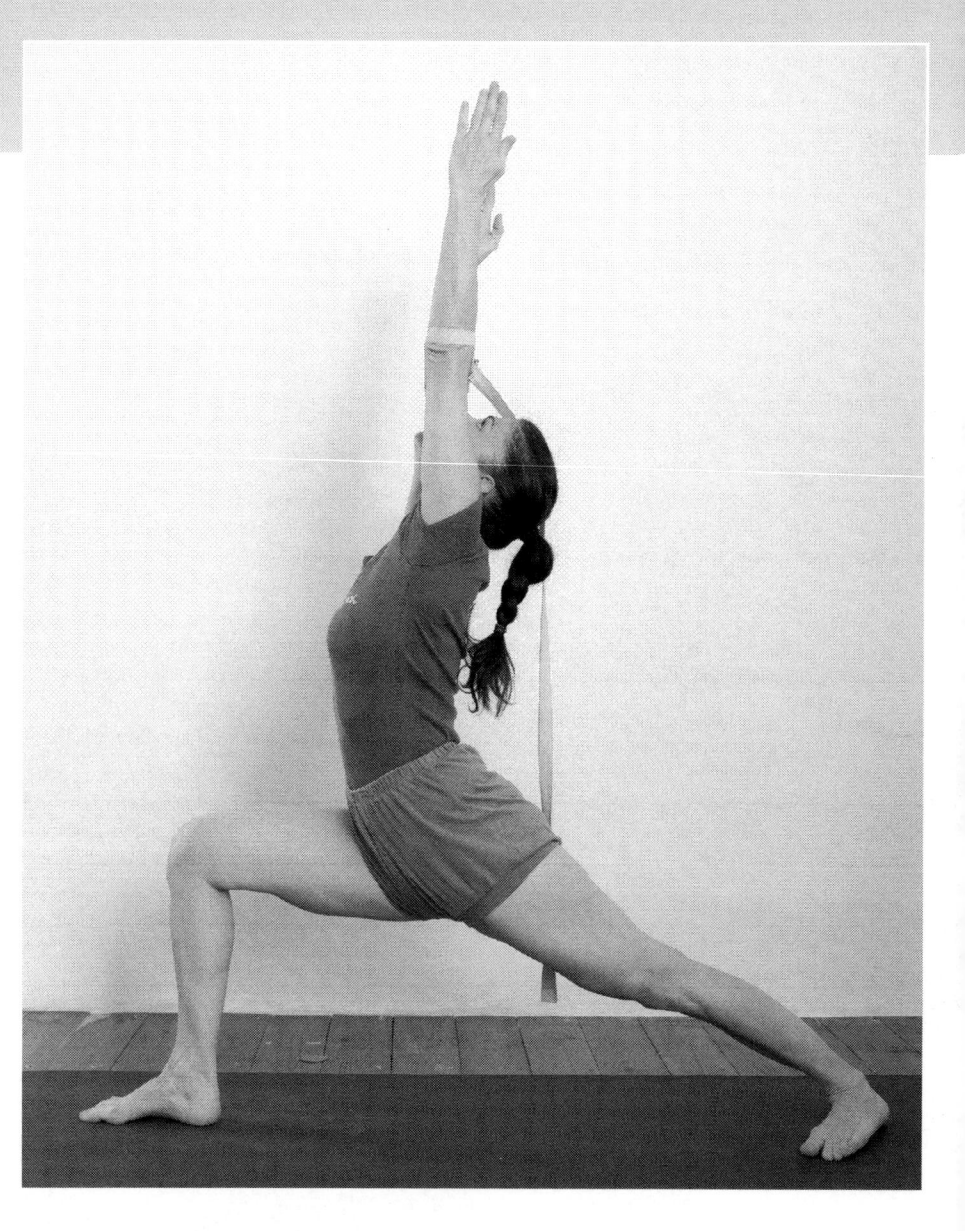

⟶ To do the pose on the right side:

› Spread your legs. Loop a belt around the elbows and set it to shoulder width.

› Lift the arms and press the bones of the outer elbows outward to stretch the belt. Extend the inner arms up from shoulders to palms.

› Turn to the right and bend the right leg to Virabhadrasana I.

Effects
the resistance of the belt helps to stretch the arms up. This variation is especially effective for people who find it hard to straighten the elbows, roll the shoulders back and/or to tuck the shoulder blades in. It is also beneficial for people whose arms are weak.

Applicability
Virabhadrasana II (when practiced with the arms stretched up), Virabhadrasana III.

Virabhadrasana I
Variation 9

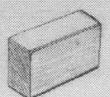

Activating the arms: Holding a block

Props
block

→ Hold a block between the bases of your palms (refer to Urdhva Hastasana on page 21).

> Spread the legs, lift the arms and press the bases of the palms against the block.

> As you bend into Virabhadrasana I, keep lifting the block.

Note: it is often beneficial to combine the above two variations: holding a block with a belt around the elbows.

Effects
Pressing against the block strengthens the arms; it also stabilizes the shoulders and helps to stretch the arms.

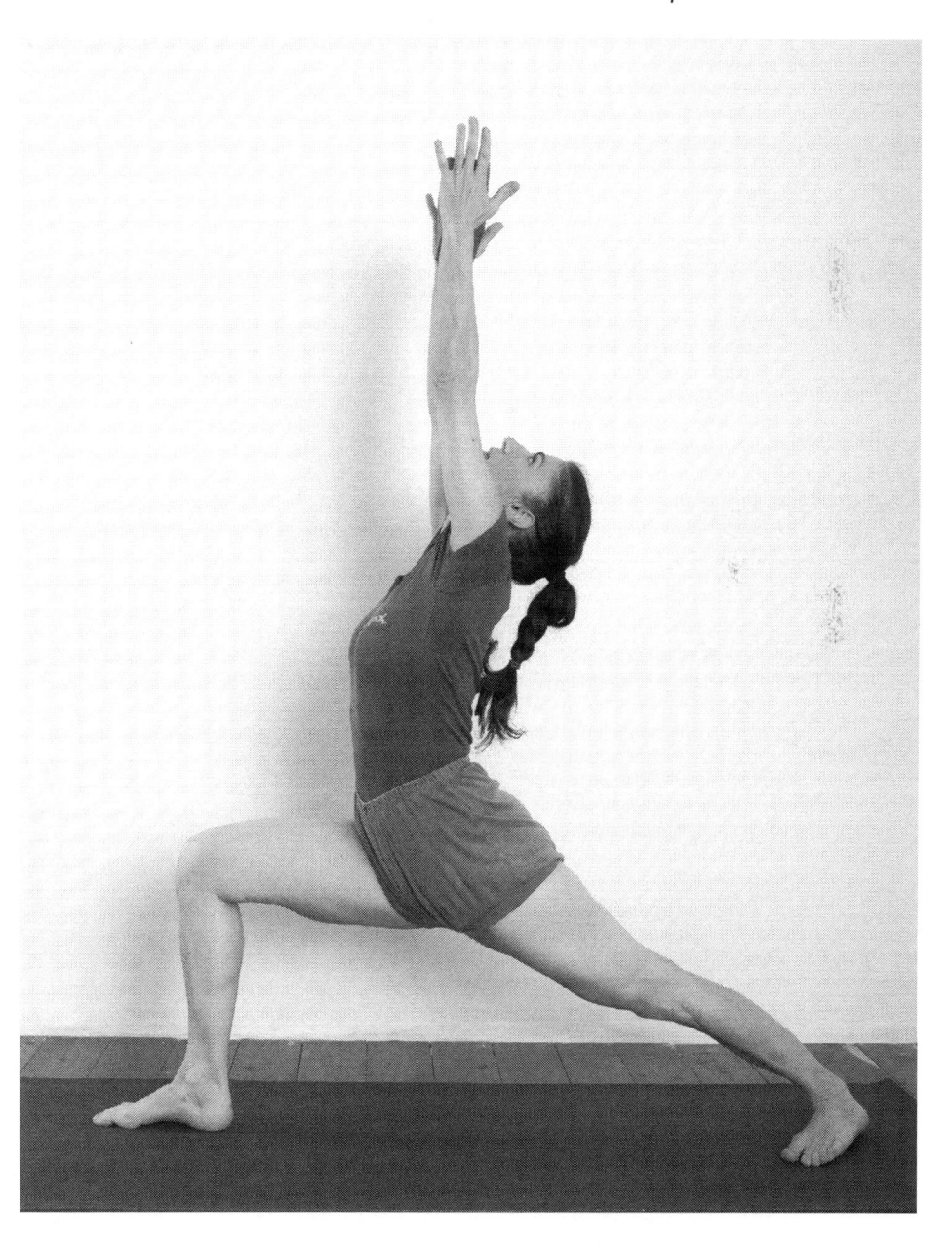

Applicability
Virabhadrasana II (when practiced with the arms stretched up), Virabhadrasana III.

Virabhadrasana I
Variation 10

Stretching upward: Holding a ceiling rope

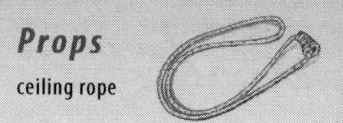

Props
ceiling rope

→ To do the pose on the right side:

> Stand under a ceiling rope. Move the right leg forward and the left leg backward.

> Make sure the center of your trunk is positioned directly below the rope. Lift the heels slightly and catch the rope high up. Keep holding the rope as you lower the heels back to the floor – this will give you the initial upward stretch.

> Now bend the right leg into the pose and simultaneously slide the left leg backward. As your buttock goes down, let your hands slide down the rope while you maintain a slight grip.

> Roll the shoulders back, tuck the shoulder blades in and look up.

> When you reach the final pose, keep pulling the rope to lift the trunk.

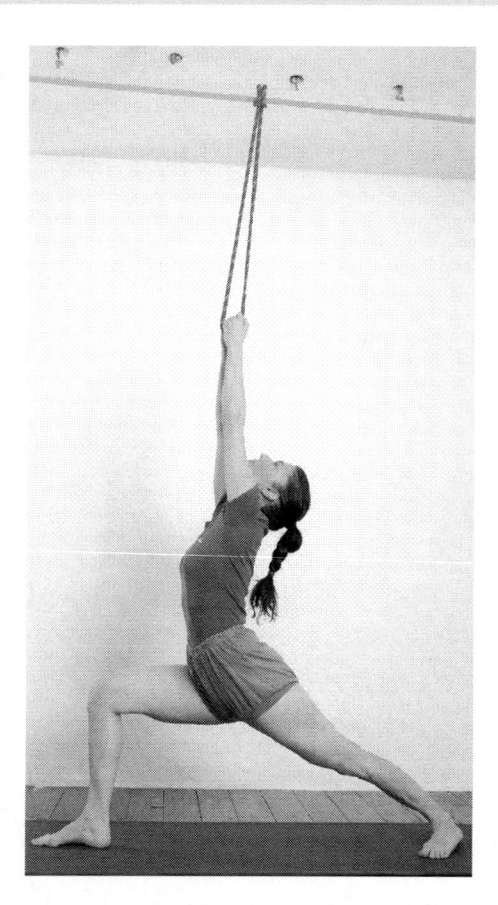

Effects

This is a wonderful way to do the pose with tremendous length in the spine and opening of the chest. It is strongly recommended for people suffering from lower back pain and it is a good way to do the pose during pregnancy. The chest is fully lifted and opened which facilitates smoother and fuller breathing.

Applicability

Urdhva Hastasana (see page 23) and Vrksasana (see page 28).

Virabhadrasana I
Variation 11

Moving the thoracic vertebrae in: Arms behind the back

⟶ Do the pose with palms joined behind the back (Paschima Namaskarasana). Other options are to interlock the arms as in Gomukhasana, to hold arms behind the back at the elbows (Paschima Baddha Hasta) or to interlock fingers behind the back (Paschima Baddhanguliyasana) (see Utthita Trikonasana on page 93 for the various arm positions).

Effects
Moving the arms behind the back helps to roll the shoulders back, tuck the shoulder blades in and move the thoracic dorsal spine into the chest. These actions open the chest. Also, these variations stabilize the arms so that one can concentrate on the actions of the legs and the pelvic region.

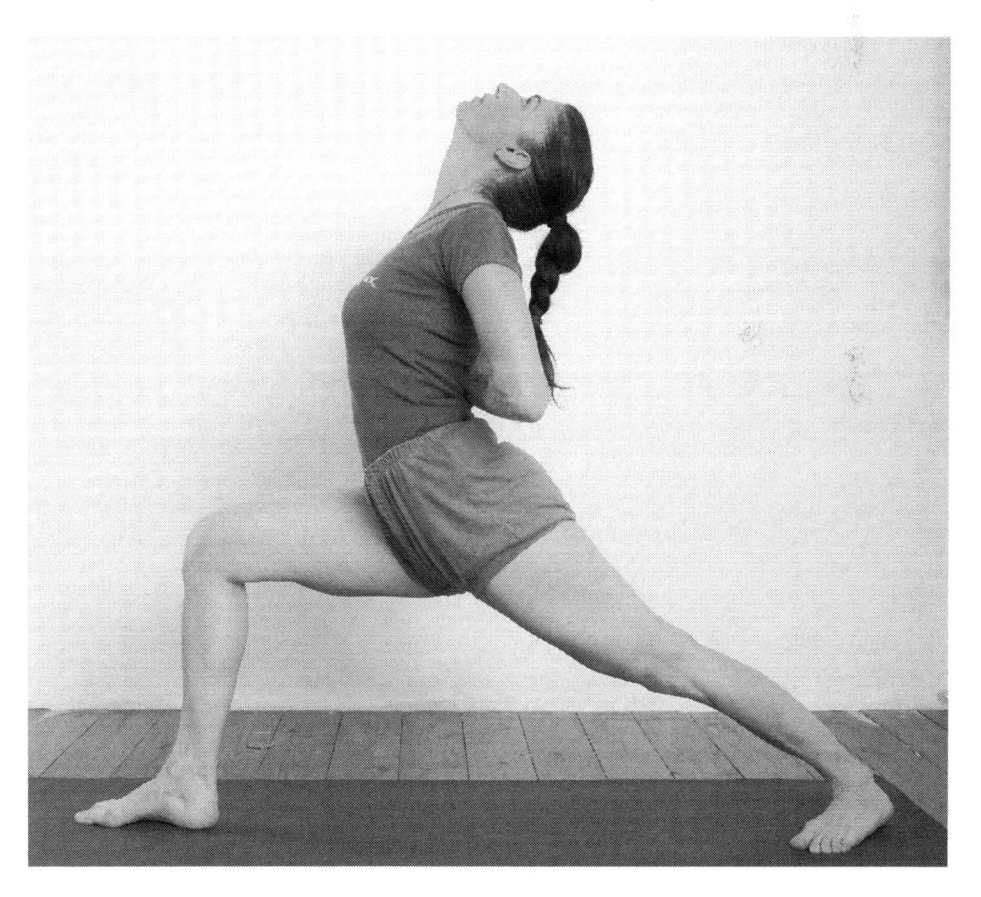

Applicability
Most standing poses.

Virabhadrasana III

This pose requires balance and strength. Following are a number of variations that develop the body and prepare it for the independent performance of this challenging pose.

Tips

✓ Imagine you are doing the pose in water and the water level is at the height of your front groins. When you enter the pose just lie on that water and imagine that your abdomen is floating on it. Move the shoulders blade in as if you wish to dip your chest slightly in the water. Extend and lift the triceps and look forward above the water level. With this image, even Virabhadrasana III can become a meditative pose!

Virabhadrasana III
Variation 1

Learning to balance: Supporting the hands

Props
wall
chair or partner

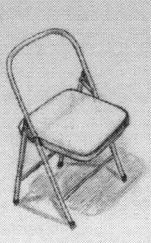

The first challenge of Virabhadrasana III is to balance on one foot. Supporting the hands on a wall is a simple way to learn to balance. It also helps to strengthen the standing leg and stretch the lifted leg.

⟶ To do the pose on the right side:

> Do Ardha (half) Uttanasana, placing the fingertips on the wall at pelvis height. ❶

> Lift the left leg and stretch it straight back. The lift should originate at the hip joint. Keep both sides of the pelvis at the same level.

> Rotate the left thigh from outside in. Broaden the left gluteus (buttock) muscle away from the sacrum and extend it back towards the heel.

> Extend the inner left leg from the groin to the inner heel and keep it parallel to the floor.

> In the right (standing) leg: Move the front thigh muscle back (into the bone); tighten and lift the outer thigh.

> Draw the shoulder blades in and look forward at the wall ❷.

> forearms on the backrest of a chair ❷ (or by holding a firm bar or a trestler - if available).

> After a while move the fingers slightly away from the wall and balance in the pose.

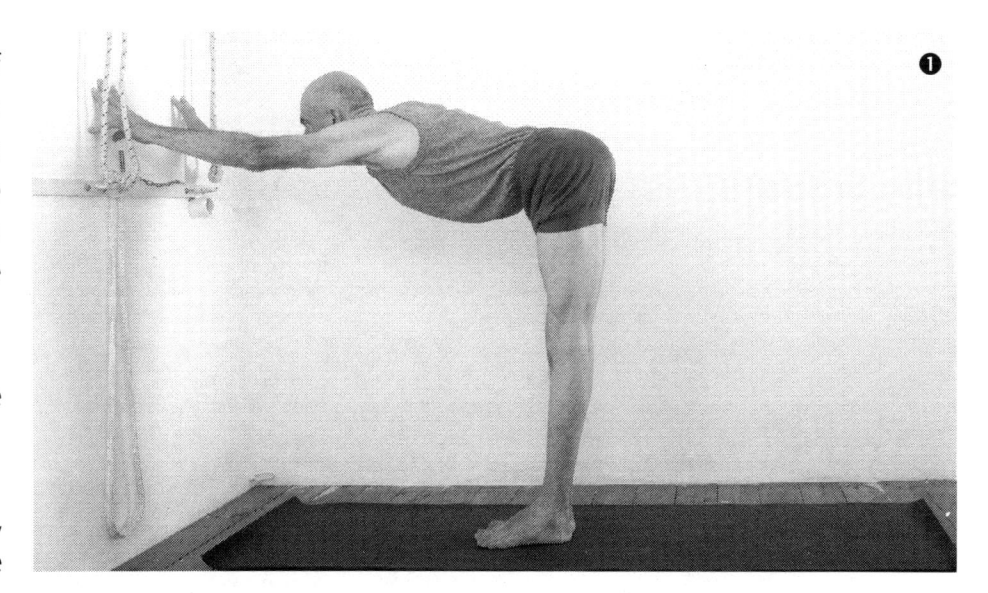

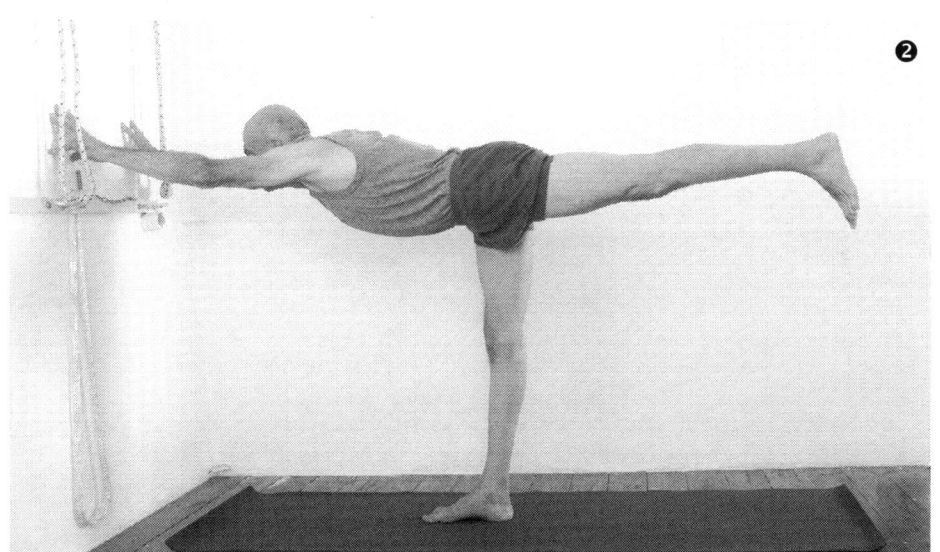

Effects

This variation strengthens the legs and helps to learn the correct alignment of the lower body. The wall support provides stability, enabling one to balance easily and concentrate on the actions of the legs and pelvis.

Virabhadrasana III
Variation 1 (cont.)

Learning to balance: Supporting the hands

Props
wall
chair or partner

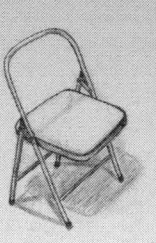

A similar version of the pose can be done by placing the outer wrists or forearms on the backrest of a chair ❸ (or by holding a firm bar or a trestler - if available).

> Once you are in the pose lift the arms off the chair and balance.

It can also be done with the help of a partner ❹.

> Partner: Once you sense that the practitioner is stable, gradually reduce the support you provide; if the practitioner is ready, let him/her balance on their own.

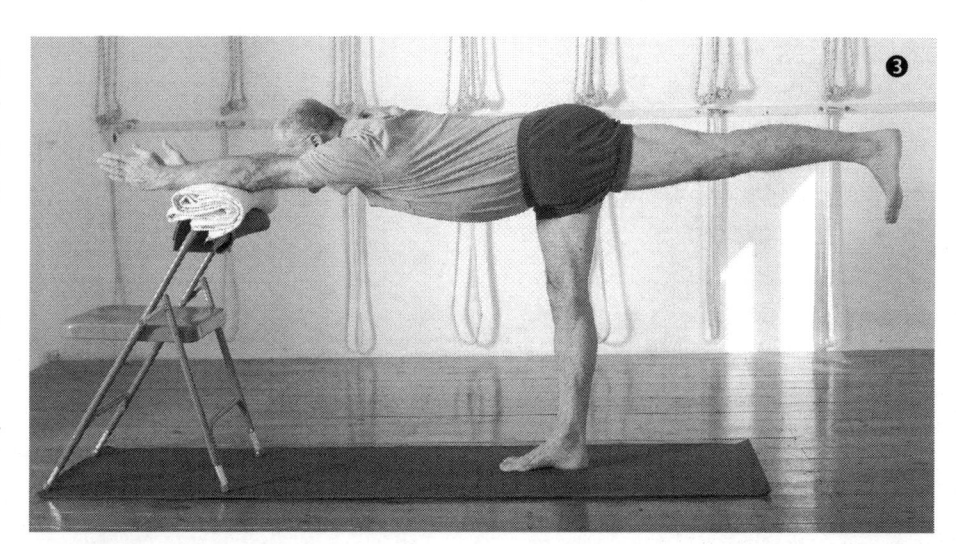

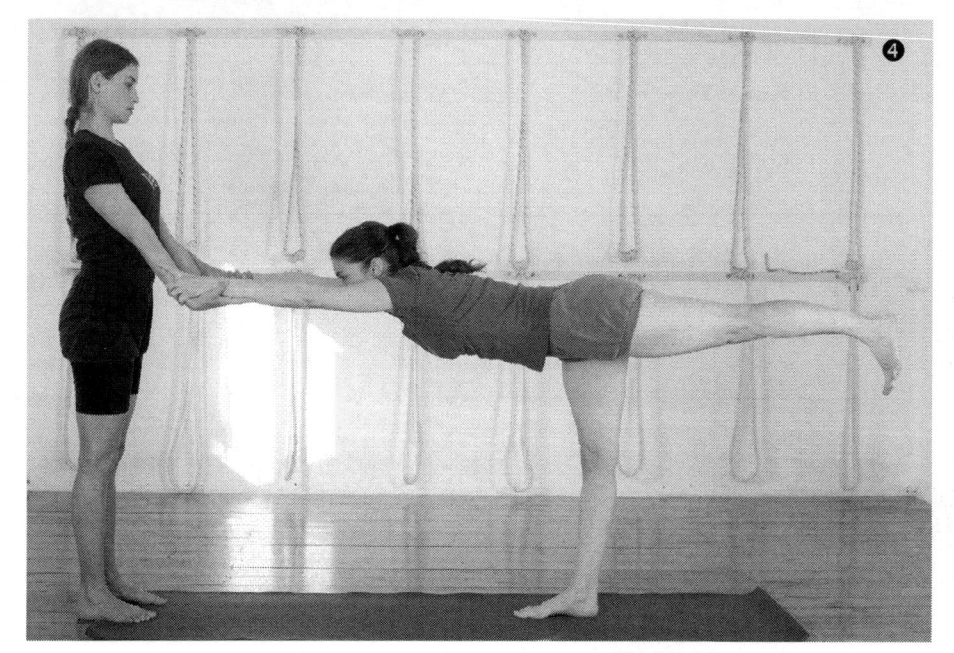

Tips

✓ In Virabhadrasana III most of the body is not in the field of vision, hence it is difficult to assess the alignment. A partner can check your alignment and guide you; for example he/she can move the lifted leg to its correct position, help you to find the correct alignment of the pelvis, to extend the buttock of the lifted leg and so on.

Virabhadrasana III
Variation 2

Horizontal alignment: Supporting the pelvis with a chair

Props
chair
blankets (optional)
wall

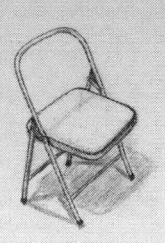

Achieving and maintaining the alignment of the pelvis in Virabhadrasana III is a great challenge. Supporting the pelvis provides stability and orientation.

⟹ To do the pose on the right side:

> Place the chair with its backrest toward you, touching the front groins.

>> *Note:* If the top of the backrest is lower than your front groins, put on it one or more blankets to make it higher.

> Lean forward to rest your pelvic bone on the back rest and hold the seat.

> Extend the arms forward.

> Lift the left leg and extend it backward.

> You can combine this variation with the previous one and put the hands against the wall ❶, or other suitable support.

>> *Note:* Tall people may prefer to use the chair in folded position in order to increase the height of the support ❷. If the chair tends to unfold, tie a belt around the legs of the chair to prevent it from opening under the body pressure.

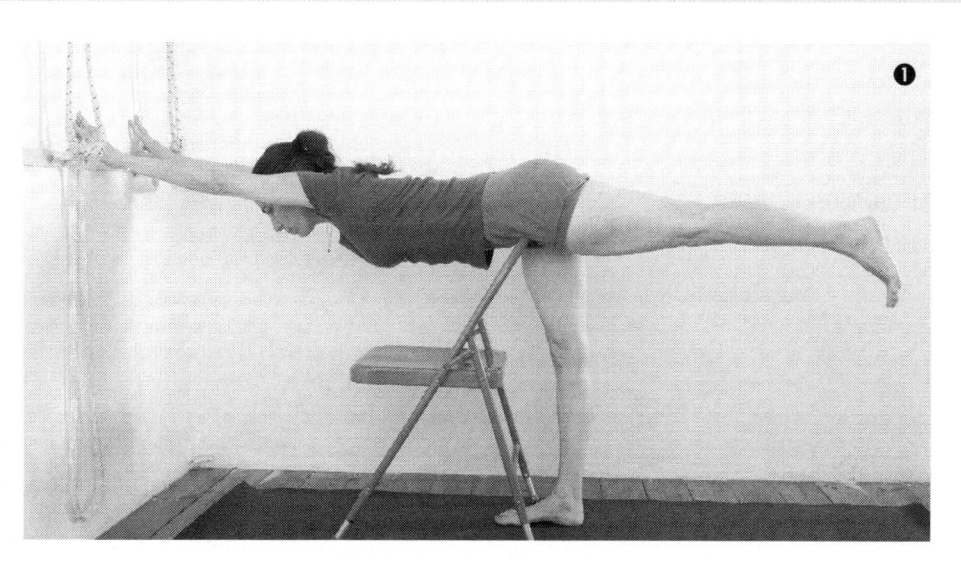

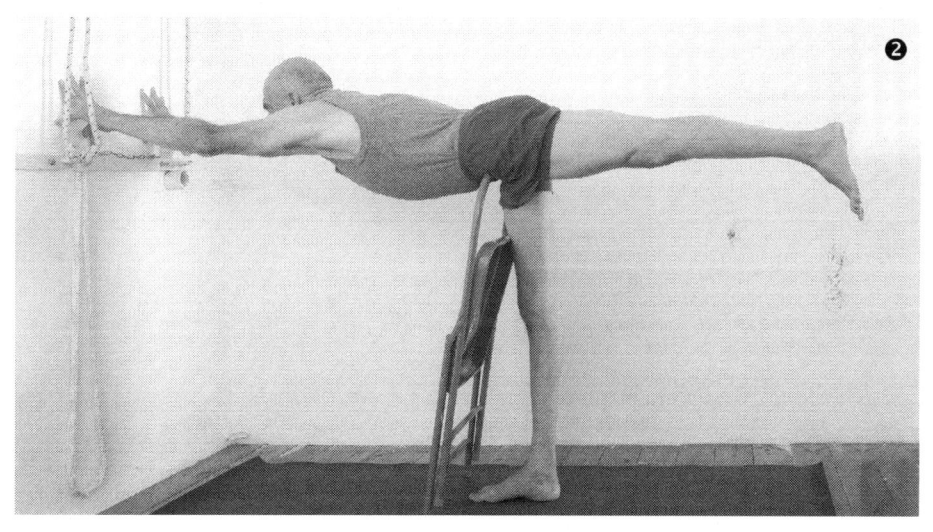

Tips
✓ The buttock of the lifted leg tends to contract and to roll upward. Learn to extend it toward the heel and to broaden it away from the tailbone.

Effects
The touch of the backrest tells you if both sides of the pelvis are level. It also supports the whole pose; with the addition of a wall to support the hands, the pose becomes restorative.

Applicability
Parsvottanasana

Virabhadrasana III
Variation 3

Props
2 blocks

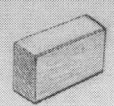

Aligning the back (lifted) leg: Hands on blocks

This is a more advanced preparation for the pose. It enables you to check the pelvic alignment. To do the pose on the right side:

⟹ Place two blocks in front of you, bend forward to Ardha Uttanasana and place the palms on the blocks. The blocks should be placed exactly below your shoulders ❶.

❯ Lower your head and lift the left leg. Look under the body at the left leg and check that
- It is parallel to the floor
- Its front thigh and toes are facing down.

❯ Check that both sides of the pelvis are at the same height.

❯ Now, lift the head and the arms and join the palms in front of the chest in Namaskar Mudra ❷.

❯ Then stretch the arms forward into the pose ❸. To maintain balance, emphasize the stretch of the left leg.

Effects
The support for the hands allows concentrating on the positioning and the stretch of the lifted leg.

Tips on the Back leg of Virabhadra III

✓ Lift the back leg from the thigh and make its ankle very heavy.

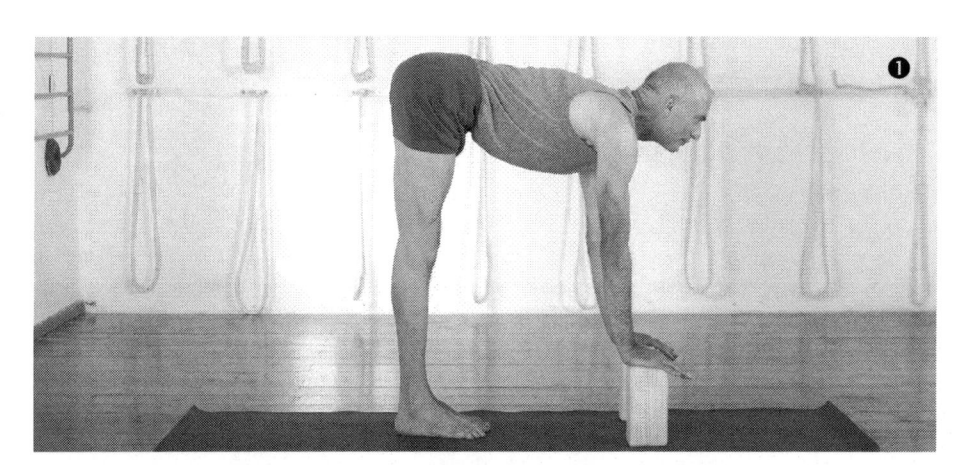

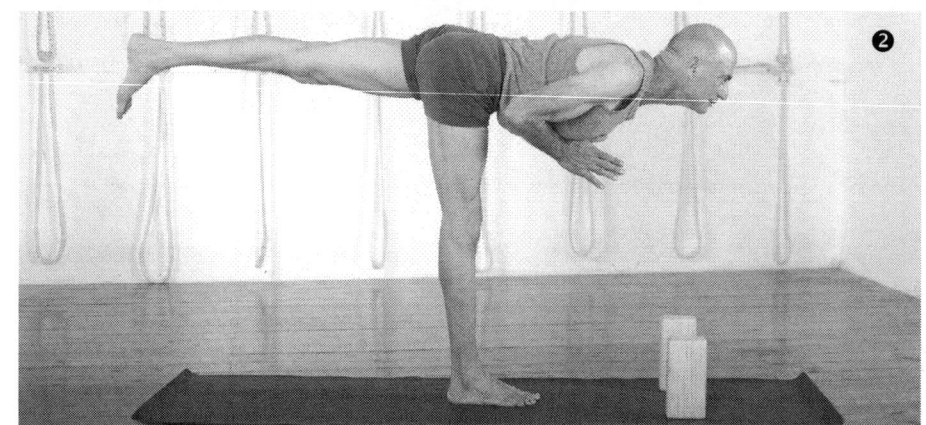

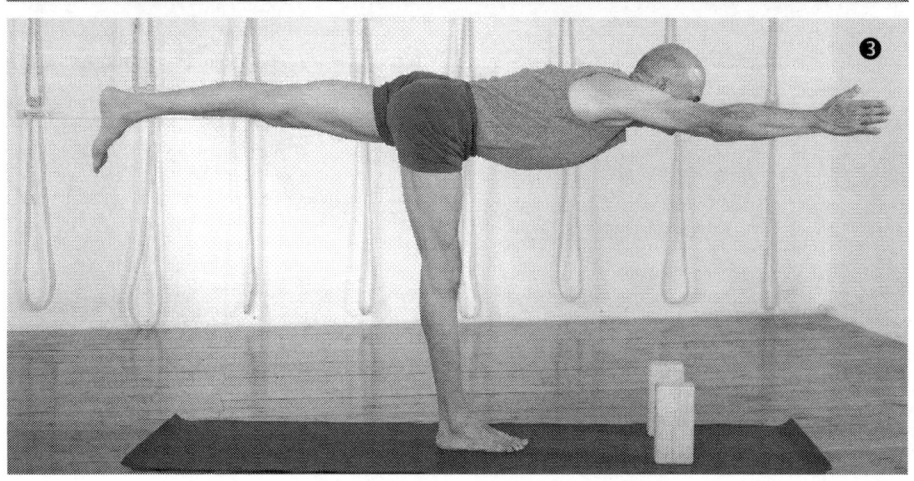

✓ Focus on the arch of the foot! Stretch the sole from the middle of the arch forward to the toes and backward to the heel. This will keep the back leg active, and will help you balance.

✓ As long as you are focused on the arch of the back foot you will not lose your balance. Note how the minute your mind wanders away from it, balance is lost!

If you find it difficult to balance, use the wall to support the back leg:

› Stand in Ardha Uttanasana with the palms on blocks and your back to the wall.

› Lift the left leg to Virabhadrasana III as described above and place its foot against the wall. Adjust the distance from the wall such that the standing leg is vertical when the back foot rests on the wall.

› Check that the trunk is parallel to the floor then raise the upper body and stretch into the pose ❹.

› Try to lift the hands and stretch them forward (be playful about losing balance. Learn from it!)

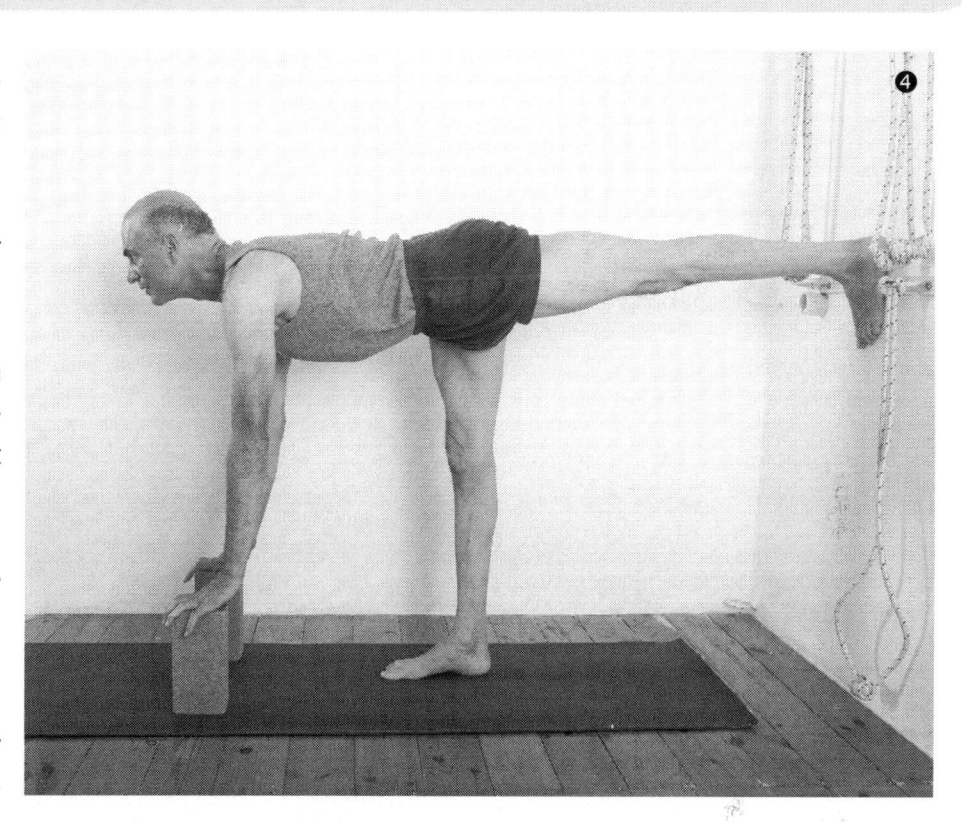

Tips

✓ Usually props help us to do the poses, but sometimes they can be used to make the pose even harder! By failing you may learn more than by succeeding. Attempting to stretch the arms forward clarifies the action of the standing leg: the front thigh of the standing leg should push strongly backward while its outer thigh should be tightened and lifted. You can learn these actions even if you fail to hold the pose with the lifted leg against the wall.

Virabhadrasana III
Variation 4

Props
belt

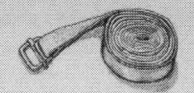

Compacting the standing leg: Belt from foot to pelvis

⟶ To do the pose on the right side:

› Loop a belt around the heel of the standing leg and the pelvis. Bend the leg and tighten the belt ❶.

> *Note:* Follow the instructions given for Variation 6 of Uttanasana on page 61, but place only around the heel of the right leg.

› Enter the pose From Ardha Uttanasana as shown in the previous variation.

› Lift the left leg to Virabhadrasana III ❷.

Effects
The belt creates compactness in the leg and pelvis. It also helps to stabilize the standing leg and maintain the balance.

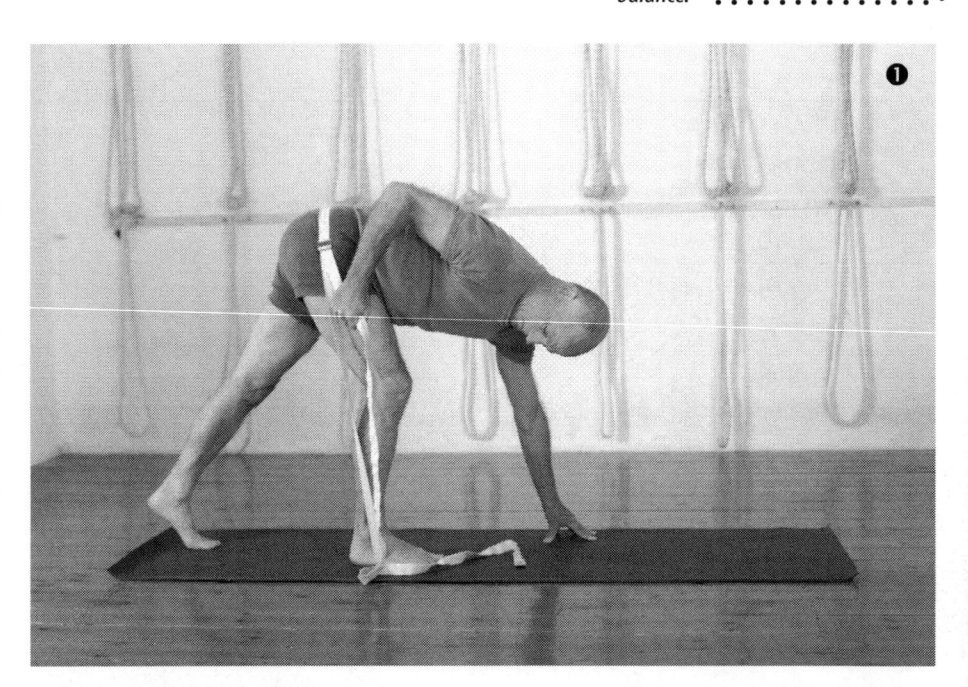

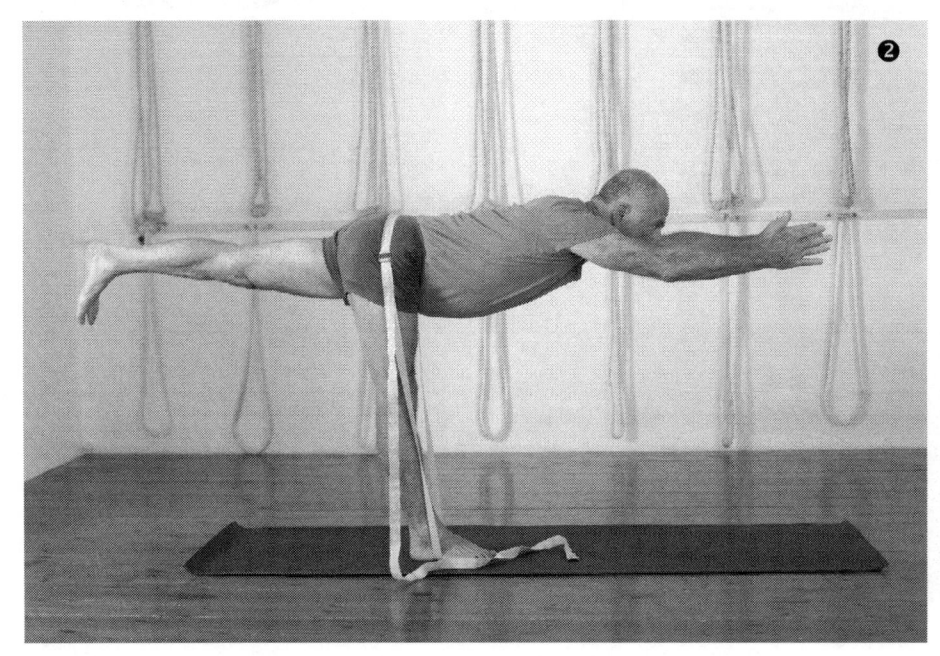

122 Props for Yoga / Chapter 1 / Virabhadrasana III

Virabhadrasana III
Variation 5

Learning to stretch horizontally: Entering from Urdhva Hastasana

→ To do the pose on the right side:

> Stand in Tadasana and lift the arms to Urdhva Hastasana ❶.

> Now simultaneously lower the trunk and lift the left leg ❷.

> Until your body is parallel to the floor ❸.

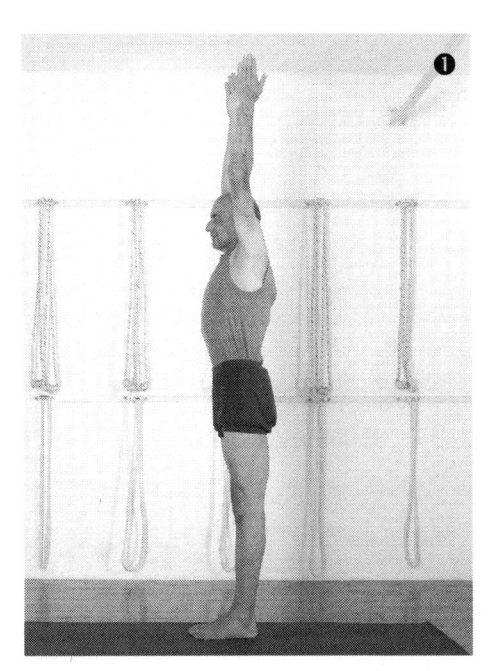

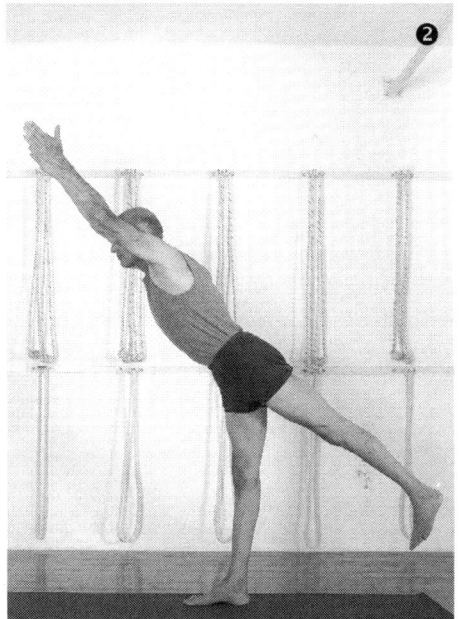

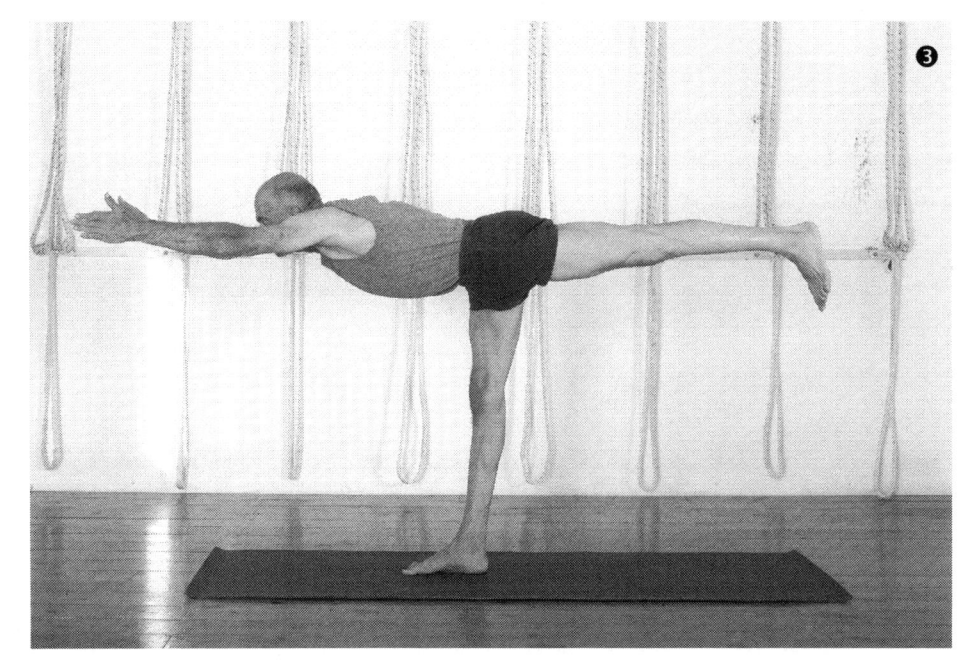

Tips

✓ Imagine there is a surface at the height of your hips (see tip on page 116) and you are just laying the body on that surface.

Props for Yoga / Chapter 1 / Virabhadrasana III   123

Virabhadrasana III
Variation 6

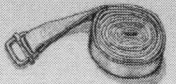

Opening the chest: Arms behind the back

Props
belt

Use the belt like in Virabhadrasana I Variation 8 on page 112.

Effects
Holding and stretching the arms behind the back helps to roll the shoulders back and open the chest; it makes the entire pose easier to hold.

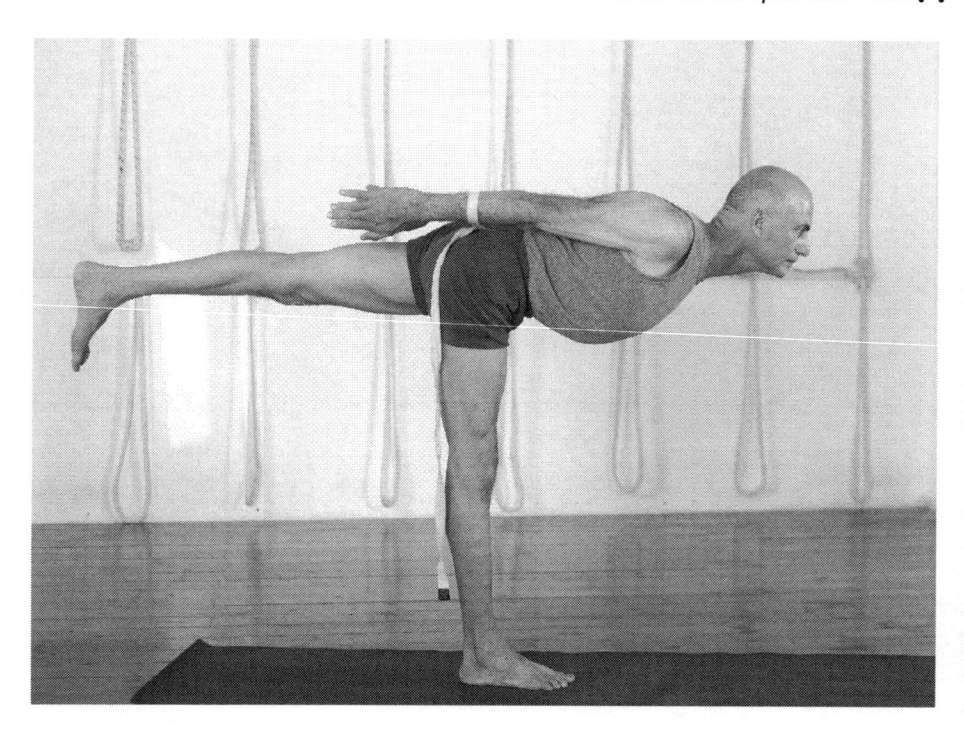

Virabhadrasana III
Variation 7

Stabilizing the pose: Belt on back leg

Props
belt

Adapt the instructions from Virabhadrasana I Variation 2 on page 106

Effects
Pulling the back leg up makes the pose much easier to hold. It also helps to roll the shoulders back and open the chest.

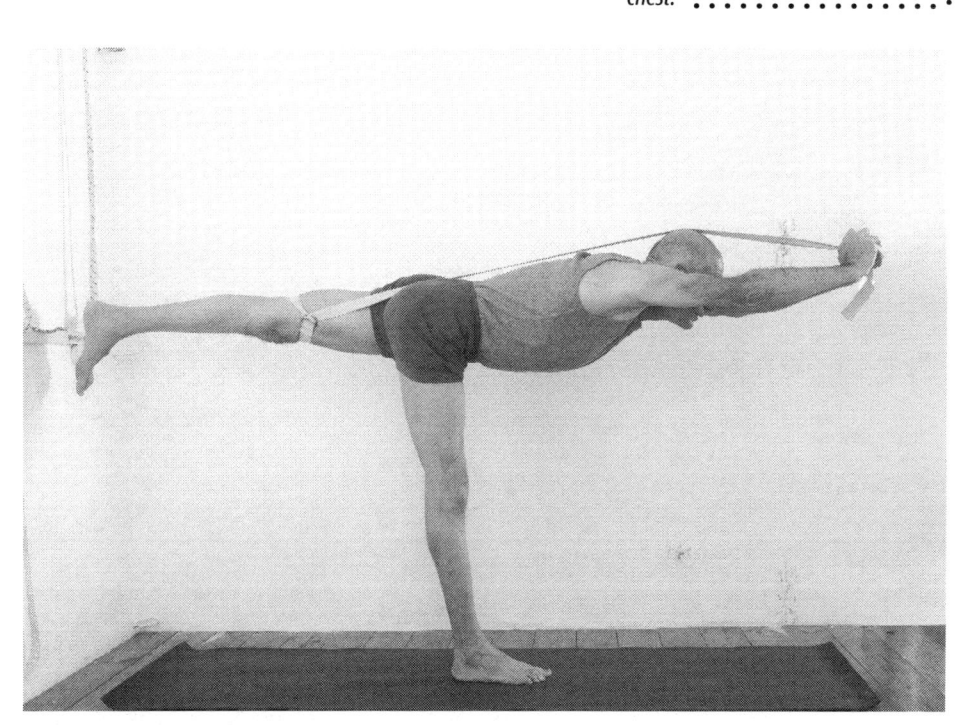

Applicability
Virabhadrasana I, Parsvottanasana (in which the belt can guide you to the proper alignment).

Virabhadrasana III
Variation 8

Floating in Virabhadra III: Holding wall ropes

Props
2 ropes
2 upper wall hooks

If you have upper wall hooks, you will be able to 'float' in Virabhadrasana III. To do the pose standing on the right leg:

→ Hold two ropes and stand at an appropriate distance from the wall.

› Bend the trunk forward while lifting the left leg.

› Press the left foot against the wall, extend the spine forward and look forward.

Effects

This is a very good opening for the shoulders. The pull of the ropes helps to lift and open the chest. The pose can be held effortlessly, as if floating in the air.

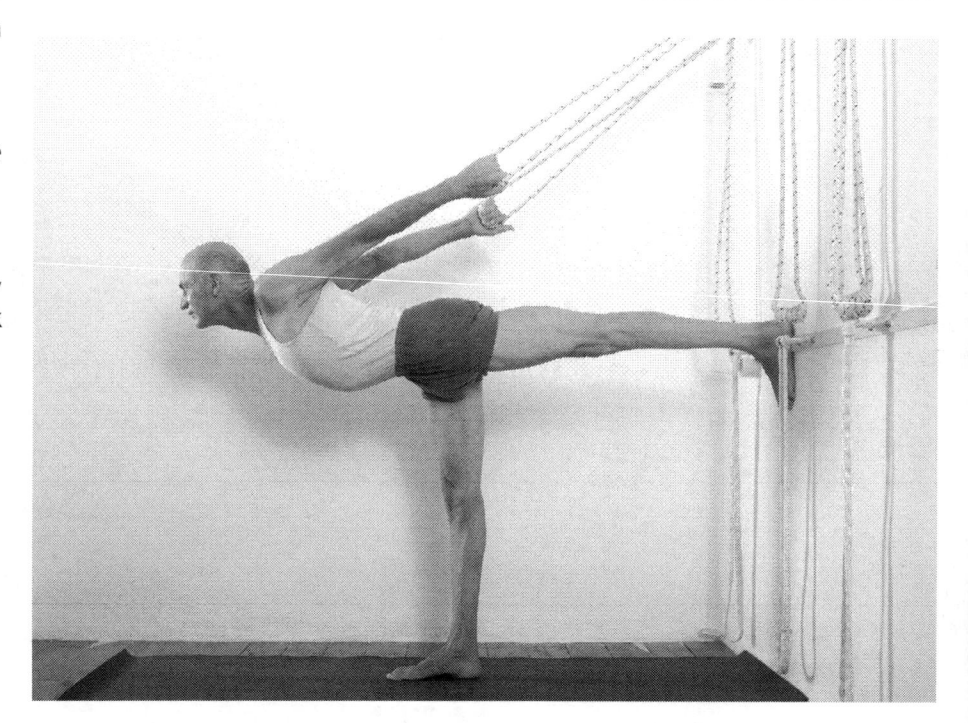

Virabhadrasana III
Variation 9

Restorative Virabhadra III: Hands on wall, back leg on stool

Props
tall chair or stool
wall
blanket (optional)
block (optional)

In this variation the wall and the chair provide complete support for the body, which turns this challenging pose into a restorative and restful one.

Note: The height of the chair should match the height of your lifted leg. If it is lower, place some blankets on it; if it's higher, stand on a block.

Effects
The wall and the stool take the load, thus it is possible to stay and improve the alignment of the body. Pregnant women should practice this variation of the pose.

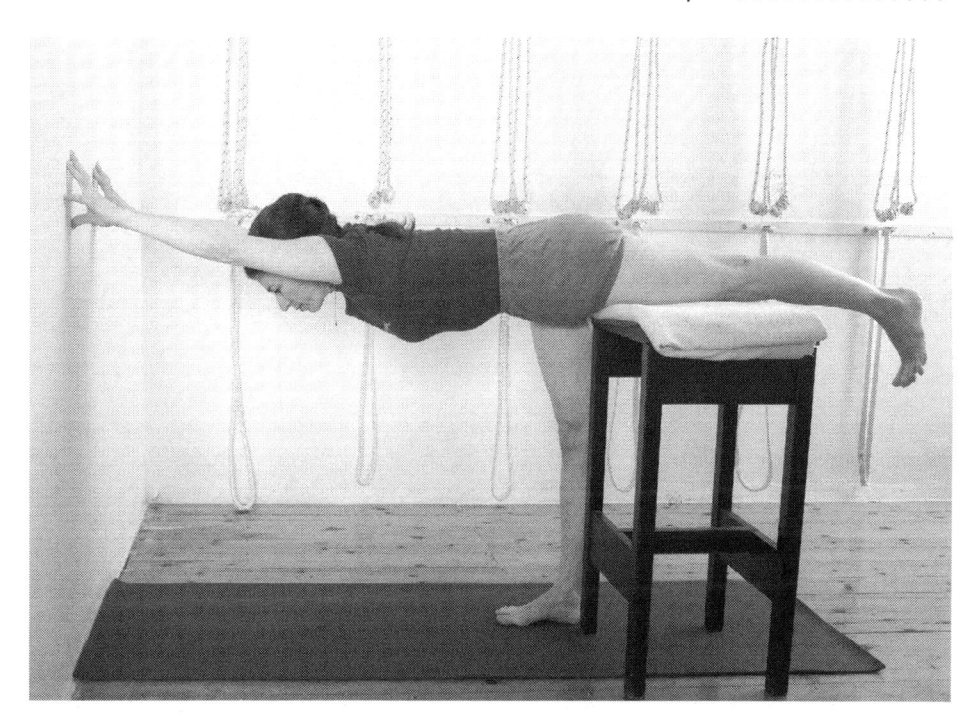

Parsvottanasana

Parsva means side; the challenge of this pose is to turn the body 90° to the side and to achieve an even alignment of the pelvis while bending forward. Variation 1 of Virabhadrasana I, demonstrating a way to enter a side pose, is applicable to Parsvottanasana and is useful in learning the sideways turn. We show here some additional variations which are specific for Parsvottanasana.

Parsvottanasana
Variation 1

Shifting weight to the back leg: Hands on wall

Props
wall
2 blocks (optional)

⟶ To do the pose on the right side:

› Stand in Tadasana facing a wall at a distance of about 60 cm (2 feet) from it.

› Step the left leg backward. Stretch up and then bend forward and place the finger tips against the wall.

› Look forward to check that both hands are placed at the same height and equidistant from the centerline of your body.

› Push the wall to press the left heel firmly on the floor. Press the outer left foot to the floor and turn the left thigh from outside in.

› Move both front thighs back and up (toward the pelvis) ❶.

› After staying for a while, move the hands down and place them at equidistance from the right foot ❷. Do this only if you can maintain the pressure of the left heel on the floor and keep both legs straight (Use blocks to support the palms if necessary).

› Concave the back, move the chest forward and then bend further down to place the head on the shin ❸.

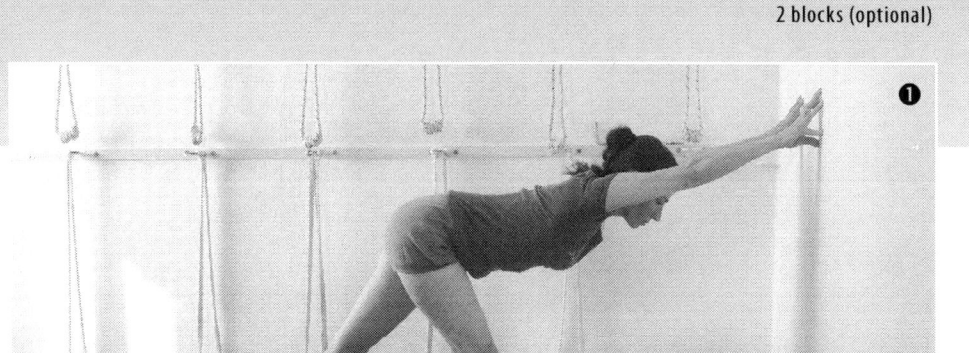

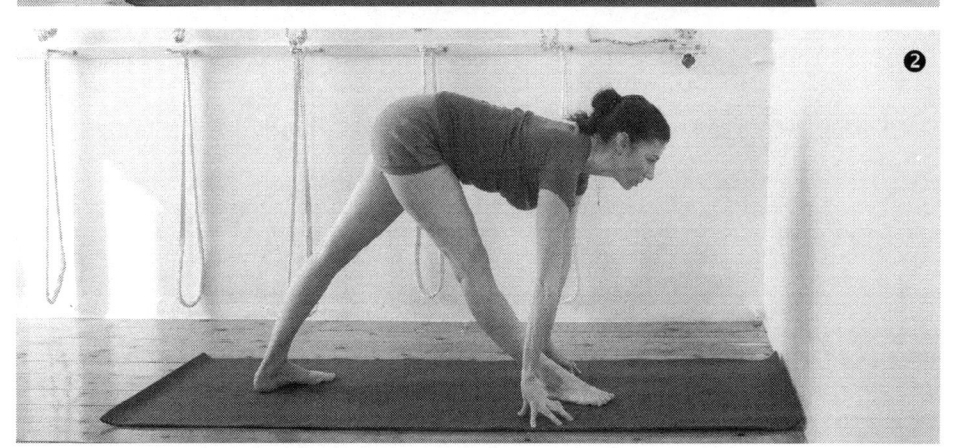

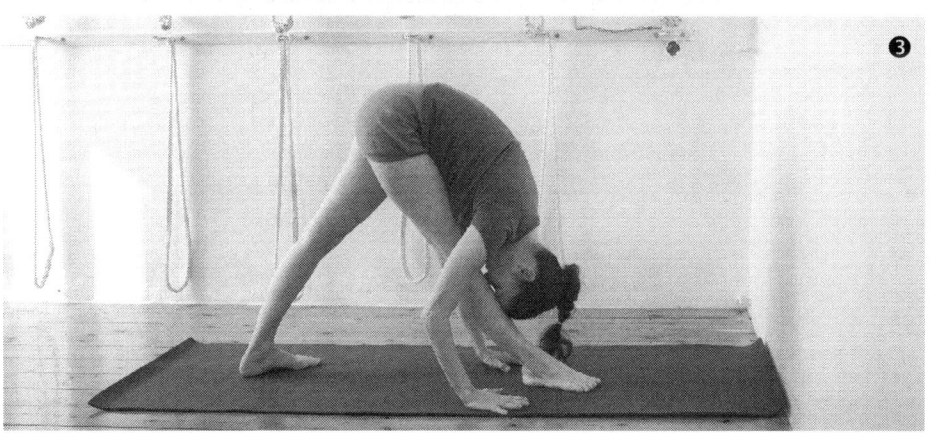

Effects

The wall helps to shift weight to the back leg and to find the correct alignment of the pelvis. Pushing the wall helps to press the back heel down and to extend the calf muscle of the back leg. People who cannot place the palms on the floor with straight front leg should do the pose in this manner (or use blocks to support the palms).

Parsvottanasana
Variation 1 (cont.)

Shifting weight to the back leg: Hands on wall

Props
wall
2 blocks (optional)

To ensure that the legs' spreading is not changed while shifting to the left side you can change to the left leg in the following way:

> Place your palms next to the right foot to mark its position.

> Move the right leg backward and join the right foot with the left one. You are now in Adho Mukha Svanasana.

> Step the left leg forward to the line of the palms, lift the trunk and place the palms on the wall to do on the pose on the left side.

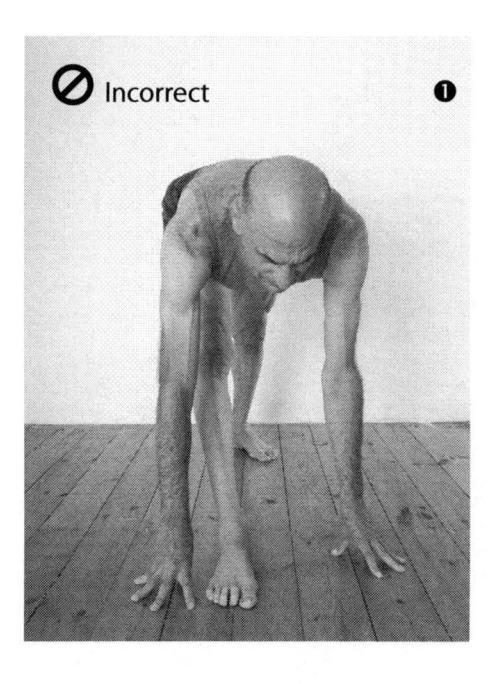

Incorrect ❶

Tips

✓ When doing the pose with the right leg forward, turn the pelvis from left to right until both sides of the pelvis are aligned. Do this by moving the left hip forward and down and the right hip backward and up.

✓ When placing the hands on the floor watch their position: if the left hand if farther back from the foot than the right hand, it means that the pelvis hasn't turned enough (see ❶).

Parsvottanasana Variation 2

Pelvis alignment: Supporting the front groins on a chair

Props
chair
bolster (optional)

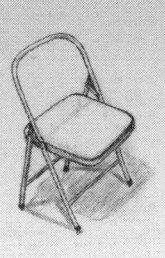

In this variation, the chair is placed against the front groins. To use the chair with the right leg forward:

⟶ Fold the chair and hold it in front so that the backrest touches your front groins; step backward with the left leg.

› Make sure that the left groin touches the chair as much as the right one.

› Bend half way forward and hold the legs of the chair; concave the back and look forward ❶.

› Exhale, bend further down and place the forehead on the chair. Keep rotating the pelvis from left to right to touch the backrest with the left side ❷.

› A bolster can be placed on the chair for cushioning and relaxation.

Effects
The feedback from the chair enables to check that the pelvis is sufficiently rotated and to keep the groins at an even height. The legs of the chair provide stable anchoring for the action of the hands while bending forward.

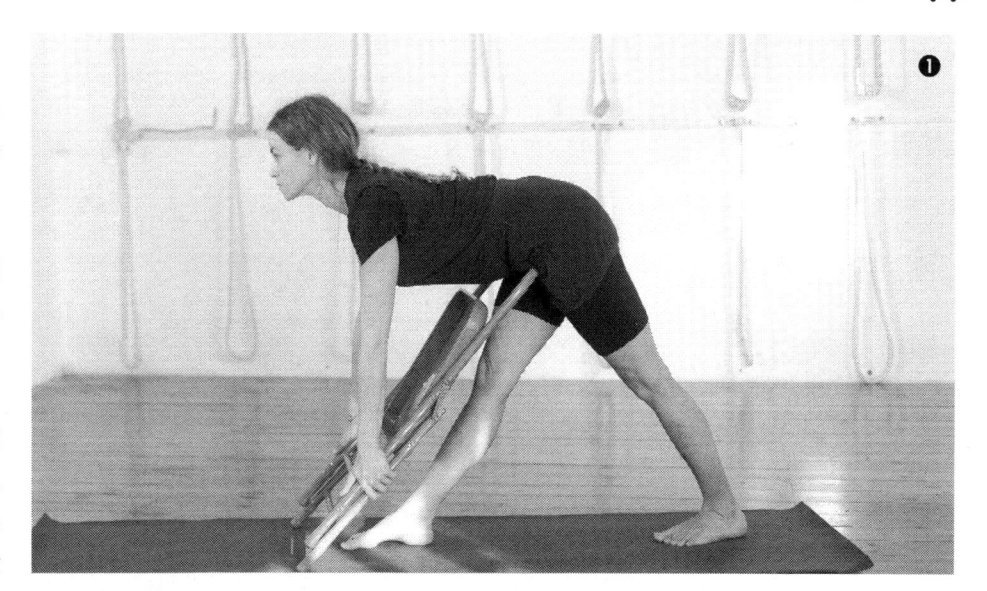

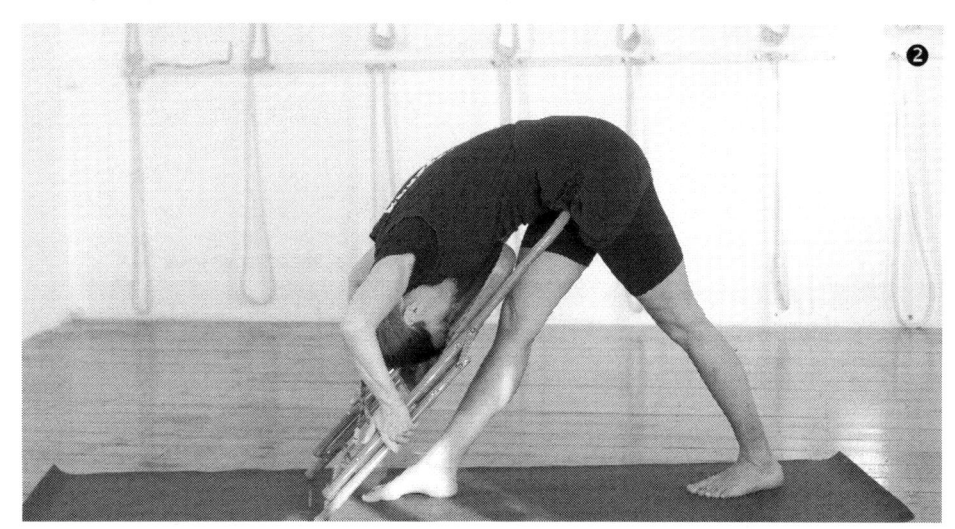

Parsvottanasana
Variation 3

Props
wall

Anchoring the back leg: Foot against the wall

⟶ To do the pose on the right side:

> Place the left heel against the wall, step the right leg forward ❶.

> Bend into the pose while pressing the left heel against the wall ❷.

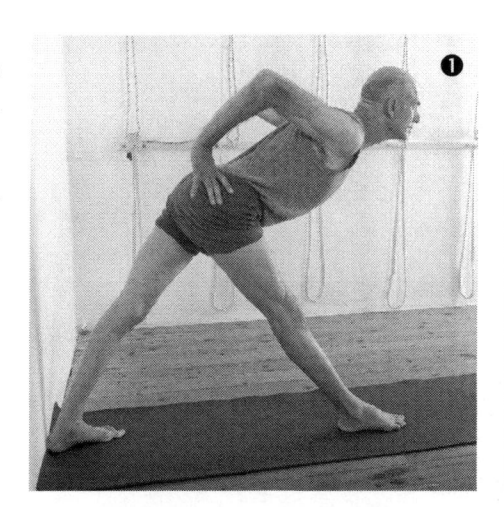

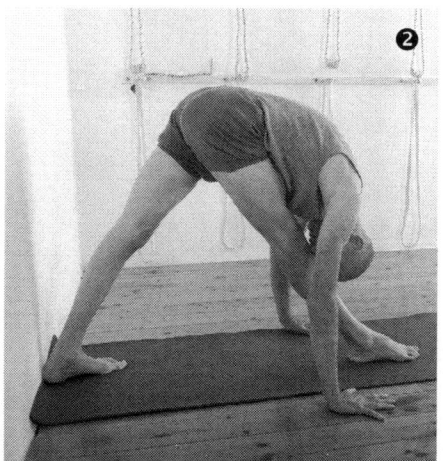

Another interesting option is to place the whole outer foot against the wall. To do the pose on the right side:

> Step the right leg diagonally forward ❸; the angle between the line of your body and the wall should be about 20º (this is equivalent to turning the right foot 70º inward).

> Press the left outer foot to the floor and against the wall and bend into the pose ❹.

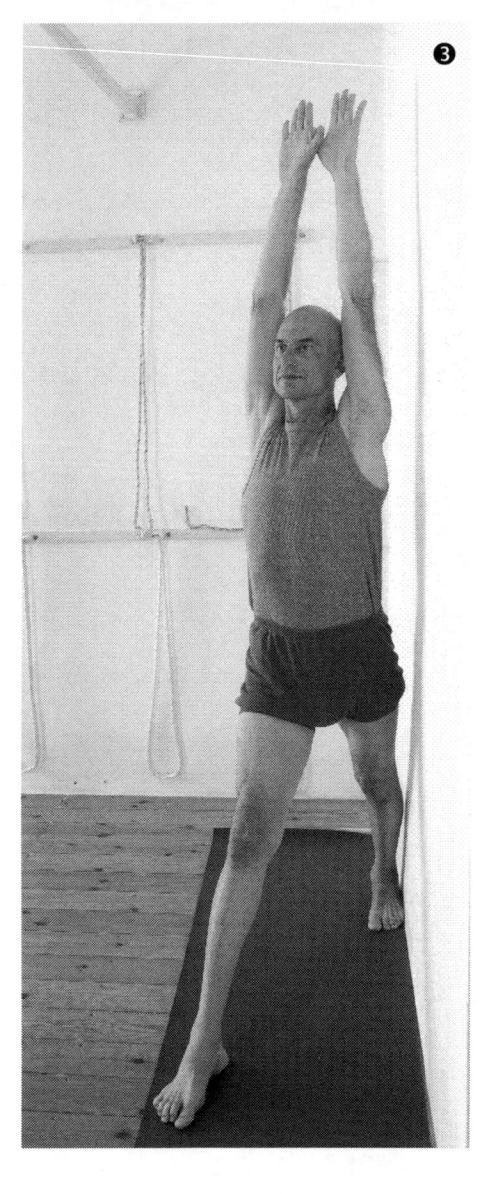

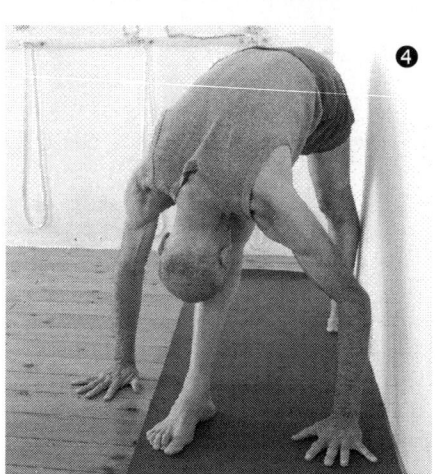

Effects
Pressing the back heel to a wall stabilizes the pose and activates the back leg. The second option emphasizes the action of the outer foot. When turning the thigh inward, the outer foot tends to lift which in turn causes the arch and the entire inner leg to drop. Therefore, it is important to bring awareness to the outer foot.

Applicability
All standing poses (especially Parivrtta Trikonasana).

Parsvottanasana
Variation 4

Intensified forward bend: Hands catching the back knee

After bending into the pose, move the arms back and catch the back leg behind the knee.

Effects
Pulling against the back knee helps to stabilize it and move the body closer to the front leg. It also develops balance.

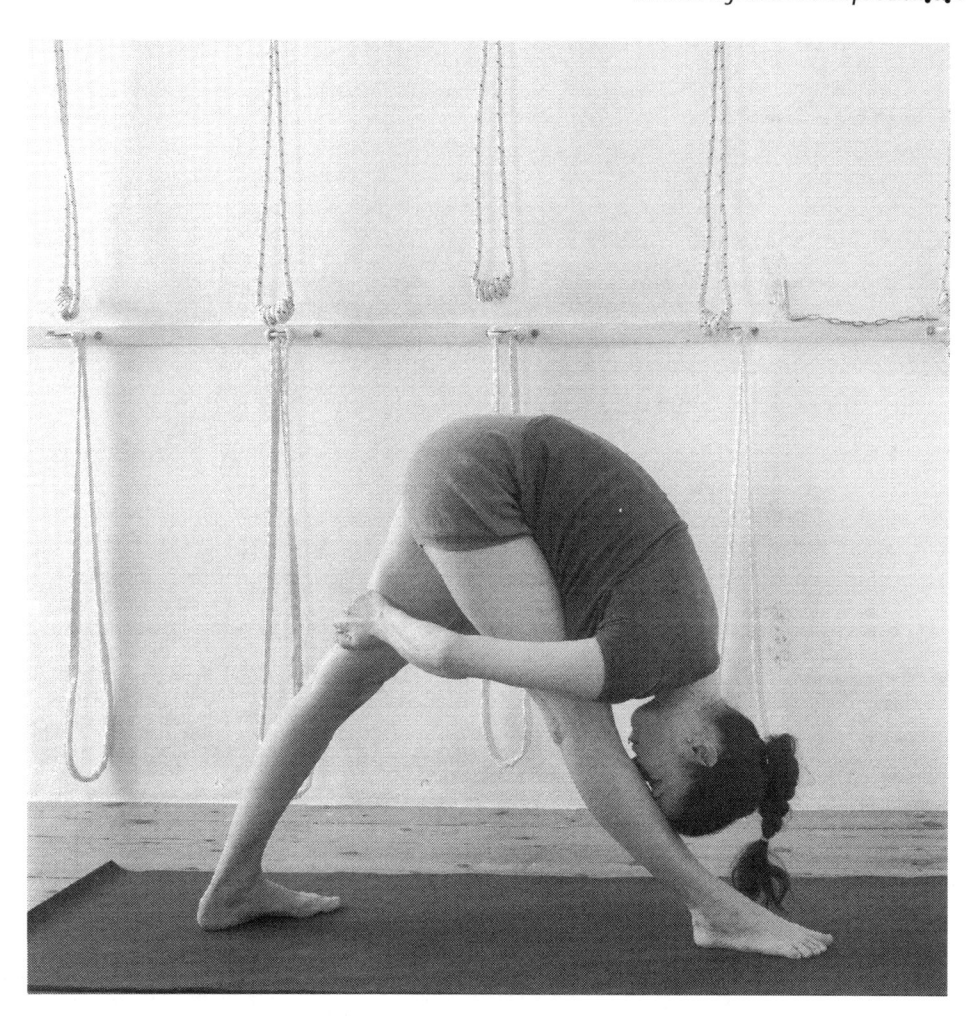

Parsvottanasana
Variation 5

Stabilizing the pelvis: Pulling the front groins with belt

Props
belt
partner

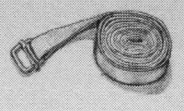

⟶ Instructions for the helper:

› Place a belt on the student's front groins.

› Stabilize the back leg of the student by gently placing your toes on the heel of the student.

› Pull the belt as the student enters the pose ❶.

› After a while, signal that you are going to release the belt and do it slowly.

> **Note:** When placing your toes on the student's heel, be careful not to pinch it.

› You can do a similar variation on your own, using a wall rope. Loop a rope in a wall hook (it can be a door handle) and move away from the wall until the rope is stretched ❷.

Effects
The external force applied by the partner clarifies the direction of the movement of the legs (front thighs are moving back and up); the practitioner can then use his/her cellular memory, and attempt to maintain the same quality when performing the pose on his/her own.

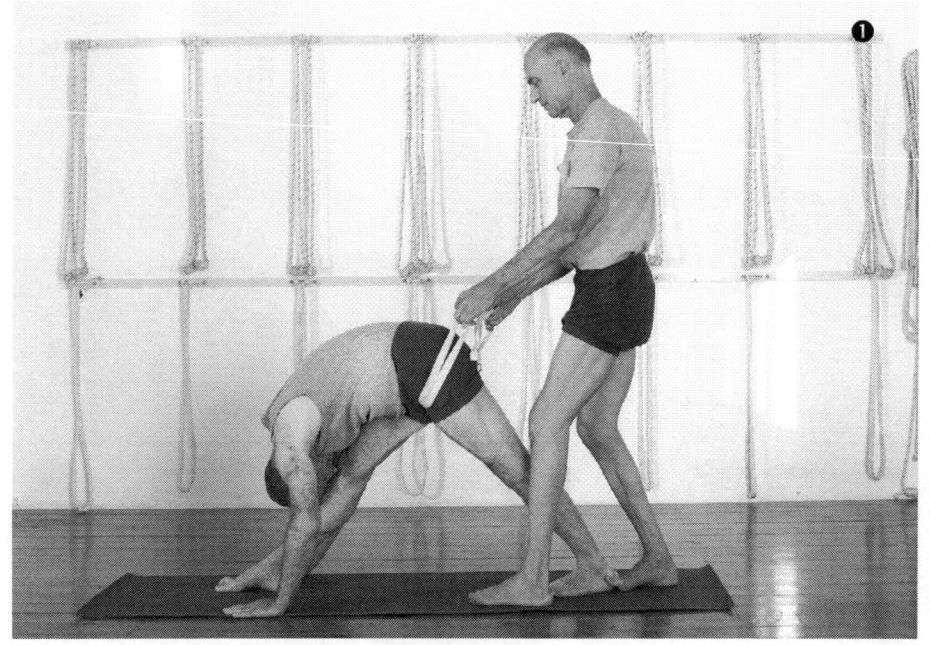

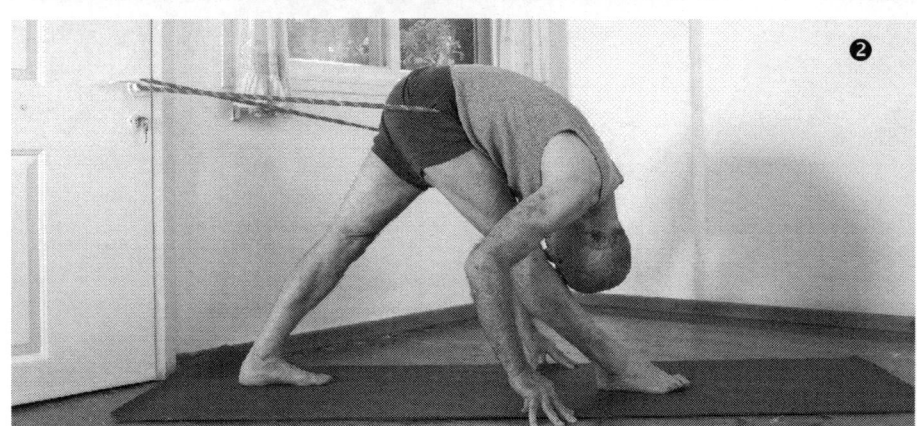

Parsvottanasana
Variation 6

Opening the shoulders: Hands in Gomukhasana

The classic way to do the pose is with the palms joined at the back in Paschima Namaskar. Some people may find this difficult and can prepare their shoulders first by interlocking the fingers or holding the arms at the elbows behind the back.

Another option is to do the pose with the arms folded in Gomukhasana. In this variation: first change the legs without changing the interlock of the arms; then release the pose, change the interlock of the arms and do the pose again on both legs.

These variations with arms behind the back were shown for Utthita Trikonasana (on page 93).

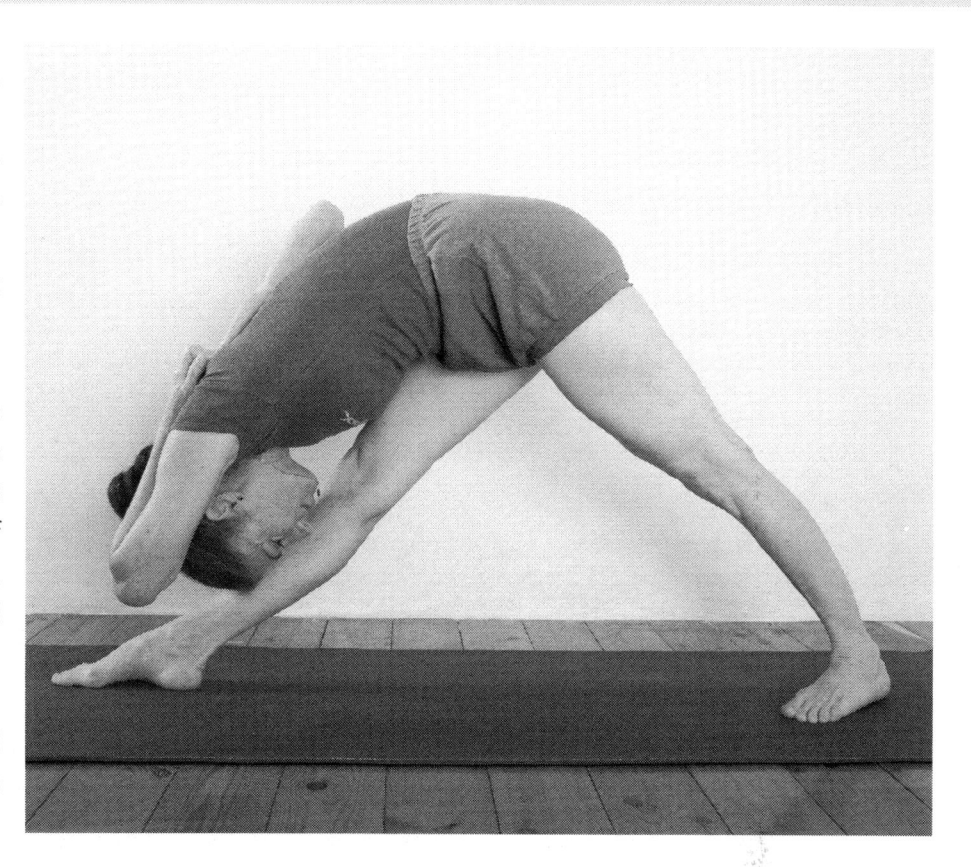

Prasarita Padottanasana

Prasarita Padottanasana is a symmetrical forward bend. When the crown of the head can be placed on the floor comfortably, the pose becomes very relaxing. It is a good preparation for Sirsasana and a good way to rest after practicing standing poses.

Prasarita Padottanasana Variation 1

Insuring symmetry: Using floor lines

Floor lines can be used to check that the feet and palms are placed at equidistance from the centerline:

⟶ Choose the centerline and position the feet and palms at equal distance from it (count the number of floor lines on each side to ensure it).

› Look at your legs and check that both inner knees and thighs are lifted equally.

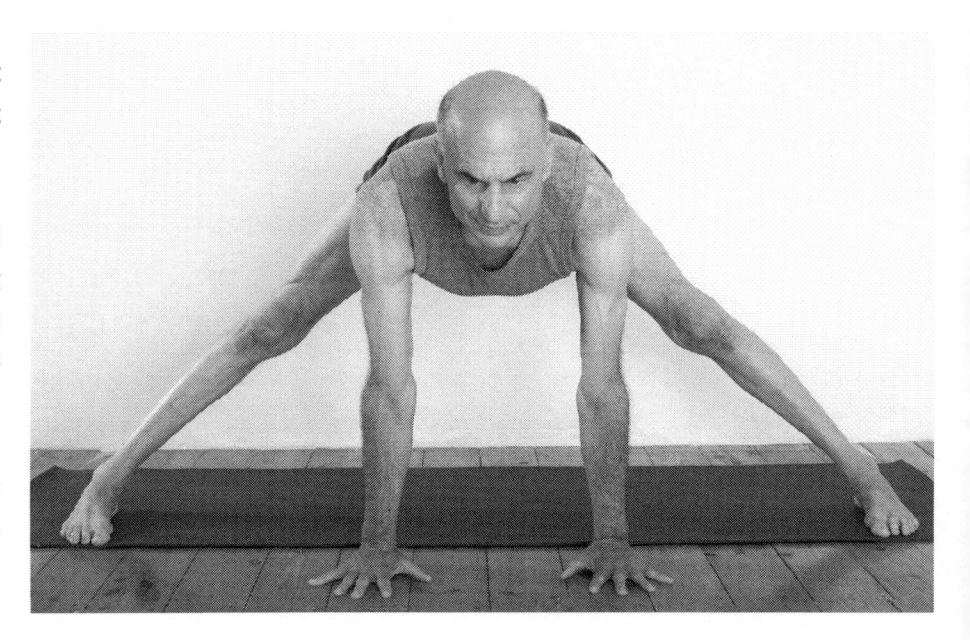

Prasarita Padottanasana Variation 2

Activating the thighs: Buttocks against the wall

Props
wall
2 blocks (optional)

→ Stand with your back to the wall a few centimeters away from it.

> Bend halfway into the pose and place the palms on the floor or on blocks.

> Now step back until the backs of the heels, the legs and the buttock bones are touching the wall.

> Press the front thighs backward until no space is left between the backs of the legs and the wall.

> If floor lines perpendicular to the wall are available, this variation can be combined with the previous one.

Effects

The wall teaches the correct positioning of the legs since it doesn't allow the buttocks to lean backward. This challenges the front thighs which have to push strongly backward.

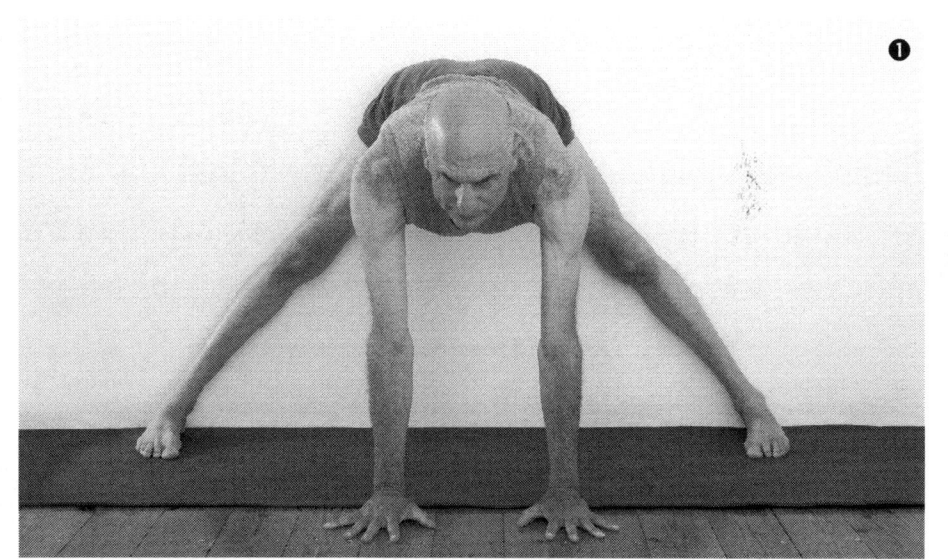

❶

❷

A partner sitting in front can push the thighs back and up.

→ Instructions for the helper:

> Sit on a sticky mat (to prevent slippage) in front of the student.

> After the student bends into the pose, place the soles of your feet on the student's front groins and gently press his/her buttock bones against the wall.

> Make sure you press both feet equally.

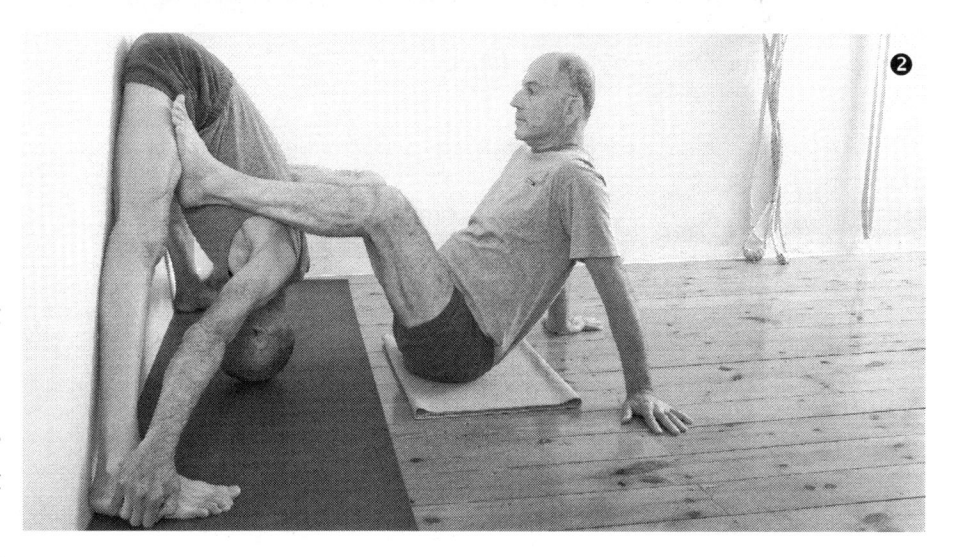

Tips

✓ Feel the contact of the buttock bones with the wall; verify that the two buttocks are leveled and are pressing the wall with equal force.

Props for Yoga / Chapter 1 / Prasarita Padottanasana 137

Prasarita Padottanasana Variation 3

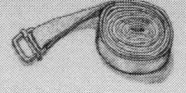

Activating the legs: Bracing the outer ankles with a belt

Props
long belt
(or two connected belts)

→ Spread the legs to the required distance and loop a belt around both feet (most people need a long belt for this).

› Tighten the belt and work the feet against its resistance. Press down the outer feet.

› Bend into the pose while keeping the same leg action ❶.

The belt can also be looped from feet to top of the pelvis:

› Enter the first stage of the pose (the concave back phase).

› Loop the belt around the feet and the sacral band; slightly bend the knees and tighten the belt ❷.

› Then straighten the knees against the resistance of the belt. Bend down to place the head on the floor ❸.

› A bandage or rolled mat can be placed between the belt and the sacrum.

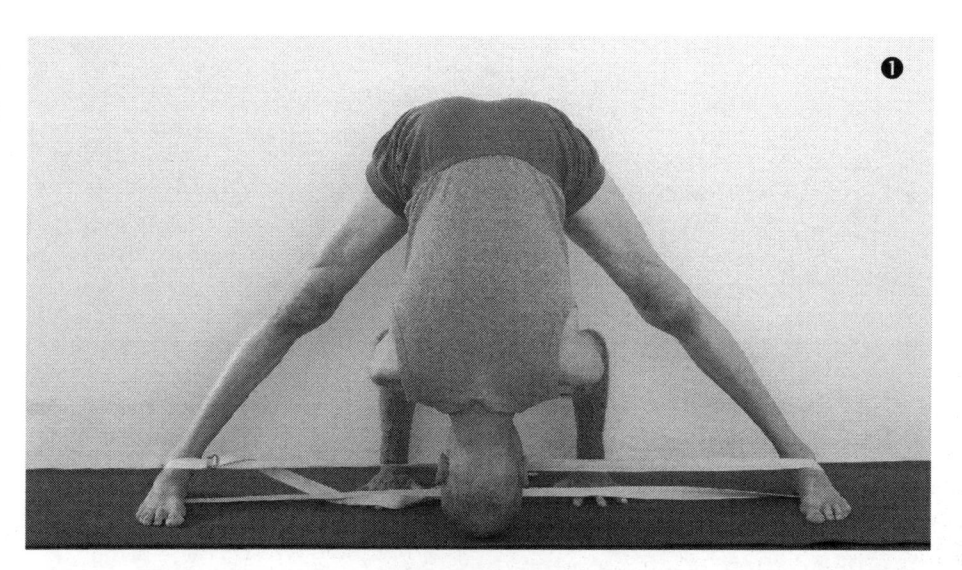

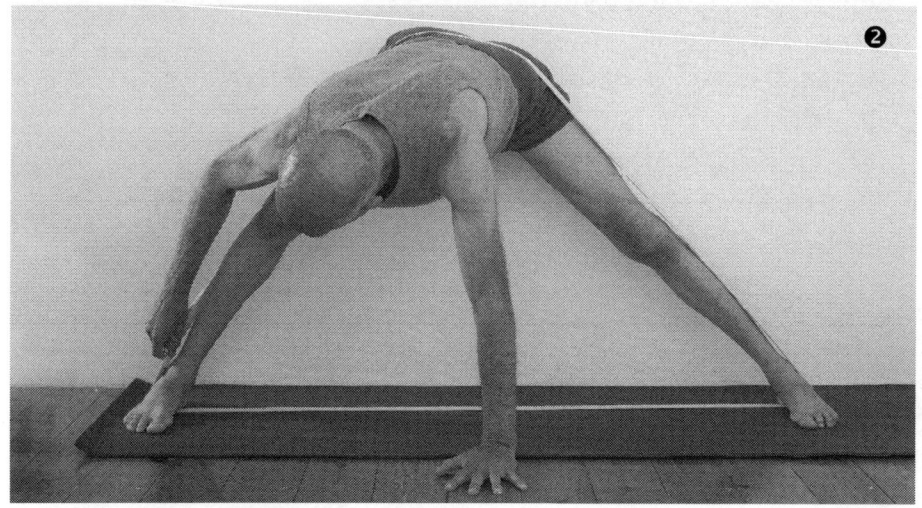

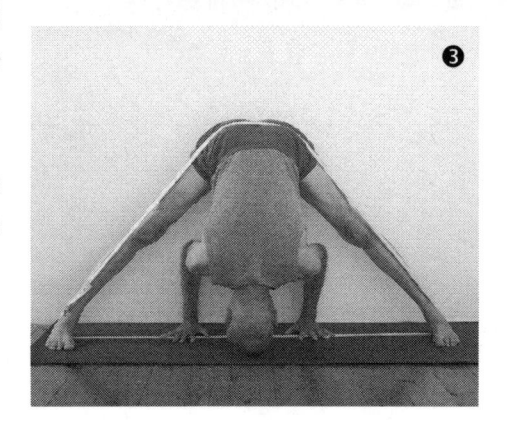

Effects

The belt makes it easier to press the outer feet to the floor. It provides compactness, activates the legs and resists the tendency of the feet to slide outward.

The variation with the belt around sacrum creates a triangular framework for the legs, so it also helps to draw the femur heads and the sacrum into the pelvis. Working against the belt helps to lift the inner thighs and groins.

Prasarita Padottanasana
Variation 4

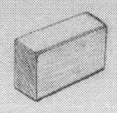

Activating the legs: Pressing outer feet against wall/block

Props
wall
block

Here is another way of anchoring the legs:

Effects
Similar to the previous variation.

→ Stand next to a wall, such that one outer foot is pressed against the wall.

› Spread your legs into the pose and place a block next to the outer foot of the other leg. Now the block marks the proper position of the foot ❶.

› In order to prevent the block from sliding, fold the end of the mat over the block.

› Then place the foot against the block (on top of the folded mat) and bend into the pose ❷.

› Lift the inner ankles and push them against the wall and the block.

> *Note:* If your mat is not long enough for folding it over the block, use additional mat, or place the mat slightly away from the wall.

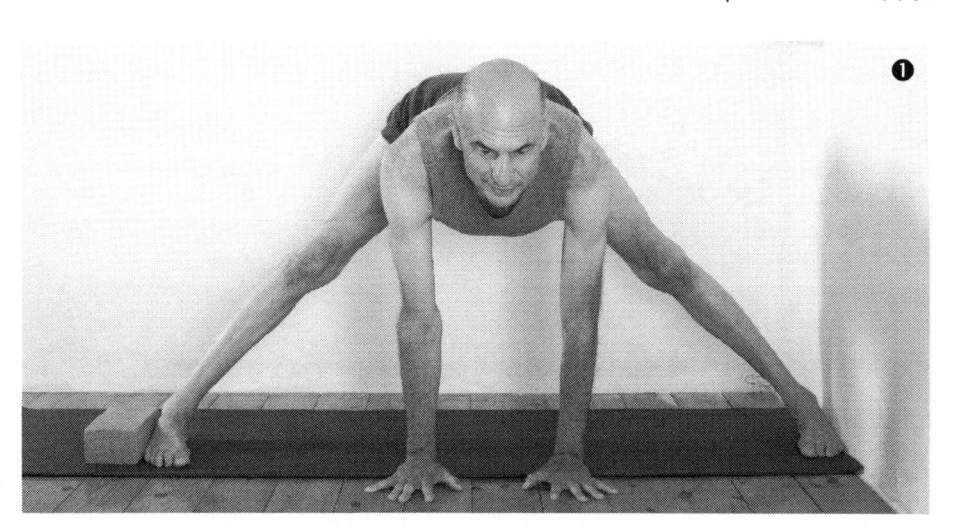

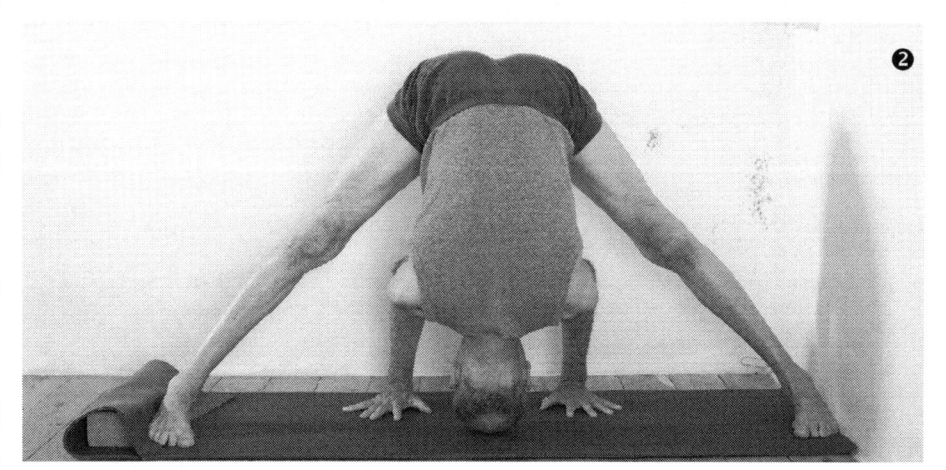

Prasarita Padottanasana
Variation 5

When the head does not reach the floor: Tilting the pelvis forward

There are two ways to go about it:

⟶ Passive work:

> To get the soothing effect of the supported head, use a bolster, a block, a folded blanket or even a chair under the head.

> Over time, gradually decrease the height of the head support.

⟶ Active work:

> Move the palms forward and roll forward until the head reaches the floor (or a folded blanket placed on the floor).

> To prevent the body from rolling forward, press the palms or forearms on the floor and take some of the weight onto the arms.

> Now, without lifting the head, move the thighs back. Slide the head on the floor toward the legs in order to approach the final pose.

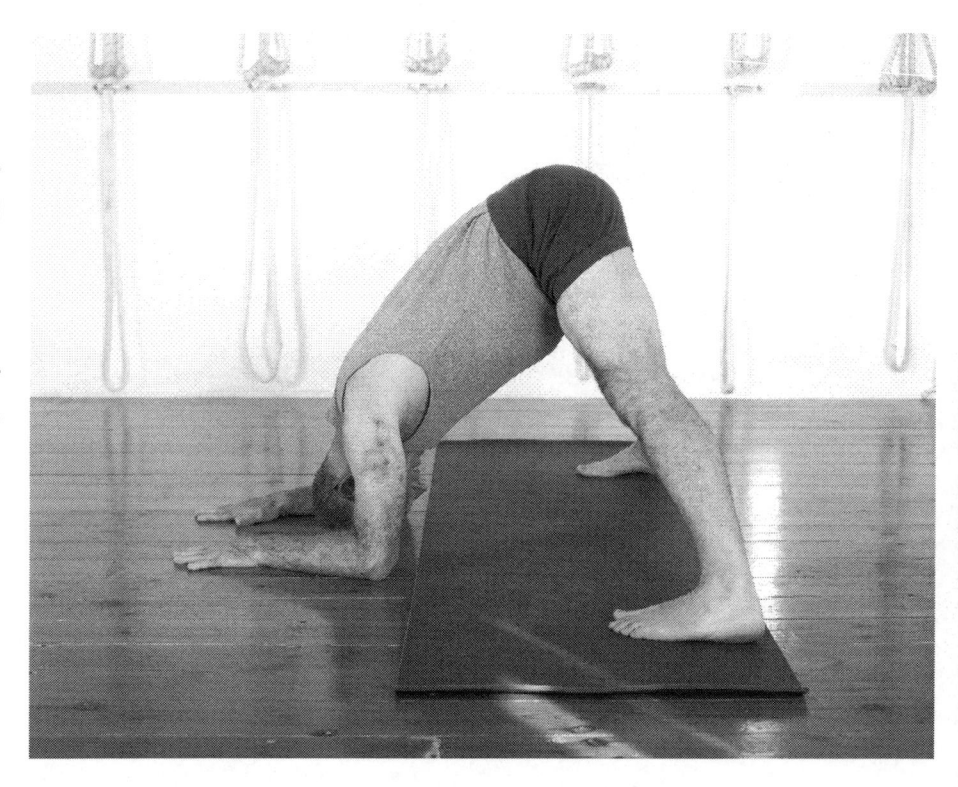

140   Props for Yoga / Chapter 1 / Prasarita Padottanasana

Prasarita Padottanasana Variation 6

Creating space in the pelvis: Pulling the inner groins

Props
partner
2 ropes (or belts)

In Prasarita Padottanasana the inner legs should spread and lift in order to widen the pelvis and create space in the organs of the lower abdomen. A partner can help to learn these actions.

⟹ Instructions for the helper:

> After the student has bent forward to Ardha Prasarita Padottanasana (concave back), place a rope around each of the student's groins.

> Place the first rope and arrange it so as to remain without having to hold it ❶.

> Then place the second rope on the other groin.

> Now catch both ropes and pull diagonally up ❷.

> Look at the student and make sure that your pull lifts and widens both sides of the pelvis equally.

> Hold the ropes for a while, then signal the students that you are about to release the ropes and then do it slowly.

Note: This variation can be more effective when two helpers pull in two opposite directions.

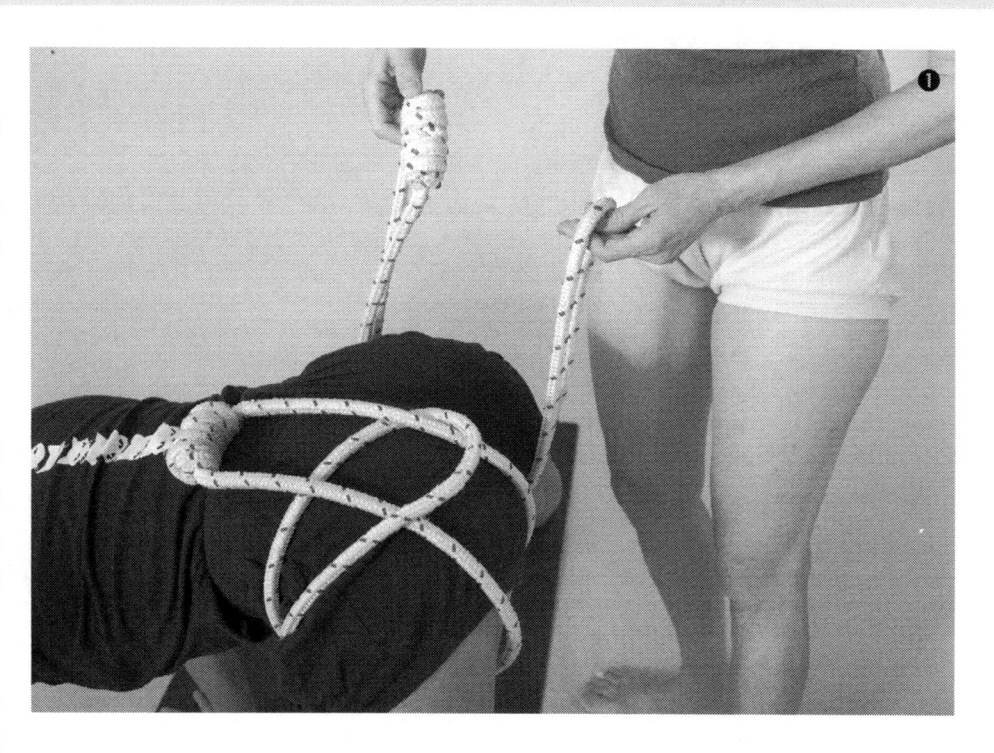

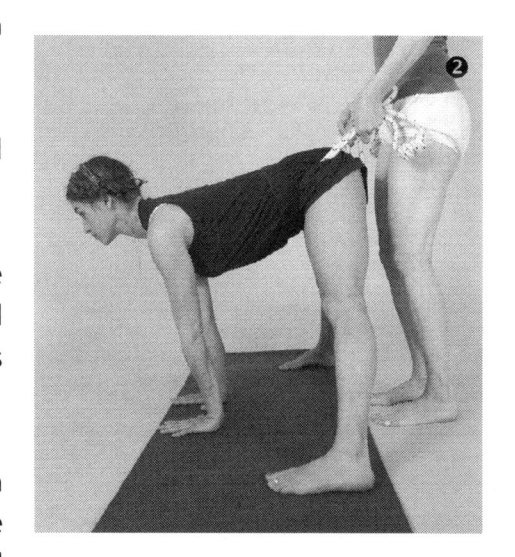

Effects

The pull creates tremendous space in the pelvic area and this is the feeling the pose should bring about. The practitioner can then use his cellular memory to maintain the same quality in the classic pose. The first part of this variation - Ardha Prasarita Padottanasana (concave back) – is recommended for pregnant women.

Tips

✓ Lift the inner legs toward the outer legs and resist with the outer legs. Without moving the legs, make the triangle formed by the inner legs wide and high.

Prasarita Padottanasana Variation 7

Intensifying the downward stretch: Standing on blocks

Props
2 blocks
2 mat pieces

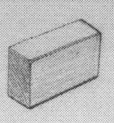

→ Place two blocks at the appropriate distance; place on each block a piece of sticky mat to prevent slippage.

› Stand on the blocks and do the pose.

› After bending down, catch the ankles or the blocks and pull the trunk down.

Effects
The blocks support the bones of the legs and provide anchoring for the action of the arms. People with a long trunk relative to their legs can stretch better in this way.

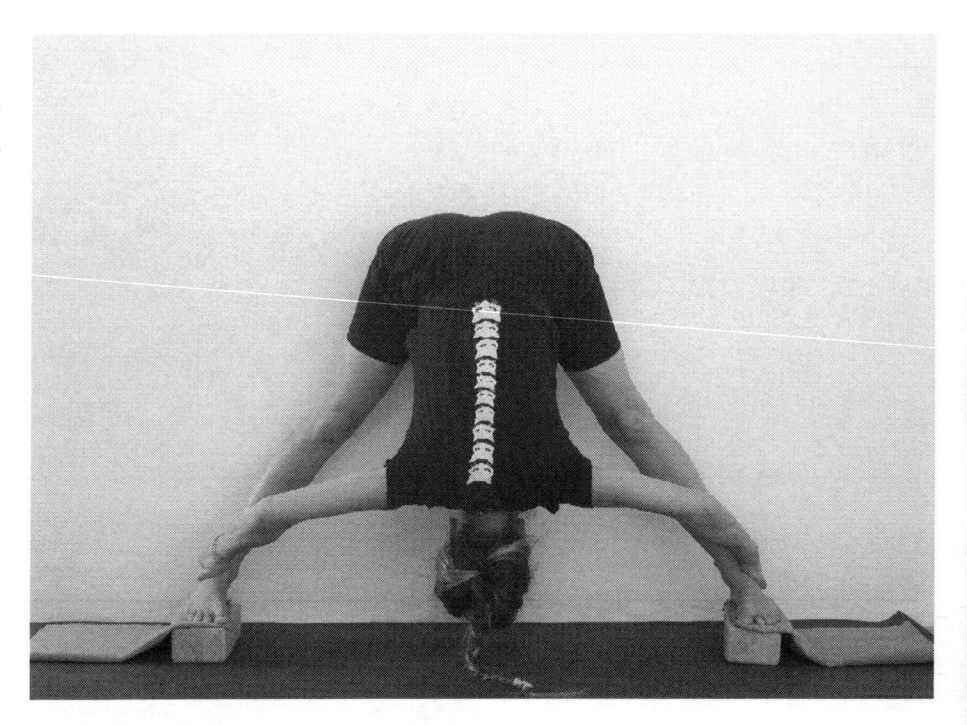

Appendix 1: A Practice Sequence

Yoga practice is significantly affected by the order in which asanas are performed in a particular session. Correct sequencing is chosen according to the purpose and intention of the session; and takes into account one's current physical and mental condition as well as the external conditions (such as the current weather).

From time to time, it is interesting and enjoyable to conduct a session around one type of prop. For example, a sequence with a chair, with blocks, with a long belt, with wall ropes, etc... This appendix presents an example of a sequence that uses blocks. The following volumes of this guide will provide additional sequences.

The following sequence includes inversions and backbends and is intended to energize the body and uplift the mind. With each asana we give the corresponding page number where the variation can be found in the book. Explanatory comments are provided for those variations that are not included in this volume.

Characteristics of this sequence are:

> **Duration:** 60 min.

> **Level:** Intermediate to advanced

> **Type:** Dynamic

> **Types of Asanas included:** Standing poses, inversions and backbends

Props

wall

block | Most of the sequence uses 2 blocks; for some variations a third block is required.

belt

blankets | 5-6 blankets are required for *Sarvangasana*

bolsters | 2 bolsters can be used as a support for *Adho Mukha Virasana* (step 25 in the sequence), but this is optional – you can do it without bolsters.

chair | A chair and an eye cover can be used for *Savasana* – again, this is optional.

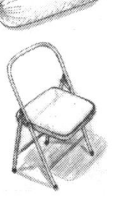

1. Adho Mukha Svanasana

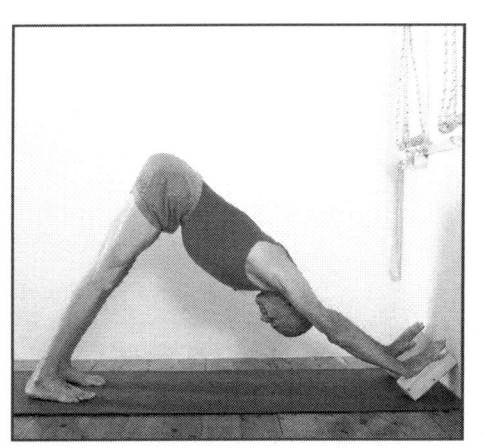

See page 32

2. Uttanasana

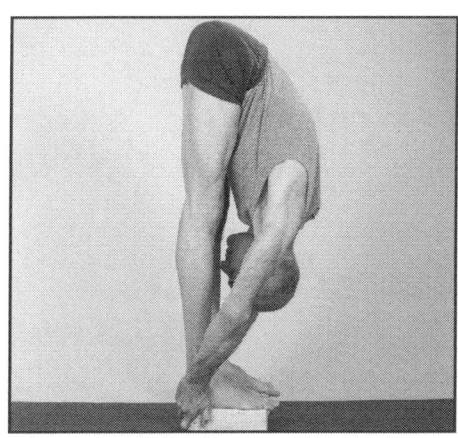

See page 60

3. Adho Mukha Svanasana

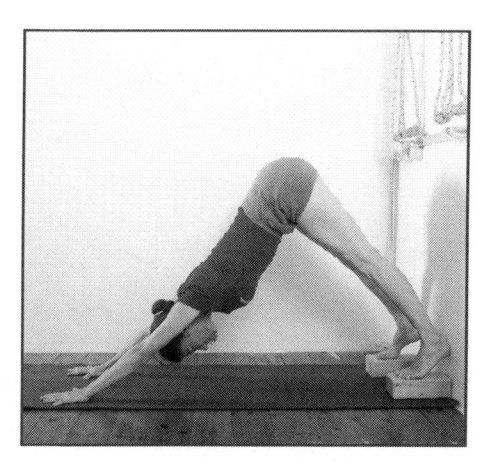

See page 39

4. Uttanasana shoulder strech

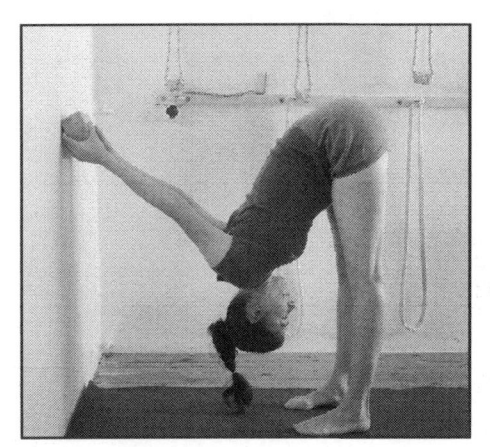

See page 63-64

5. Adho Mukha Svanasana

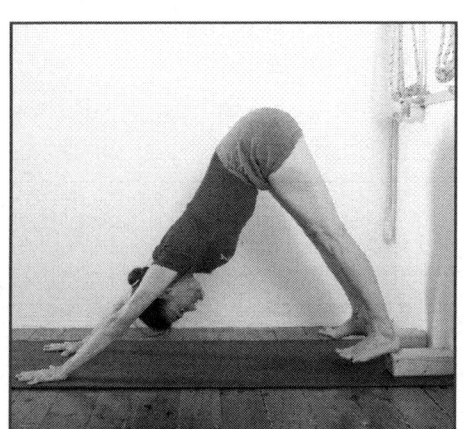

See page 39

6. Adho Mukha Vrksasana

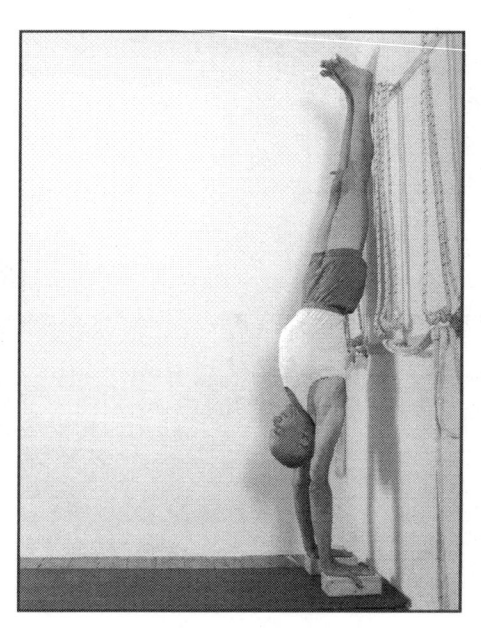

Adho Mukha Vrksasana: The palms are placed on blocks; this gives support for the bones of the arms and makes the pose easier to hold (although it is slightly more difficult to jump up into the pose).

144 Props for Yoga / Chapter 1 / Apendix 1

7. Adho Mukha Vrksasana

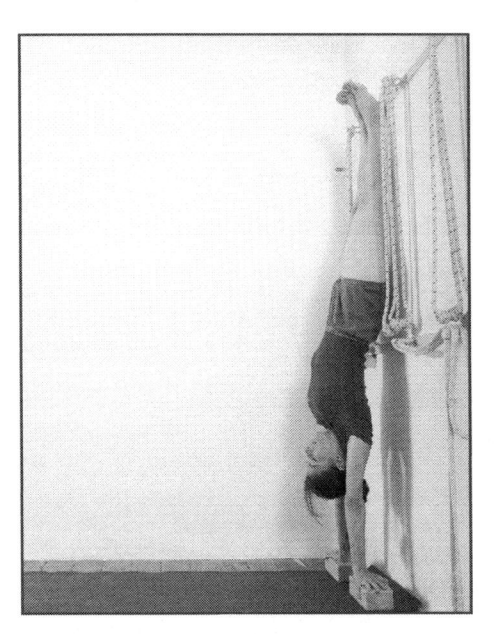

8. Utthita Trikonasana

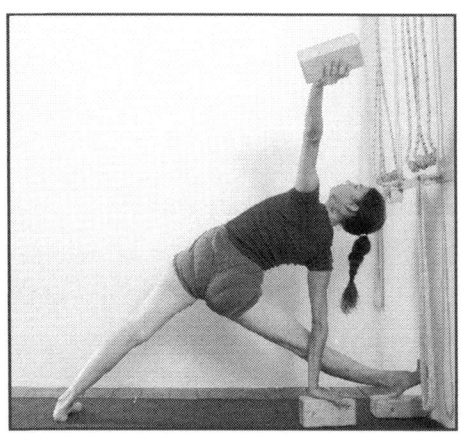

See page 88

9. Utthita Parsvakonasana

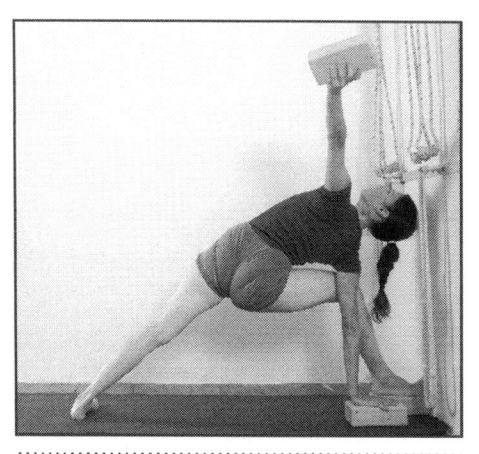

10. Virabhadrasana II

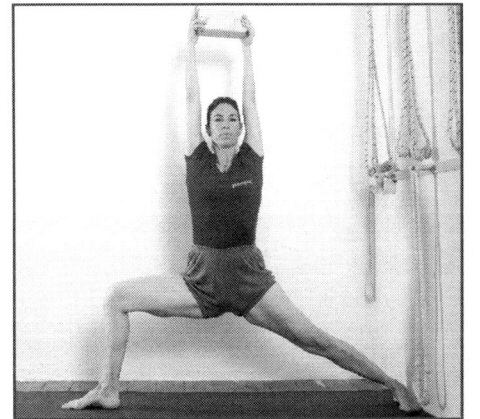

See page 102

11. Virabhadrasana I

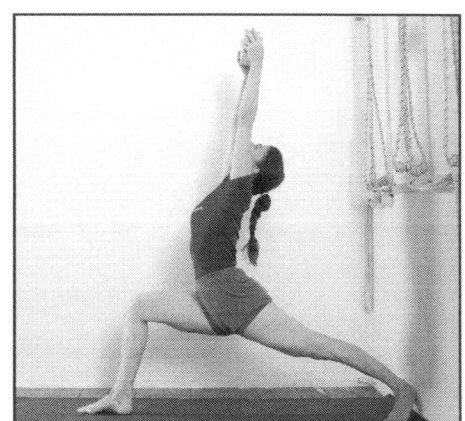

See page 108

12. Pincha Mayurasana

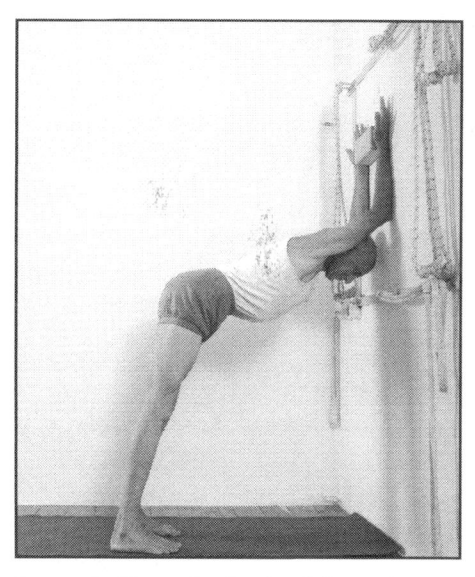

(prep. 1): Place the back of the palms on the wall and hold a block in between them (turning the palms this way turns the outer elbows inward). Place the elbows at shoulder width. Move the shoulder blades in as you concave the back. Keep the buttocks moving down toward the heels to avoid overarching the lumbar spine. Create movement in the shoulders by moving the sternum away from the wall and the head toward the wall.

13. Pincha Mayurasana

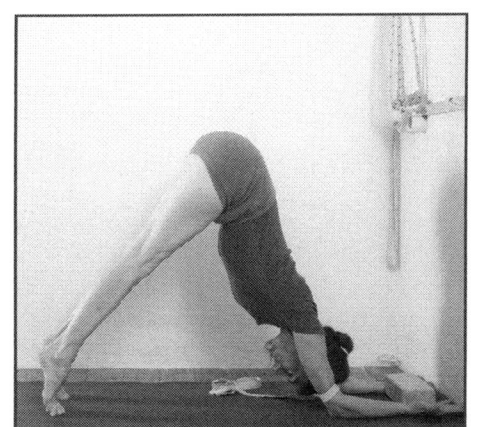

(prep. 2): This preparation is similar to the previous one. It is closer to the final pose, because you have to push against the floor, resisting gravity. Use two blocks if needed (one flat and one standing) to match the width of your shoulder girdle (shown in next variation). Forearms should be parallel to each other at shoulder width. Use a belt for the elbows if they tend to widen out. Concave the back, lift the heels and step forward. The more you step forward, the greater the challenge of concaving the back.

14. Pincha Mayurasana

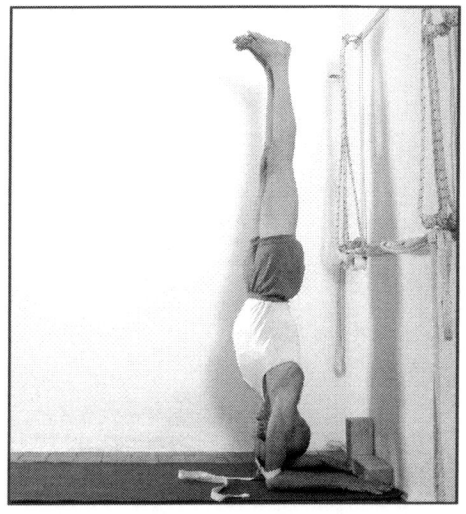

When the previous preparation is done near the wall, you can jump directly from there to Pincha Mayurasana; use the wall to help you find the balance, and then balance without the wall.

15. Sirsasana

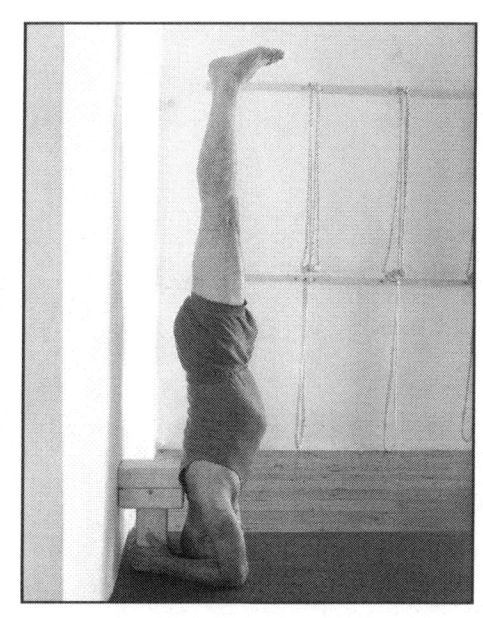

Prepare the blocks for Sirsasana as shown here: The two upper blocks support the thoracic dorsal spine; this teaches how to move the vertebrae of this region in (there are several other arrangements of blocks that achieve different effects; they will be shown in the next volume of this guide).

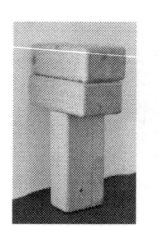

16. Urdhva Mukha Svanasana

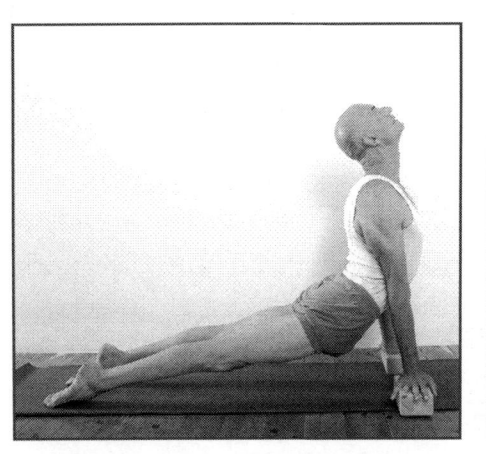

Turning the palms outward helps to roll the shoulders back and thus to open the chest. This is especially useful for people with stiff shoulders.

17. Chaturanga Dandasana

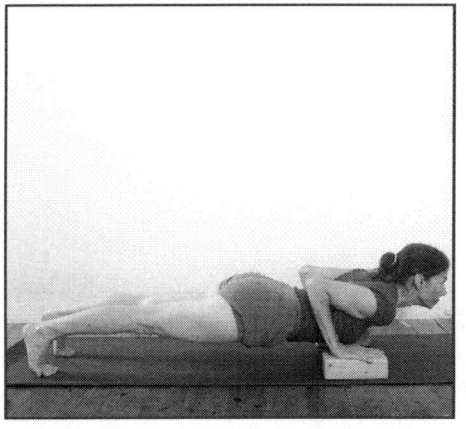

18. Urdhva Mukha Svanasana

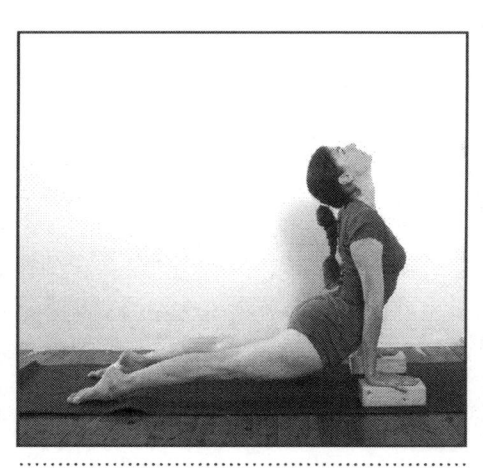

19. Ustrasana

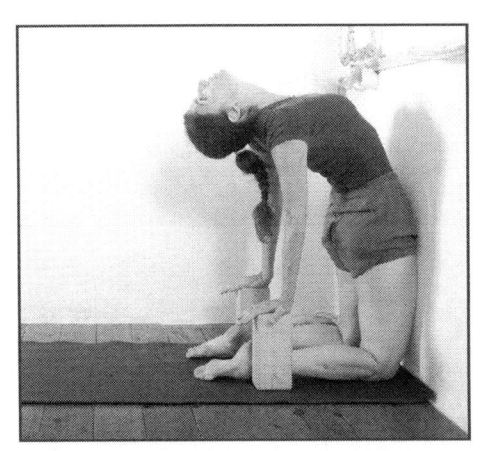

Kneel facing the wall; place your hands on the pelvis. Move the tailbone in and press the pubic bone firmly against the wall. Arch back into the pose while keeping contact between the pubic bone and the wall. Move the hands back and place the palms on the blocks. Push against the blocks to lift and open the chest. You can then move the palms to the feet, as in the final pose.

20. Ustrasana

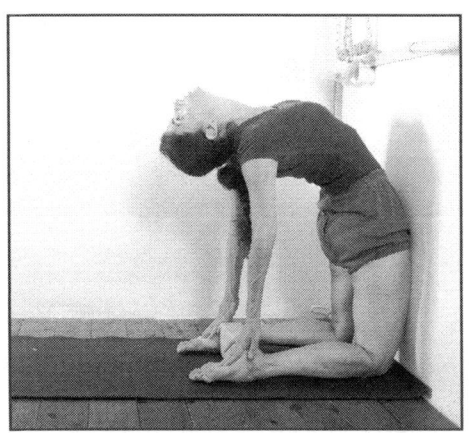

Press the feet firmly against the block. This charges the legs, thus creating a firm base for arching the back.

21. Urdhva Dhanurasana

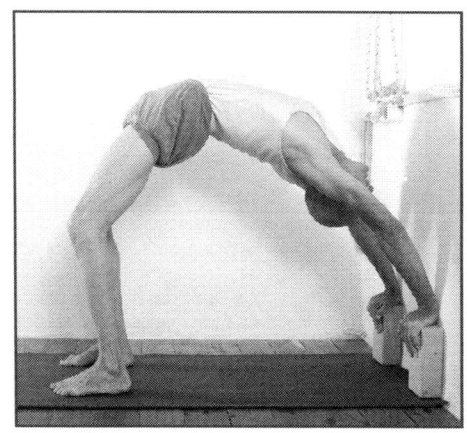

The standing blocks give significant height for the hands; this is a good way to start working on Urdhva Danurasana – especially for people with stiff shoulders. One can create the arch shape (Danur) even when shoulder movement is limited.

22. Urdhva Dhanurasana

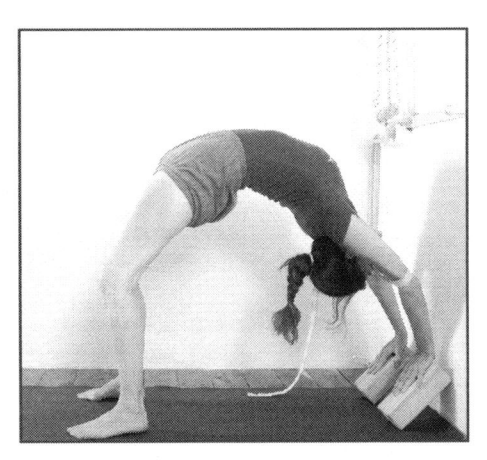

This could be a second step; the slanting blocks are useful for people with sensitive or painful wrists, because they decrease the load on the hands and the movement required in the wrist. The slanted surface helps to press the palms in order to lift the body. The belt on the elbows (optional) helps to stabilize the arms.

23. Urdhva Dhanurasana

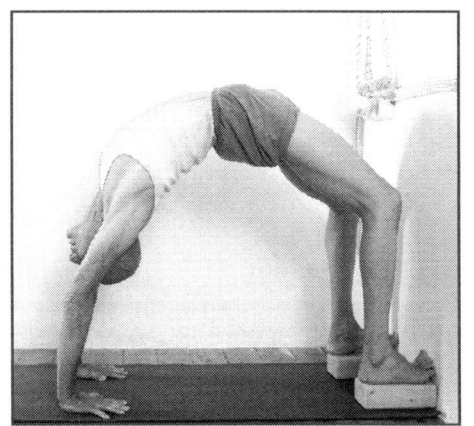

Lifting the feet in Urdhva Danurasana helps to lift the pelvic girdle and to soften the abdomen.

24. Adho Mukha Svanasana

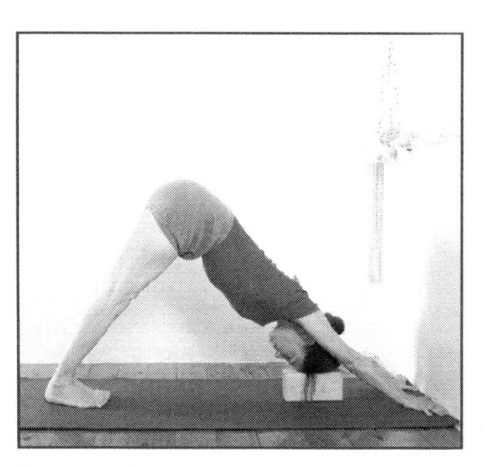

See page 52

Props for Yoga / Chapter 1 / Apendix 1 147

25. Adho Mukha Virasana

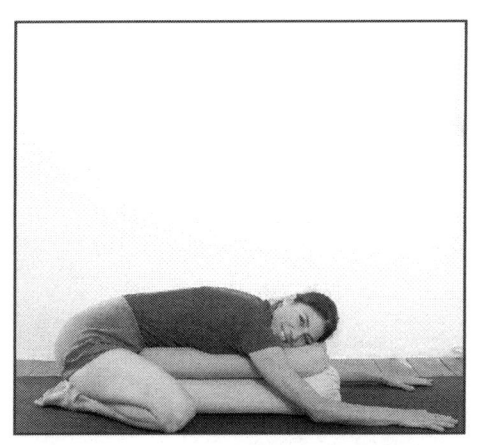

26. Dwi Pada Supta Pavana Muktasana

27. Urdhva Prasarita Padasana

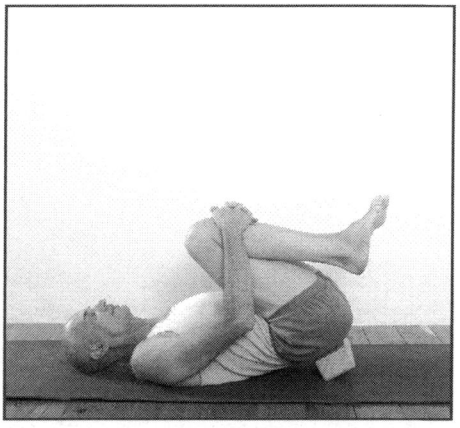

This pose is a good release for the back and gives rest for the brain. The two bolsters are optional. However, if available, resting on the bolsters will makes the pose even more soothing and pleasant. If no bolsters are available, doing without is also beneficial.

The slanted block under the sacrum rounds out and extends the lower back, releasing it after the backbends.

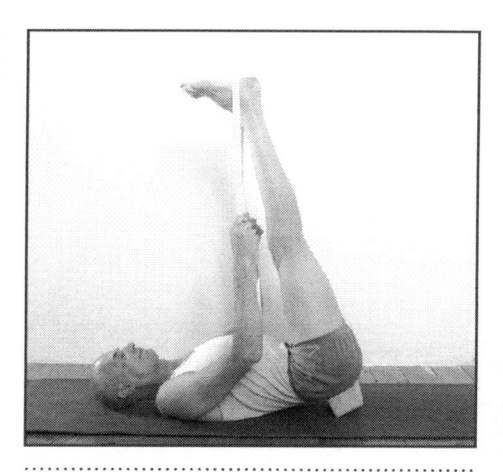

28. Bharadvajasana I

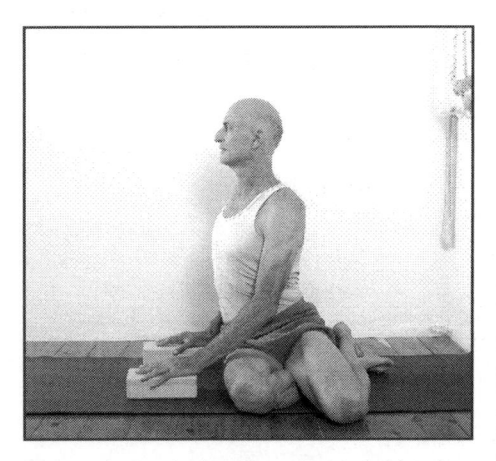

29. Salamba Sarvangasana

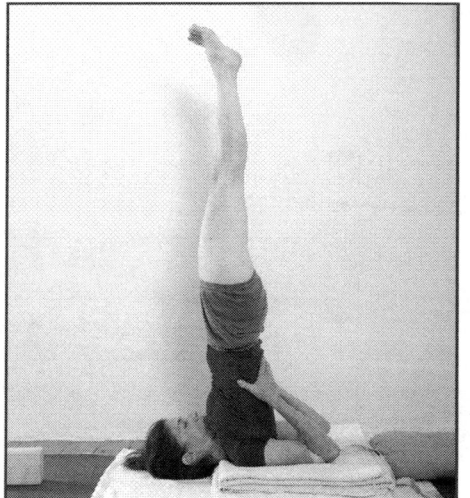

30. Halasana

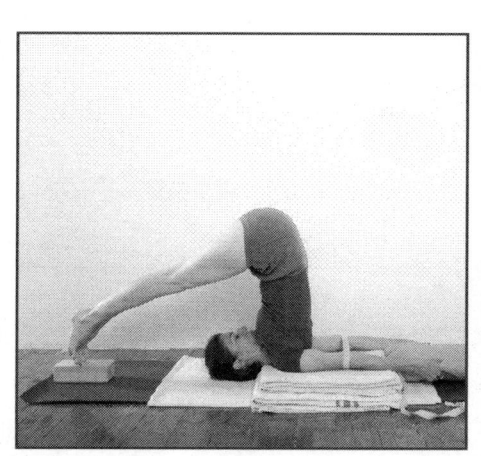

This variation is done to release the lumbar spine. Allow the trunk to tilt sideways and turn the trunk from its base. The blocks that support the palms help to lift the chest.

This setup of props for the Sarvangasana cycle helps to check and correct the alignment of the body:
- Spread one blanket on the mat (for head cushioning) and stack five folded blankets on it to create a platform.
- Place a block in the middle of the mat, where the feet should be in Halasana; and a bolster on the other side of the platform.

By using the block and the bolster as shown, you can easily check whether your alignment is correct. Make sure the toes land on the middle of the block. Feel the bolster and check that the arms are aligned with it.

31. Karnapidasana

The knees should be at shoulder level. When doing the pose on the floor, the knees are placed on the floor, next to the ears. Since we do Sarvangasana on a platform, the knees hang in the air (unless you collapse the pose to force them to the floor). Placing blocks on both sides of the head provides support for the knees and make the pose more relaxing.

32. Paschimottanasana

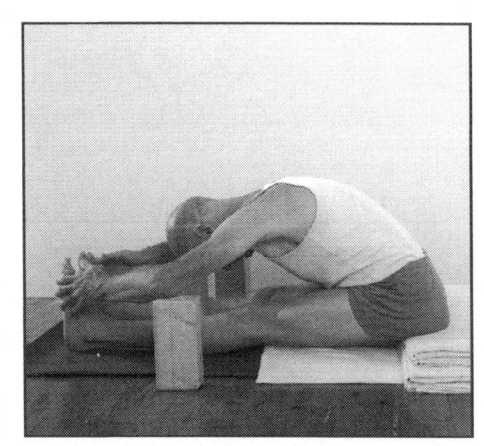

This variation is done not for stretching but to release the back (after the backbends) and to pacify the brain as a preparation for Savasana. Sit on the Sarvangasana platform and support the forehead and the elbows on blocks.

33. Savasana

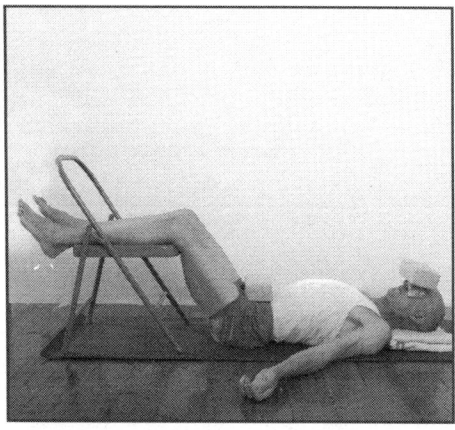

Backbends are active and energizing; this is good! But at the end of the session you need to bring the mind to a quiet, passive state. This variation is an effective way to calm down after this dynamic sequence. The chair and the eye cover are optional. However, if available, supporting the lower legs on a chair lengthens and broadens the lower back and the abdomen. The eye cover and the block on top of it deeply relax the brain and bring about a sattvic (calm, passive, pure) state of mind.

Index:

Two sets are provided below:

> Listing by Prop   > Listing by Asana Name or Specific Action

Index 1: Listing by Prop

belt	Asana	Variation	Page No.
	Adho Mukha Svanasana	2 - Ensuring symmetry: Using a middle line	31
		4 - Stretching back and up: Partner pulls backward with belt	34
		12 - Releasing the neck: Partner pulls the trapezius muscles	43
		17 - Stabilizing the arms: Belt around elbows	48
		19 - Moving the shoulder blades in: Starting with forearms on the floor	50
		22 - Passive extension of the spine: Wall rope around front groins	53
	Parsvottanasana	5 - Stabilizing the pelvis: Pulling the front groins with belt	134
	Prasarita Padottanasana	3 - Activating the legs: Bracing the outer ankles with a belt	138
	Tadasana	2 - Activating the knees: Block between knees	6
		3 - Activating the thighs: Block between thighs	7
		4 - Turning the upper thighs in: Belt on each groin	8
		5 - Stabilizing the pelvis: Belt around pelvis	9
		10 - Activating the arms: Belt around forearms	14
		11 - Moving the trapezius down: Shoulder traction	15
		12 - Sensitizing the top chest: Belt around chest	17
	Urdhva Hastasana	2 - Activating the arms: Belt around forearms, block between palms	21
	Uttanasana	6 - Compact legs: Belt around feet and pelvis	61
		7 - Folding deeply into the pose: Belt around back and legs	62
	Utthita Trikonasana	3 - Activating the back leg: Foot on belt	70
		4 - Activating the back leg: Pulling the leg with belt	71
		5 - Lifting the inner groin: Partner pulls the back leg	72
		6 - Turning the legs: Two belts on the upper thighs	73
		12 - Ensuring lateral alignment: Back against the wall	81

belt (cont.)

Asana	Variation	Page No.
Utthita Trikonasana (cont.)	15a - Bending from the hips: Partner pulls the front hip	86
	15b - Pulling the front groin while stabilizing the back leg	87
Virabhadrasana I	2 - Opening the chest: Belt attached to the back leg	106
	7 - Experiencing lightness: Helpers lift the groins	111
	8 - Activating the arms: Belt around the elbows	112
Virabhadrasana II	1 - Squaring the front leg: Belt from knee to back leg	96
Virabhadrasana III	4 - Compacting the standing leg: Belt from foot to pelvis	122
	6 - Opening the chest: Arms behind the back	124
	7 - Stabilizing the pose: Belt on back leg	125

blanket

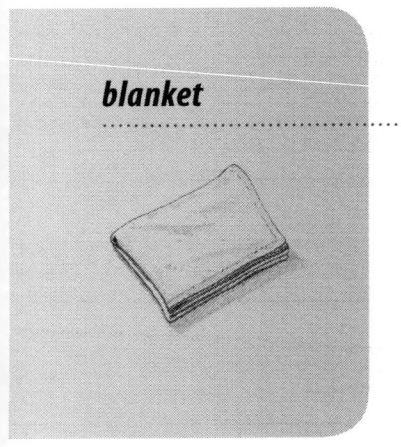

Asana	Variation	Page No.
Adho Mukha Svanasana	20 - Moving the middle back in: Starting with the head low	51
	21 - Relaxing the brain: Head support	52
Uttanasana	10 - Relaxing the brain: Top of the Head on block	66
Virabhadrasana III	9 - Restorative Virabhadra III: Hands on wall, back leg on stool	127

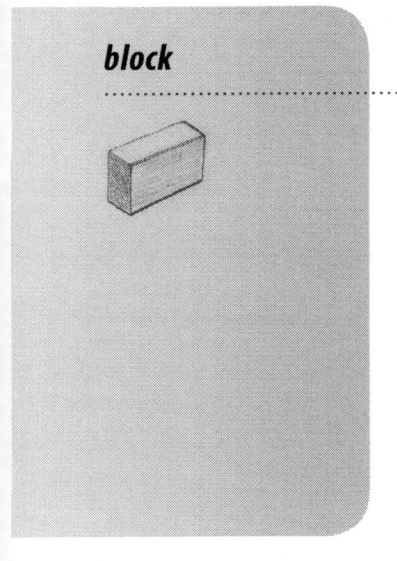

block

Asana	Variation	Page No.
Adho Mukha Svanasana	3 - Shifting weight to the legs: Supporting the palms	32
	7 - Action and counter-action: Partner pushes against back groins	38
	8 - Sensitizing the buttocks: Elevating the feet	39
	9 - Lifting the entire pose: Feet and palms on blocks	40
	10 - Activating the front thighs: Heels on blocks' edges	41
	13 - Spreading the fingers: Using wall and blocks	44
	18 - Stabilizing the arms: Elbows on blocks or inverted chair	49
	21 - Relaxing the brain: Head support	52
	22 - Passive extension of the spine: Wall rope around front groins	53

152 Props for Yoga / Chapter 1 / Index 1

block (cont.)

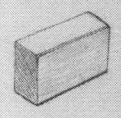

Asana	Variation	Page No.
Practice Sequence		143
Prasarita Padottanasana	4 - Activating the legs: Pressing outer feet against wall/block	139
	7 - Intensifying the downward stretch: Standing on blocks	142
Urdhva Hastasana	2 - Activating the arms: Belt around forearms, block between palms	21
	3 - Extending the armpits: Facing the wall, palms on blocks	22
Uttanasana	1 - Checking the symmetry: Buttocks against the wall	56
	5 - Stand high; bend low: Standing on a raised platform	60
	6 - Compact legs: Belt around feet and pelvis	61
	8 - Creating movement in the shoulders: Holding a block behind the back	63
	10 - Relaxing the brain: Top of the Head on block	66
Utthita Trikonasana	2 - Anchoring the back foot: Outer foot against the wall	69
	10a - Activating the front leg: Heel on block	77
	11 - Opening the groins: Diagonal alignment	79
	13 - Broadening the trunk and relaxing the eyes: Facing the wall	83
	16 - Active work for hyper-extended knee: Pressing the foot against the wall	88
	17 - Stabilizing hyper-extended knee: Supporting the calf with block	89
	18 - Turning the chest: Upper hand holds weight	90
	20 - Rolling the shoulders back: Bottom palm on block	92
	21 - Moving the shoulders back: Arms behind the back	93
Virabhadrasana I	3 - Arching back: Hands against the wall	107
	4 - Activating the back leg: Supporting the heel	108
	6 - Moving the tailbone in: Pubic bone against a wall corner	110
	9 - Activating the arms: Holding a block	113
Virabhadrasana II	2 - Squaring the front leg: Supporting the knee with a block	97
	6 - Lifting the chest: Holding a block	102
Virabhadrasana III	3 - Aligning the back (lifted) leg: Hands on blocks	120
Vrksasana	3 - Widening the pelvis: Facing the wall	27

Bolster

Asana	Variation	Page No.
▷ Adho Mukha Svanasana	21 - Relaxing the brain: Head support	52
	22 - Passive extension of the spine: Wall rope around front groins	53

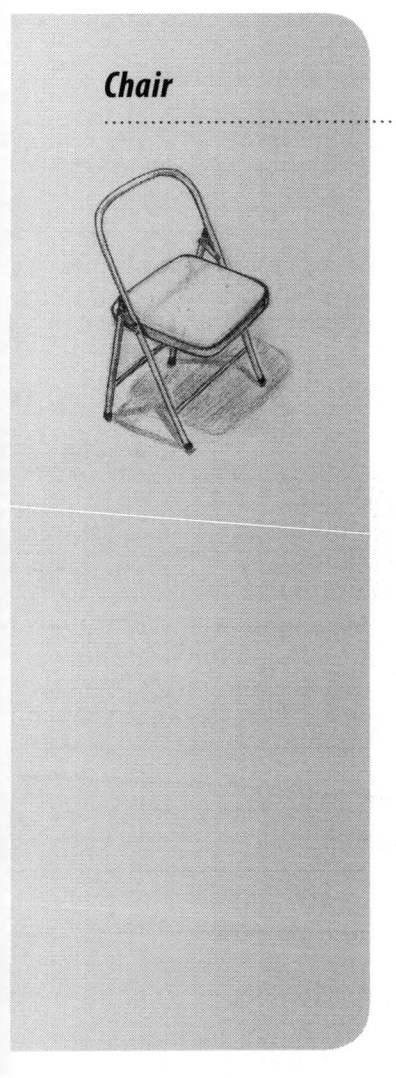

Chair

Asana	Variation	Page No.
▷ Adho Mukha Svanasana	3 - Shifting weight to the legs: Supporting the palms	33
	8 - Sensitizing the buttocks: Elevating the feet	39
	18 - Stabilizing the arms: Elbows on blocks or inverted chair	49
▷ Parsvottanasana	2 - Pelvis alignment: Supporting the front groins on a chair	131
▷ Tadasana	9 - Extending the calves: Standing on a slant	13
▷ Uttanasana	3 - Stabilizing the legs: Leaning over the backrest of a chair	58
	4 - Extending the calves: Standing on a slanted surface	59
	5 – Stand high; bend low: Standing on a raised platform	60
	7 - Folding deeply into the pose: Belt around back and legs	62
▷ Utthita Trikonasana	19 - Turning the chest: Hands holding a chair from behind	91
▷ Virabhadrasana I	5 - Reducing muscular effort: Front thigh rests on chair	109
▷ Virabhadrasana II	3 -Reducing muscular effort: Resting the buttock on a chair	98
▷ Virabhadrasana III	1 - Learning to balance: Supporting the hands	118
	2 - Horizontal alignment: Supporting the pelvis with a chair	119

Partner

Asana	Variation	Page No.
▷ Adho Mukha Svanasana	4 - Stretching back and up: Partner pulls backward with belt	34
	5 - Rooting the heels: Sitting on the "dog"	36
	6 – Moving in the sacrum: "Two dogs"	37
	7 - Action and counter-action: Partner pushes against back groins	38
	11 - Widening the shoulder girdle: Partner helps to turn the arms	42
	12 - Releasing the neck: Partner pulls the trapezius muscles	43
▷ Parsvottanasana	5 - Stabilizing the pelvis: Pulling the front groins with belt	134

partner (cont.)

Asana	Variation	Page No.
Prasarita Padottanasana	2 - Activating the thighs: Buttocks against the wall	137
	6 - Creating space in the pelvis: Pulling the inner groins	141
Tadasana	7 - Thighs back, buttocks in: Two opposite pulls	11
Utthita Trikonasana	5 - Lifting the inner groin: Partner pulls the back leg	72
	12 - Ensuring lateral alignment: Back against the wall	82
	15a - Bending from the hips: Partner pulls the front hip	86
	15b - Pulling the front groin while stabilizing the back leg	87
Virabhadrasana I	7 - Experiencing lightness: Helpers lift the groins	111
Virabhadrasana II	5 - Aligning the chest above the pelvis: Partner holds the back arm	101
Virabhadrasana III	1 - Learning to balance: Supporting the hands	118

rope

Asana	Variation	Page No.
Adho Mukha Svanasana	12 - Releasing the neck: Partner pulls the trapezius muscles	43
	22 - Passive extension of the spine: Wall rope around front groins	53
Prasarita Padottanasana	6 - Creating space in the pelvis: Pulling the inner groins	141
Tadasana	7 - Thighs back, buttocks in: Two opposite pulls	11
	11 - Moving the trapezius down: Shoulder traction	15
Urdhva Hastasana	4 - Extending the entire body upward: Holding a ceiling rope	23
Utthita Trikonasana	12 - Ensuring lateral alignment: Back against the wall	82
	22 - Stretching the top arm: Holding a rope	94
Virabhadrasana I	7 - Experiencing lightness: Helpers lift the groins	111
	10 - Stretching upward: Holding a ceiling rope	114
Virabhadrasana II	4b - Aligning the chest above the pelvis: Back hand holds a wall rope	100
Virabhadrasana III	8 - Floating in Virabhadra III: Holding wall ropes	126
Vrksasana	4 - Extending the body upward: Holding a ceiling rope	28

Wall

Asana	Variation	Page No.
▷ Adho Mukha Svanasana	3 - Shifting weight to the legs: Supporting the palms	32
	5 - Rooting the heels: Sitting on the "dog"	36
	8 - Sensitizing the buttocks: Elevating the feet	39
	10 - Activating the front thighs: Heels on blocks' edges	41
	13 - Spreading the fingers: Using wall and blocks	44
	15 - Wrist stretch: palms against the wall	46
	18 - Stabilizing the arms: Elbows on blocks or inverted chair	49
	20 - Moving the middle back in: Starting with the head low	51
	22 - Passive extension of the spine: Wall rope around front groins	53
▷ Parsvottanasana	1 - Shifting weight to the back leg: Hands on wall	129
	3 - Anchoring the back leg: Foot against the wall	132
▷ Practice Sequence		143
▷ Prasarita Padottanasana	2 - Activating the thighs: Buttocks against the wall	137
	4 - Activating the legs: Pressing outer feet against wall/block	139
▷ Tadasana	13 - Aligning the spine: Spine on a wall edge	18
▷ Uttanasana	1 - Checking the symmetry: Buttocks against the wall	56
	2 - Increasing the thighs action: Back of legs against the wall	57
	7 - Folding deeply into the pose: Belt around back and legs	62
	8 - Creating movement in the shoulders: Holding a block behind	64
	9 - Resting in half-inverted pose: Back against the wall	65
▷ Utthita Trikonasana	10a - Activating the front leg: Heel on block	77
	10b - Stretching the front leg: Sole against the wall	78
	12 - Ensuring lateral alignment: Back against the wall	81
	13 - Broadening the trunk and relaxing the eyes: Facing the wall	83
	14 - Extending the sides of the trunk: Front hand on wall	85
	16 - Active work for hyper-extended knee: Pressing the foot against the wall	88
▷ Virabhadrasana I	3 - Arching back: Hands against the wall	107
	6 - Moving the tailbone in: Pubic bone against a wall corner	110
▷ Virabhadrasana II	2 - Squaring the front leg: Supporting the knee with a block	97
	4a - Activating the back arm: Back palm against the wall	99
▷ Virabhadrasana III	1 - Learning to balance: Supporting the hands	117
	2 - Horizontal alignment: Supporting the pelvis with a chair	119
	9 - Restorative Virabhadra III: Hands on wall, back leg on stool	127

Feet and Legs Actions (cont.)

Action	Asana	Page No.
Supporting the bent leg with a chair	Virabhadrasana I	109
General	Tadasana	4
Elevating the feet	Adho Mukha Svanasana	39
Standing on a slanted surface	Uttanasana	59
Turning the legs out		
Entering Utthita Trikonasana from Utthita Parsvakonasana	Utthita Trikonasana	75
Turning the front foot more than 90°	Utthita Trikonasana	74
Two belts on the upper thighs	Utthita Trikonasana	73

Palms & Fingers Actions

Action	Asana	Page No.
Relieving wrist pain - palms on a slant	Adho Mukha Svanasana	45
Spreading the fingers and palms	Adho Mukha Svanasana	44
Turning the palms	Adho Mukha Svanasana	47
Wrist stretch - Palms against the wall	Adho Mukha Svanasana	46

Hyper extended knees - correcting

Action	Asana	Page No.
Active work for hyper-extended knee	Utthita Trikonasana	88
Supporting the shin of the front leg	Utthita Trikonasana	89

Pelvis and Legs Actions

Action	Asana	Page No.
Anchoring the legs with a belt	Prasarita Padottanasana	138
Back to the wall	Prasarita Padottanasana	137
Belt around feet and pelvis	Uttanasana	61
Belt looped around the standing leg and pelvis	Virabhadrasana III	122
Buttocks against the wall	Uttanasana	56
Moving the pubic bone to a wall corner	Virabhadrasana I	110
Opening the pelvis		
Back against the wall	Vrksasana	26
Back against the wall	Utthita Trikonasana	81
Bent leg against the wall	Vrksasana	25
Diagonal leg alignment	Utthita Trikonasana	79
Facing the wall	Vrksasana	27
Facing the wall	Utthita Trikonasana	83
Partner pulling back	Parsvottanasana	134

Pelvis and Legs Actions (cont.)

Action	Asana	Page No.
Partner pulling the back leg	Utthita Trikonasana	72
Partner pulling the front groins with a rope	Prasarita Padottanasana	141
Supporting the back heel	Virabhadrasana I	108
Supporting the front groins on a chair	Parsvottanasana	131
Two helpers lift the groins	Virabhadrasana I	111
Wall rope to support the pelvis	Adho Mukha Svanasana	54

Restorative Actions

Action	Asana	Page No.
Back supported on a wall	Uttanasana	65
Head support	Adho Mukha Svanasana	52
Restorative Virabhadrasana III	Virabhadrasana III	127
Supporting the crown of the head	Uttanasana	66

Stretching Actions

Action	Asana	Page No.
Stretching with a ceiling rope	Vrksasana	28
Supporting the palms	Adho Mukha Svanasana	32
Top arm holding a ceiling or a wall rope	Utthita Trikonasana	94

Trunk and Upper Body Actions

Action	Asana	Page No.
Belt around the elbows	Virabhadrasana I	112
Holding a block	Virabhadrasana I	113
Holding a ceiling rope	Virabhadrasana I	114
Holding the arms behind the back	Virabhadrasana I	115
Maintaining Length Along the Sides of the Trunk	Utthita Trikonasana	84
Pulling the front groin of the front leg	Utthita Trikonasana	86
Pulling the front groin while stabilizing the back leg	Utthita Trikonasana	87
Front hand on wall	Utthita Trikonasana	85
Top hand holding a weight	Utthita Trikonasana	90
Using a chair	Utthita Trikonasana	91

Turning Sideways	Action	Asana	Page No.
	Entering by stepping back	Virabhadrasana I	104

Made in the USA
San Bernardino, CA
08 March 2019